Euthanasia and Patristic Tradition

Euthanasia and Patristic Tradition

Reading St John Damascene and St Symeon the New Theologian on Christian Bioethics

Ioannis Bekos

Foreword by Stanley Hauerwas

Afterword by Ulrich Volp

James Clarke & Co

James Clarke & Co
P.O. Box 60
Cambridge
CB1 2NT
United Kingdom

www.jamesclarke.co
publishing@jamesclarke.co

Hardback ISBN: 978 0 227 17698 6
Paperback ISBN: 978 0 227 17697 9
PDF ISBN: 978 0 227 90694 1
ePub ISBN: 978 0 227 90695 8
Kindle ISBN: 978 0 227 90696 5

British Library Cataloguing in Publication Data
A record is available from the British Library

First published by James Clarke & Co, 2019

Dedicated to my wife Εἰρήνη

Contents

Part Two

The Creation of Man According to the Image of God and the Prospect of Voluntary Death

Abbreviations

i) General texts

BMFD	*Byzantine Monastic Foundation Documents*, J.P. Thomas and A.C. Hero (eds), Washington, DC, 2001
CMH	*The Cambridge Medieval History IV: The Byzantine Empire Part II*, J.M. Hussey (ed), Cambridge, 1967
DS	*Dictionnaire de spiritualité ascétique et mystique: doctrine et histoire*, Paris, 1990
DTC	*Dictionnaire de théologie catholique*, Paris, 1924
EC	*The Encyclopedia of Christianity*, Vol. III, Michigan and Leiden, 2003.
EPLB	*Ἐγκυκλοπαίδεια Πάπυρος – Λαροὺς – Μπριτάννικα* (Encyclopaedia Papyros Larousse Britannica), Athens, 1983-1997
HLPSS	*Historisches Lexikon zur politisch-sozialen Sprache in Deutschland (Geschichtliche Grundbegriffe)*, Band 6, Stuttgart, 1984
PG	*Patrologiæ Cursus Completus*, Series Graeca, J.P. Migne (ed), Paris, 1857-1866
NCE	*New Catholic Encyclopedia*, Washington, DC, 2002
OCP	*The Oxford Companion to Philosophy*, T. Honderich (ed), Oxford, 1995
ODB	*The Oxford Dictionary of Byzantium*, A.P. Kazhdan (ed), New York, 1991

REE	*Θρησκευτικὴ καὶ Ἠθικὴ Ἐγκυκλοπαίδεια* (Religious and Ethical Encyclopaedia), Athens, 1962-1968
SC	*Sources Chrétiennes*, Paris, 1942-
TRE	*Theologische Realenzyklopädie*, Berlin, 1977-2000

ii) Works of St John Damascene (with English translation of the title)

Anast.	*Laudatio sanctae martyris Anastasiae* (Encomium on St and Martyr Anastasia), Kotter v, 289-303
Barb.	*Laudatio sanctae martyris Barbarae* (Encomium on St and Martyr Barbara), Kotter v, 256-78
Dial. brev.	*Dialectica-Capita philosophica (recensio brevior)* (Philosophical Chapters) (short version), Kotter i, 57-142
Dial. brev. o.	*Dialectica-Capita philosophica (recensio brevior)* (Philosophical Chapters) (short version, other chapter), Kotter i, 143-46
Dial. fus.	*Dialectica-Capita philosophica (recensio fusior)* (Philosophical Chapters) (long version), Kotter i, 51-142
Dorm. I	*Oratio prima in dormitionem sanctae Dei genitricis Mariae* (First Sermon on the Dormition of the Holy Mother of God), Kotter v, 483-500
Dorm. II	*Oratio secunda in dormitionem sanctae Dei genitricis Mariae* (Second Sermon on the Dormition of the Holy Mother of God), Kotter v, 516-40
Dorm. III	*Oratio tertia in dormitionem sanctae Dei genitricis Mariae* (Third Sermon on the Dormition of the Holy Mother of God), Kotter, v, 541-555
Expos.	*Expositio Fidei* (An Exact Exposition of the Orthodox Faith), Kotter ii, 7-239
Ficus	*Oratio in ficum arefactam et in parabolam vineae* (Sermon of the Dead Ficus and the Parable of the Vineyard), Kotter v, 102-110
Haeres.	*Liber de Haeresibus* (Heresies), Kotter iv, 19-67
Imag.	*Contra imaginum calumniatores orationes tres* (On the Divine Images), Kotter iii, 65-200
Instit.	*Institutio elementaris* (Elementary Introduction of Doctrines), Kotter i, 20-26
Manich.	*Contra Manichaeos* (Against Manichaeans), Kotter iv, 351-98
Nativ. M.	*Homilia in nativitatem domini* (Sermon on the Nativity of Theotokos), Kotter v, 169-82

Sabbat. *Oratio in Sabbatum sanctum* (Sermon on Great Saturday), Kotter v, 121-46

Sarac. *Disputatio christiani et saraceni* (Dialogue between a Saracen and a Christian), Kotter iv, 427-38

Trisag. *Epistola de hymno Trisagio* (On the Trisagios Hymn), Kotter iv, 304-32

Volunt. *De duabus in Christo voluntatibus* (On the Two Wills in Christ), Kotter iv, 173-231

iii) Works of St Symeon the New Theologian
(with English translation of the title)

Cat. *Catéchèses* (Catechetical Discources), B. Krivocheine and J. Paramelle (eds), i (Cat. 1-5), SC 96, 222-469; ii (Cat. 6-22), SC 104, 12-393; (Cat. 23-34), SC 113, 12-303

Cent. 1 *Chapitres Théologiques, Gnostiques et Pratiques* (Practical and Theological Chapters 100), J. Darrouzés (ed), SC 51 *bis*, 40-101

Cent. 2 *Chapitres Théologiques, Gnostiques et Pratiques* (Theological and Gnostic Chapters 25), J. Darrouzés (ed), SC 51 *bis*, 102-19

Cent. 3 *Chapitres Théologiques, Gnostiques et Pratiques* (Theological and Practical Chapters 100), J. Darrouzés (ed), SC 51 *bis*, 120-87

Eth. *Traités Ethiques* (Ethical Orations), J. Darrouzés (ed), i (Eth. 1-3), SC 122, 170-441; ii (Eth. 4-15), SC 129, 8-459

Hymn *Hymnes* (The Divine Hymns), J. Koder, J. Paramelle and L. Neyrand (eds), i (Hymn. 1-15), SC 156, 156-301; ii (Hymn. 16-40), SC 174, 10-493; iii (Hymn. 41-58), SC 196, 10-309

Life *Un grand mystique byzantin: Vie de Symeon le Nouveau Théologien (949-1022) par Nicétas Stéthatos* (The Life of St Symeon the New Theologian), I. Hausherr and G. Horn, OC, 12 (1928), 1-128

Theol. *Traités Théologiques* (Theological Orations), J. Darrouzés (ed), SC 122, 96-1

iv) Works of Michael Psellos

Chron. *Imperatori di Bisanzio (Cronografia)* (Chronographia), D. del Corno, S. Impellizzeri and U. Criscuolo (eds)

	(Milano: Fondazione Lorenzo Valla, 1984)
Phil. Ps	*Philosophica Minora* (Philosophical Works) (Bibliotheca Scriptorum Graecorum et Romanorum Teubneriana series), J.M. Duffy and D.J. O'Meara (eds) (Leipzig: B.G. Teubner, 1989)
Theol. Ps	*Theologica* (Theological Works) (Bibliotheca Scriptorum Graecorum et Romanorum Teubneriana series), P. Gautier, L.G. Westerink and J.M. Duffy (eds) (Leipzig: B.G. Teubner, 1989)

Foreword
by Stanley Hauerwas

I am honoured to write in support of Ioannis Bekos' work. I do so, however, as one whose training has been primarily in the philosophical and theological traditions of the West. As one so formed I am, therefore, in a certain way overwhelmed by the resources Bekos has brought to his criticisms of the development of modern bioethics, as well as his constructive account of Christian anthropology. His ability to show the connections, for example, between St John Damascene's understanding of the hypostatic union and how Christians should understand death makes his work unique and important in the field of bioethics.

Reading Bekos reminds me of a seminar I once conducted on the work of Reinhold Niebuhr. A Russian Orthodox priest who was visiting as a Fulbright scholar was in the class. He had told me that he thought Orthodox theology was in good shape but he thought it needed a better social ethic. I responded that I doubted that was the case. My judgement was confirmed in one of the seminar sessions when he asked in reference to Niebuhr's account of freedom of the individual – 'What does this word, "individual" mean?' I tried to explain, referring him to liberal political theory in which 'individual', drawing on mathematical precedent, had simply meant 'a free-standing entity'.

I could see, however, he was having trouble comprehending what I was trying to explain. So, I tried another approach. I said probably the closest word in his tradition to suggest what 'individual' might mean was 'person'. His face lit up and he said, 'Oh, you mean "Trinity"'. I told him that was a perfectly reasonable conclusion given his tradition, but that is not what 'individual' means in the politics of the West. However, that is precisely what Bekos means by 'individual' which is why he quite rightly argues that his account of what it means to be an individual is a challenge to how that word is used in contemporary bioethics in liberal social orders.

Equally impressive is Bekos' use of the theology of St Symeon to inform and shape our understanding of death. I simply know of no work comparable to Bekos' thick account of death in which our relationship to God is not forgotten. Moreover, his suggestion that in the Orthodox tradition self-knowledge is prioritised to self-preservation is a stunning insight that I look forward to seeing him develop. For I take it he is quite right to suggest that such an understanding of self-knowledge does challenge the fundamental presuppositions of bioethics in the West.

Though Bekos is completely at home in the theology of the Orthodox tradition, his knowledge of philosophical alternatives in the West is impressive. His characterisation and criticism of such an important philosopher as Jonas is testimony to his command of philosophical developments in the West. His constructive use of Levinas, MacIntyre and Manent is equally adept. I was quite taken, moreover, by his use of Foucault to show how the development of bioethics involves power dynamics often unacknowledged.

Finally, Bekos' focus on euthanasia to illustrate his philosophical and theological arguments works well to show the implications of what some might consider his anthropological 'theory'. His understanding of 'voluntary death' in terms of our ultimate destiny to be in union with God will not easily be understood by those advocates of the bioethics Bekos critiques. However, I am sure, like all significant positions, given time his arguments will be rightly appreciated for their power. For when it is all said and done, 'Trinity' is the first and last word we have to say as Christians. We are in Bekos' debt for helping us, even those of us who are 'Westerners', to recover that fundamental truth.

Stanley Hauerwas
Gilbert T. Rowe Professor of Theological Ethics
Duke Divinity School
Durham, NC, United States

Acknowledgements

The research endeavour that resulted in this book was not simply an academic engagement. It was also an opportunity for communication and friendship with many influential people who often had different views on a variety of issues. Their presence in my life is a gift of God and such a gift cannot but enrich my life in all its aspects. This research would not have been completed or even started without the support and encouragement of numerous people to whom I am deeply indebted.

I arrived at Geneva after finishing my theological studies and completing four years of teaching Christian theology and ethics in Athens. Many thanks are due to the Faculty of Theology of the University of Athens that laid the foundations of my theological training and oriented me towards my doctorate studies in theology at the University of Geneva and the Institute for Postgraduate Studies in Orthodox theology at the Orthodox Centre of the Ecumenical Patriarchate in Chambésy, Geneva. I owe special thanks to, among others, Professor Vlasios Phidas and late Professor Konstantinos Scouteris. My thanks are also owed to the Greek Ministry of Education, the Hellenic American Educational Foundation and Athens College for granting me a four-year sabbatical and providing the necessary financial support for me to complete my doctorate studies.

There was also another person who had a deep influence on my choice to focus on and deal with Christian ethics. Professor Stanley Hauerwas of Duke University is a friend and an inspiring interlocutor regarding theology and its impact on human life. I am profoundly grateful not only for his writings and friendship, but also for the comments that he provided at a very crucial stage of this book.

The directors of my work are among those to whom I owe a debt of gratitude. The late Professor Metropolitan of Ephesus Chrysostomos Konstantinidis of the Orthodox Institute and Professor François Dermange of the Autonomous Faculty of Protestant Theology of the University of Geneva read, reread and constructively criticised the various drafts of my book and offered me the privilege of engaging with them in theological discussions that went far beyond the completion of this study.

I was fortunate to have the opportunity to profit from my engagements with distinguished scholars on bioethics at the Kennedy Institute of Ethics and the Center for Clinical Bioethics of Georgetown University in Washington, DC, where I was appointed visiting researcher during the summer of 2003. I would like to thank, in particular, the late Professor Edmund Pellegrino and Professor John Keown, and the director of the Center for Clinical Bioethics, Sister Carol Taylor, for their support and fruitful discussion on issues relevant to my research.

I owe many thanks to Metropolitan Nikolaos Hatzinikolaou of Mesogea and Lavreotiki, who helped me to see the importance of writing a theological work on euthanasia and granted me access to the library of the Hellenic Center for Biomedical Ethics.

I also thank and acknowledge the contribution of Professor Vlasios Phidas, dean of the Orthodox Institute, who, from the very beginning of our association, trusted me unreservedly and who also provided much encouragement, discussing and commenting on aspects of my book. My thanks are also owed to the Reverend Antonios Pinakoulas with whom I discussed certain aspects of my research and whose knowledge and inspired thought helped me to develop my work. Also, I would like to thank the Reverend Dr Demetrios Bathrellos for his long-lasting friendship and encouragement, as well as for reading and commenting on parts of my book.

I also acknowledge with thanks the all-round support of those serving at the Orthodox Center and the Orthodox Institute at Chambésy, and particularly former Metropolitan Jeremy of Switzerland, former Bishop Makarios of Lampsakos and Dr Gary Vachicouras.

Finally, my deepest gratitude goes to my wife, Dr Irene Kassini, for her willingness to read and comment on many parts of my book and above all for her love and patience in every aspect of my life.

General Introduction

To take a specific religious and spiritual tradition as one's point of orientation, in order better to grapple with the ethical dilemmas with which modern society is concerned, is perhaps not regarded as a useful pursuit in this era. Nevertheless, such an approach may challenge well-established perceptions, according to which the religious traditions, such as the Christianity, constitute an obstacle towards the foundation of a common morality.[1] This book will argue that the Christian tradition has at least the same power claims and therefore that it may participate in the public dialogue along with all those ideologies that have the benefit of being arbitrarily considered closer to the truth and more compatible with modern and postmodern society.

The description of the way in which such a claim might successfully be made is the first aim of this book. The framework for achieving this aim is the discipline of bioethics, which is a popular discipline that enjoys academic respect, as it has assumed the responsibility of establishing rules for exercising the dominant role, over the last decades, of medicine and technology over human life and death. Since my intention is to criticise the dominant reality, this will be more successful if it targets concurrently the study of a specific bioethical dilemma such as euthanasia.[2]

---

1. The designation of the moral norms that all humans may share (Veatch, 'Is There a Common Morality?', p. 189).
2. For the rest of this book the use of the term 'euthanasia' signifies all forms of deliberate administration of death by those moral agents involved in the medical context such as the physician, the patient and the relatives.

Having completed an in-depth criticism of sovereign bioethics – and by this what is meant is the kind of bioethics that shapes the relevant discussions in the public arena, and unjustifiably imposes particular values, boundaries and conditions on the discussion relevant to bioethical dilemmas – it is helpful to see what the Christian tradition, and, more particularly, the tradition of the Church Fathers,[3] could contribute to an ethical dilemma like euthanasia. This is the second aim of this book. The intention is not only to make a contribution to theology, but also to demonstrate to a person of the modern world the value of appealing to content-rich accounts of human existence that ignore neither universal aspects of the human condition nor modern reality.

On this level we find elements that are true of human life regardless of political, religious or other ideas, elements that can be detected throughout the history of mankind. In a discussion on bioethics, it is valuable to study a description of this level of the human condition, because, first, the ideological confrontation as to what is ethical and what is not is thus transferred to the account of those elements that are inevitably related to the behaviour of all representatives of all views. Moreover, the issue of a shared understanding of human existence is not being sought through the Sisyphean struggle of formulating common values in a world characterised by a pluralism of values, but through the description of the diachronic fundamentals of human existence as they are verified through historical experience and their continuous presence in each worldview, and in each era.

With this description in mind, the reliability of each view regarding specific ethical dilemmas is not being judged on its religious or secular presuppositions, but on whether it takes into consideration and it successfully manages human reality. In such a questioning framework, the study of the patristic tradition is being judged on its readiness not to ignore human reality, since its main preoccupation is man and his concerns.

Undoubtedly, the question that readily emerges is concerned with the way that the description of human existence outside each available anthropological framework is possible. Such an endeavour presupposes the existence of a method that will approach human existence without the illumination of a normative tradition being necessary. Moreover, for the study of a modern ethical dilemma like euthanasia, the use of this method is only valuable if it is organically connected with human life and the reality of human death.

---

3. From now onwards, the reference to 'Christian tradition' signifies the Christian tradition upon which the theological aspect of this book is based, namely the Greek patristic tradition, unless otherwise noted.

I. A Diachronic View of Human Existence: Bioethics and the Question of Euthanasia

The 'descriptive theory of decision' by Panajotis Kondylis[4] meets the requirements described in the General Introduction. To justify this selection, we draw on some points from his last and most systematic work to date – *The Political and Man: The Fundamentals of Social Ontology*[5] – that incorporates his major arguments, which he developed in some of his previous writings. A presentation of the descriptive theory of decision will follow.

A cornerstone of Kondylis' thought is his belief that, in order to understand the behaviour of an individual, superindividual factors must be taken into consideration, because the results of all human activities, decisions and actions originate in an ontological zone outside the individual actions of the active persons.[6] Kondylis places these superindividual factors in the so-called 'sociontic field' (*sozialontische Feld*), which 'consists of factors or powers, the constitution and spectrum of which direct the action of each active in each society'.[7] There are three factors, or powers, that are primarily interrelated and contribute to what is happening in a society: the social relation (*die soziale Beziehung*), the politic (*das Politische*) and the human being (*der Mensch*).

The social relation coincides with the very being of a given society and is a component of its very meaning,[8] whereas the politic is the particular social relation that makes society its object as a totality that must have cohesion as well as order.[9] The human being pertains to the

4. Kondylis, *Macht und Entscheidung.*
5. Kondylis, *Das Politische und der Mensch.*
6. Ibid., pp. 155-56. This is in direct contrast to contract theories (i.e. *The Theory of Communicative Action* of Jürgen Habermas) that establish the individual action as a superior explanatory principle.
7. Ibid., p. 194. Kondylis, in adopting the concept of the sociontic field, aims to show that the perception of each social reality takes place in a such a 'field' and not in a vacuum which is 'more fluid, more movable, more multiform than everything that can be grasped by the different social sciences with the help of their conceptual weaponry, which is designated each time from the logic of their foundation' (ibid., pp. 185-86).
8. Ibid., p. 206. The definition of the social relation is based on the perception that 'whatever happens in a society and can be called social, is being conduced through visible and invisible human interrelationships and is born from the dynamic of these relationships' (ibid.).
9. The politic has as its object generally accepted rules and represents the social as it is used in more general terms. Here, when we talk about people's decisions and actions, they refer to the social totality and they raise the most general social claim (ibid., pp. 209-10).

anthropological side of the sociontic field, i.e. the explanation of the way in which human nature is connected with the social relation and the politic. Here, socio-ontologically-directed anthropology does not treat the contents but the boundaries of the social relation which are marked out by the anthropological reality – the integral sociability and the integral mortality of the human being which means the possibility of being killed.[10] This is where the connection between Kondylis' thought and euthanasia, the topic of this book, begins. We will talk more about this in one of the following chapters. For the moment we will discuss the anthropological fact of mortality in a little more detail.

For Kondylis, the sustentation or the interruption of the vital functions constitute what is most fundamental and primary for man. In a way, someone may detect in mortality the deepest and most unique need of human existence. Thus:

> the fact that life is recallable whereas death is irreversible gives life a superior position to death to the degree to which the intensity and range of social actions must be viewed in the light of their irreversible character, which is their proximity to death. Life can not become a criterion of death, since the dead person does not know what life is, whereas death may become a criterion of life, since the living may imagine death at any moment – death as he or someone else is dying or being killed.[11]

Neither mortality nor death would be important for us if death occurred everywhere and always in the same manner, as a 'natural death', and as a result of the malfunction and the deterioration of the vital functions, and without the intervention of other people or the indirect or direct impact of social factors. Kondylis' point – that it is not a mere expected reality but something that gives practical possibilities to the active subject – is of great interest. Man can use these possibilities 'at some, usually chosen, moments, both for other subjects and for himself, since everyone knows or finds what he should do to cause his own death or someone else's death, when this is sought'.[12] If the last statement reminds us of the issue of euthanasia as an option for modern man, then this is not accidental. For Kondylis, the anthropological fact of mortality reveals the extreme expression of the range in the social relation that is characterised through the dipole of friendship/enmity, which corresponds, on one hand, to the sacrifice of someone's

10. Ibid., p. 215.
11. Ibid., pp. 240-41.
12. Ibid., p. 241.

life for the other (self-sacrifice) and, on the other, the idea of someone killing somebody else (murder). In this framework of understanding, euthanasia comes somewhere between the two poles, i.e. it is only an intermediate point in this dipole.

The position that euthanasia occupies within the friendship/enmity dipole depends on the particular crystallisation of modern reality that is defined according to the specific anthropological content that accompanies it. As, since we are interested in the issue of euthanasia in modern society, we are also interested in a person's perception of euthanasia and the implied argumentation interwoven into that perception, as well as in how the 'indicated' practices of management of the specific ethical dilemma are formulated.

However, postmodern society is a society which thinks that we can truly subscribe to a common morality free of any particular anthropology – something that allows it to lay claim to general power. Sovereign bioethics and all the discussions relative to bioethical dilemmas are conducted within this climate. How justified is such a reality?

It should have become clear that this particular book is oriented towards criticising such a reality in order to show the importance of a content-rich anthropology for modern society and thus work towards a more rational confrontation of modern ethical dilemmas. To accomplish this, we must emphasise the fact that sovereign bioethics, like all theories of human existence, has a polemical character – it fights for self-preservation and sovereignty by exerting power claims over others – for it moves within the dipole of friendship/enmity, and therefore has friends and enemies. Then we need to show its partially subjective character with regard to the alleged representation of common ideas and values, something that will completely justify the expression of power claims in public life by particular spiritual traditions, such as the Christian tradition. Lastly, it is necessary to show the contents of the anthropology that represents bioethics. This will be made with reference to the issue of euthanasia.

Such an undertaking cannot be accomplished by an enrolee theory, such as a normative theory, but rather only by a theory devoid of any normative or axiomatic principle – all theories with normative[13] positions

---

13. Kondylis, in using the term 'normative', or 'normative principles' or 'normative values', does not refer only to the common ethical commandments. Instead, he refers to each 'world-construction' or worldview (*Weltanschauung*) that is shaped by the desire for self-preservation and the broadening of the power of a human being or of a collective entity (Kondylis, *Macht und Entscheidung*, pp. 11-12).

follow a procedure towards the submission of the various 'worlds' to the real world and, as such, they tend to ignore the resultant multiformity.[14] On the contrary, Kondylis proposes the descriptive theory of decision. He argues that his theory does not indicate what is right and what is wrong, but rather that it describes the framework of human thought, and consequently essential elements of the human existence.

In the descriptive theory of decision (DTD), a decision (*de-cisio*, *Ent-scheidung*) is defined as an action or procedure of abruption and breakaway, from which an ideology or worldview that suitably safeguards a person's ability for orientation and self-preservation has arisen.[15] The cornerstone of DTD is the belief that the character of these kinds of decisions presupposes power claims that always aim towards the broadening of power of the subject or the subjects of decisions as a precondition for their self-preservation.

The DTD starts from the undeniable and irreversible character of historical multiformity, detects the cause of this in the action or the procedure of abruption and decision, and tries to explain the abruption and the decision by pointing out the necessity for the transformation of the objective from self-preservation to power claims. Thus, it can explain the emergence of different and peculiar 'worlds', namely the different theories of the human existence.

Given the innate orientation of all theories of human existence towards self-preservation and power claims, the existence of universal and objective ethical theories is beyond consideration and therefore all theories are fundamentally subjective. Then, an assumption is made that, as this is true of all proposed theories of human existence, the emergence of bioethics and its domination over modern ethical discussion is polemical in character. These two consequences of the descriptive theory of decision are of fundamental importance for this book, for the exclusion of 'particular' moralities from the current debate of bioethics is shown to be unjustified, given that all theories are basically subjective and polemical. Thus, the application of DTD, on the one hand, repudiates the widespread belief that a knowledge of human existence itself is not necessary but rather detrimental to dealing with current moral issues; while, on the other hand, it opens the door to a thorough-going consideration of each issue, such as, for instance, the question of euthanasia, given that the current debate on euthanasia does

14. Ibid., pp. 38-39. The purpose of Kondylis' theory is, among others, to challenge any previous theories on decision that are based either on the 'existential proper' or on the acceptance of an 'objective proper'.

15. Ibid., p. 14.

not take into account the character of human existence. In particular, these findings from the application of DTD in bioethics are made more explicit through an analysis of the 'project of common morality'.

The common morality project is based on the assumption that, in a fragmented world, bioethicists must designate the moral norms that all humans should share.[16] This assumption presupposes that the distinction between the 'common' and the 'particular' makes sense, where the former is considered as objective and the latter as subjective. It also implies that common morality is justified to reign over human life, given that the 'objectivity' that it enjoys safeguards the 'ethical interests' of all human beings. The application of DTD reveals the fallacy of making a distinction between the 'common' and the 'particular' through identifying the common ground shared by all theories relevant to human existence – all theories serve their own needs of self-preservation through presenting their subjective principles as objective and therefore as appropriate for power claims over human life.

This 'discovery' establishes the common ground that bioethics and the history of human existence share; it also allows us to find the measure of bioethics in this era and to gauge its character. Thus, though bioethical approaches, such as the project of common morality, are presented as being divorced from any anthropological account of human existence for the sake of universality and objectification, their actual application reveals a different picture. In particular, the current discussion around euthanasia reveals that modern bioethical thought involves a disguised system of anthropology and, therefore, in a different way, it is subjective and oriented towards power claims over human life. This anthropology is indirectly promoted in the sense that it designates the character of the discussions on bioethical issues, such as, which parameters of human existence are considered important, and, consequently, shapes human existence itself. Obviously, the distinction between the 'common' and the 'particular' is at least unjustified.

At this point we must consider the prospect of equal power claims that derive from particular traditions, including the Christian tradition. Since the Christian tradition will be examined in this book, it is important to note the relationship between Kondylis' thought and important concepts underpinning the Christian tradition.

Interestingly enough, the fundamental assumption of DTD, according to which all theories of human existence are polemical in character, is

16. The core idea of this project is the possibility of there being a pretheoretical awareness of certain moral norms by all humans (Veatch, 'Is There a Common Morality?', p. 189).

shown to be in total agreement with the Christian tradition and what Christ says about the character of this world with regard to those who want to prevail over others: 'You know that the rulers of the Gentiles lord it over them [κατακυριεύουσιν], and those in high positions use their authority over them [κατεξουσιάζουσιν].'[17] Also, the position that the friend/enemy schema represents a common anthropological norm is perfectly justified by Christ's commandments regarding human relationships: 'love one another just as I have loved you. No one has greater love than this – that one lays down his life for his friends. You are my friends if you do what I command you',[18] and: 'Love your enemies, do good to those who hate you, Bless those who curse you, pray for those who mistreat you.'[19] Moreover, the anti-idealistic position of Kondylis, which culminates in his argument that there are no ideas, but rather there are human beings who fight for their self-preservation, is consistent with the Christian morality that is developed in this book, which is a morality that is not based on ideology but rather on Christ, the incarnate Son of God. However, from a Christian point of view, the use of Kondylis' descriptive theory of decision in this book by no means assumes that such a theory can grasp human existence as a whole. The theological part of this book shows that, while DTD is also applicable to Christian

17. Matthew 20:25. The use of the prefix κατα with the Greek words κυριεύω and ἐξουσιάζω indicates that the power exercised by the rulers of this world over others has no limits.

18. John 15:12-14. See also Kondylis, *Das Politische und der Mensch*, p. 321. In the patristic tradition this particular biblical reference is associated with Christian voluntary death (see, for example, St Maximus the Confessor, *To Thalassion, Patrologiæ cursus completus* [PG 90], 725C-D), to which an extended part of this book is devoted.

19. Luke 6:27-28. The schemas of friend and enemy, friendship and enmity or peace and war are found also in patristic literature, and particularly in texts like those of Pseudo-Dionysius that continue to represent an important source for Christian theology. Thus, the work of Pseudo-Dionysius, *On the Divine Names*, refers to the establishment of peace among the living through a connatural friendship (ὁμοφυῆ φιλίαν) (PG 3, 952A) that is established through the self-existent peace that is God. In regards to the expressions of enmity among the living, this happens even when they desire peace and friendship: they grant their desire wrongly, since their actions aimed to fulfill are based on the effort to accomplish something so ephemeral (it is implied that they are not based on the self-existent peace that is God, a peace that does not change by time). (τῇ ἀποπληρώσει τῶν ἀεὶ ἀποῤῥεόντων εἰρηνεύει) (PG 3, 953A). Interestingly, Kondylis also associates the operation of the spectrum friendship/enmity with the liquidity and movement of the sociontic field. The difference between Kondylis and Pseudo-Dionysius centres on the fact that the latter recognises the possibility of overcoming the entrapment that is associated with the particular spectrum in question.

theology, it cannot encompass those aspects of human existence that refer to the divinity given that, for the Christian tradition presented in this book, divinity is, in a way, part of human existence itself.[20] Some introductory points on the theological part of this book follow.

II. Christian Individualism and the Individualistic Society of the Modern Era

If the distinction between the 'common' and the 'particular' cannot stand, a book on Christian ethics, which constitutes a 'particular' morality, itself may claim to have equal authority with the other approaches to bioethics and its own place in the public debate. Moreover, it may be possible to view it as a feasible alternative to what is generally accepted in bioethics. To be convincing, such an alternative must fulfil two conditions. First, it should not share common ground with the other theories of human existence, common ground that consists of an orientation towards self-preservation with consequent power claims over human life. Second, it should offer a persuasive alternative regarding the 'treatment' of the moral issues in the medical context and, in particular, euthanasia. This has to be adaptable within the current ideology that is dominated by individualism and the consideration of man as an autonomous being.

Regarding individualism as a characteristic of modern civilisation, this book uses the notion of individualism in accordance with the Alexis de Tocqueville's description, [21] according to which individualism:

> is a reflective and tranquil sentiment that disposes each citizen to cut himself off from the mass of his fellow men and withdraw into the circle of family and friends, so that, having created a little society for his own use, he gladly leaves the larger society to take care of itself.

Such individualism, although not identified with egoism and the passionate and exaggerated love of self that causes the seed of all the virtues to shrivel up, 'in the end will be subsumed in egoism'.[22] Nevertheless, a

20. The intimacy between divinity and humanity within human existence is discussed in detail in the second part of this book.
21. The continuing popularity of de Tocqueville's *Democracy in America* is indicative of the depth and truth of its arguments, which stir modern people 'from a sleepy complacency with the values that govern our way of life' in a democratic state (Koritansky, 'Alexis de Tocqueville (1805-1859)', p. 18).
22. Alexis de Tocqueville, *Democracy in America*, p. 585.

definition of individualism would be incomplete if it did not take into consideration the reality of mass democracy that supplements the ideas of the dignity of man and self-realisation.[23] Both these last ideas are associated closely with the arguments in favour of euthanasia. These will occupy a later part of this book.

Autonomy is the second cardinal characteristic of the modern society. Modern thought is basically characterised by the transition from self-governance to autonomy.[24] This transition is marked by the decline of heteronomy and the denial of any decisive role of God in human life. Thus, morality becomes human-centred, though it excludes the character of human existence from the centre of interest for the sake of universal principles and norms. It is within such a context that we consider the contribution of the Christian tradition.

The presentation of the theological arguments of the patristic Christian tradition in the second part of this book marks an epistemological transition from a descriptive to a normative approach with regard to human existence. Even though a Christian theological tradition is also subject to the descriptive power of the descriptive theory of decision, and as a consequence is subject to an orientation towards self-preservation and power claims, it also constitutes a disclaimer to both the self-preservation and the power claims over human life. A tradition that traces itself back to the voluntary death of Christ and those who believed in Him, such as the martyrs, would be considered a tradition oriented towards self-relinquishment rather than self-preservation and the power claims over oneself or others. Also, it should not be ignored that even Christians, to the extent that they are inescapably shaped by the secular character of this world, are subject to the descriptive

23. Kondylis, *Das Politische und der Mensch*, pp. 35 and 69-70. Kondylis develops his thought even more and talks about the 'individualising' (*Atomisierung*) of society, in which individuals (*Atome*) are considered to be 'the last elements in an operational whole that cannot be reduced to something else'. The existence of 'primarily independent, equivalent human beings of whose interaction society consists' is a prerequisite (ibid., pp. 5-6). Manent's reference to man in modern society is particularly interesting, since he sees him in confrontation with the Greek city and the Church, noting that we have 'the genesis of this radical man, the individual prior to the citizen and Christian alike' (Manent, *The City of Man*, p. 35).

24. Schneewind, *The Invention of Autonomy*, p. 483. The idea of moral self-governance can be traced back to St Paul's assertion that the gentiles are 'a law unto themselves' (Romans 2:14). On the contrary, Kant's idea of morality as autonomy 'presupposes that we are rational agents whose transcendental freedom takes us out of the domain of natural causation. It belongs to every individual, in the state of nature as well as in society' (Schneewind, *The Invention of Autonomy*, p. 515).

power of Kondylis theory. The discussion of such a bipolar character of Christian life is at the centre of interest for this book. In such a context, the elaboration of Christian individualism is considered within the parameters of Christian thought.

To avoid any misunderstanding, the choice of such a context for a theological discussion does not imply the acceptance of the fundamentals of contemporary society, particularly as expressed in the field of bioethics. It is assumed that this society, with its multicultural character, cannot assume any definite anthropological basis for ethical issues, for if it did, this would go against attempts to establish a universal morality in modern ethics. The Christian theology that is presented in this book stands at the very opposite pole to this assumption. In fact, according to such a Christian tradition, it is not possible to talk about man and the ethical issues surrounding human life if there is not a clear understanding of what man is.

The exposition of Orthodox Christian anthropology is an ongoing process. Christian theologians, while remaining deeply aware of the cultural characteristics of each era, try to properly present the Christian tradition, taking the Scriptures, the teaching of the Church Fathers and the Ecumenical Councils as a basis. This approach is by no means a process towards the secularisation of Christianity. On the contrary, it represents the consciousness of the Church that, while it constitutes the Body of Christ, it is at the same time a body of earthly human beings who live within a particular civilisation and who are influenced by contemporary ideologies. In other words, Christian theology does not ignore the role of history in human life and the inevitable dependence of all human beings, including Christians, on the particular historical (cultural, ideological) circumstances. The understanding of the character of man is a prerequisite for Christian ethics, an understanding that necessarily takes into account the relevant theological tradition as well as the contemporary cultural and ideological state of affairs. In this book this theological elucidation is developed as follows.

A book on Christian ethics that aims to discuss the issues surrounding euthanasia through the elaboration of a specific view of human existence could take as its starting point the narration of the creation of man in the Old Testament. According to this account, God created man according to His own image,[25] placed him in paradise, but warned him that if he ate from the tree of the knowledge of good and evil he would surely die.[26] Such a biblical narration clearly makes a link between, on one hand, a fundamental anthropological principle and, on the other, the entry of

25. Genesis 1:26.
26. Genesis 2:8-17.

death into human life. Therefore, the creation of man according to the image of God is the first step towards elaborating a Christian anthropology in order to be able to discuss the issues surrounding human death.

Although God created man according to His own image and placed him in paradise, man decided to abandon that life. The fall of Adam and Eve that followed changed man and his whole life. The changes that occurred in human nature, a nature shaped according to the image of God, is the second stage that needs to be examined in the theological inquiry of this book. Obviously, the creation of man according to the image of God entailed the presence of freedom in human life, and as a result of this freedom man was able to decide to reject the paradisiacal life.

Despite man's decision to leave his life in paradise, God decided to become man in order to save humankind from our fallen state and make us gods by grace. This was achieved through the death, burial and resurrection of Christ. Such redemption is continuously worked within the Church and Christian life as the faithful followers of Christ, such as the martyrs, have designated it. Therefore, the incarnation of God in Jesus Christ and its significance for understanding the character of human nature is the third stage around which the theological arguments in this book will be centred and developed.

This book develops this tripartite exposition of Christian anthropology with a view to the proper understanding of the character of Christian individualism. Within an individualistic secular society, a Christian individualism that presupposes a kind of relationship between the immanent and the transcendent sounds strange. However, it is worth making the attempt.

The writings of St John Damascene (seventh/eighth century)[27] and St Symeon the New Theologian (tenth/eleventh century),[28] two Greek

27. There is uncertainty regarding the dates both of his birth and death. Most scholars assume that he was born around 650 and died in 749 (Stiefenhofer, *Des Heiligen Johannes von Damaskus*, p. viii) or around the end of the first or the beginning of the second half of the eighth century (Kotter, '*Johannes von Damaskus*', *Theologische Realenzyklopädie* [TRE] XVII, p. 127). Others hold that he was born around 680 (Fitzgerald, 'John of Damascus', *The Encyclopedia of Christianity* [EC], Vol. III, pp. 70-71) and that he was alive at the time of the Synod of Hiereia (754) that condemned him (Christou, 'Ἰωάννης Δαμασκηνός', *Religious and Ethical Encyclopaedia* [REE] VI, p. 1221).

28. There is no agreement on Symeon's chronology. The dates of his birth range between 949 (Hausherr, *Un grand mystique byzantin*, [Life] p. xxxix, and Krivocheine, *St Symeon the New Theologian*, p. 15) and 956 (Christou, 'Εἰσαγωγή', p. 21), whereas the year of his death is considered to be either 1022 (Hausherr, *Un grand mystique byzantin*, p. xxxix, and Krivocheine, 'The Writings of St Symeon the New Theologian', p. 298), 1036 (Christou,

Fathers, have been chosen for study for the purpose of forming a Christian understanding of individualism. The former experienced a society in a transition, a society that was on a quest towards a reconsideration of the relationship between Christian teaching and the ideological orientation of public life. The latter wrote and taught within the culmination of the end result of this reconsideration, namely a secular society marked by the centrality of individualism.

By selecting these two Church Fathers one by no means underestimates the significance of the rest of the Church Fathers. On the contrary, each Church Father always builds on account the preceding patristic tradition. This is true both of John Damascene, who in a way recapitulated the theology that preceded him, and also of Symeon the New Theologian, whose ideas correspond to the teaching of some well-respected Fathers such as St Gregory of Nazianzus, St Maximus the Confessor, St John of the Ladder, St Theodore and St Symeon the Studite.[29]

John Damascene lived in a Byzantine society that, while experiencing the so-called Dark Ages, was simultaneously a society in transition. The Dark Ages of Byzantine society is evident in the drastic reduction in literary output and in the production of artwork,[30] as well as the absence of any significant theological writings.[31] In such a context, it is not accidental that during this period apocalyptic literature re-emerged, a genre that usually flourishes during times of political, economic or spiritual crisis.[32] At the same time, the iconoclastic controversy that took place in John Damascene's era is an indication that Byzantine society was really a society in transition.

'Εἰσαγωγή', p. 22), 1037 (Sotiropoulos, *Συμεὼν ὁ Νέος Θεολόγος*, pp. 20-21) and 1042 (Holl, *Gesammelte Aufsätze zur Kirchengeschichte II*, pp. 403-08). However, what is of interest for this book is not the exact dates of their birth and death but rather the characteristics of the respective historical periods in which Symeon the New Theologian and John Damascene lived.

29. Alfeyev, *St Symeon the New Theologian and Orthodox Tradition*, pp. 271-75.
30. Kazhdan, *A History of Byzantine Literature*, p. 14; Mango, 'Historical Introduction', pp. 1-6; and Moffatt, 'Schooling in the Iconoclast Centuries', pp. 85-92.
31. Phidas, *Ἐκκλησιαστικὴ ἱστορία II*, pp. 271-72.
32. The apocalypse of Pseudo-Methodius identified the Roman Empire with the last of the four world empires of the vision of Daniel and predicted an ultimate victory over the enemy, the Arabs (Haldon, *Byzantium in the Seventh Century*, pp. 367-68). The case of Anastasios of Sinai, whose work is likewise apocalyptic in character (ibid., pp. 431-33), is also very interesting as John Damascene seems to have known his *Guidebook* (*Hodegos*) (Kazhdan, *A History of Byzantine Literature*, pp. 78-79).

In particular, the emergence of iconoclasm was not accidental.[33] On the one hand, iconoclasm was an anti-spiritual movement that opposed the Greek tradition of the Empire;[34] on the other hand, iconoclasm came as a challenge to the established informal 'agreement' between the State and the Church and consequently worked against the particular character of their coexistence and cooperation. The belief that iconoclasm was simply the posing of the question of how far the divine is allowed to impinge on the human world[35] demonstrates the profound theological questions behind such a challenge. John Damascene's defence is oriented towards this challenge,[36] namely the desire for the reconsideration of the relation

33. Though the eruption of iconoclasm could be characterised as a 'historical accident' in the sense that Leo III failed to see the consequences of his actions, the fact that the impact of iconoclasm was connected with a series of political, social, institutional and theological issues (Phidas, *Ἐκκλησιαστικὴ ἱστορία I*, p. 773) may justify the argument that its character was not in fact accidental.
34. Zakythinos, '*La grande brèche dans la tradition historique de l'Hellénisme, du septième au neuvième siècle*', pp. 318-19. It has been argued that this historical period may be identified with the last great choice of the Christians of the Greek-Latin West, that of the choice of 'humanistic' Christianity, according to which the incarnate God can be described. On the contrary, 'Asiatic' Christianity chose the elevation of the divinity along with the condemnation of the material (Lemerle, *Le premier humanisme byzantin*, p. 100). The result of that choice was 'the emergence of the Byzantine Church from the iconoclastic crisis as more than ever a "Greek" Church' (Meyendorff, *Byzantine Theology*, p. 54).
35. Brock, 'Iconoclasm and the Monophysites', p. 57, and McGuckin, 'The Theology of Images and the Legitimation of Power in Eighth-Century Byzantium', pp. 47-48).
36. It is not accidental that John devotes a whole chapter of his second treatise against the iconoclasts to the unacceptable intervention of Emperor Leo III who, in 726, issued a law code, the *Ecloga*, in which he is presented, as the Emperor, to claim a kind of priesthood and, consequently, such legitimate authority on Church issues. John says that: 'The emperors do not have any right to style themselves lawgivers in the Church. . . . Political prosperity is the business of the emperors; the condition of the Church is the concern of shepherds and teachers. . . . For if we begin to erode the foundation of the Church even a little, in no time at all the whole edifice will fall to the ground' (*Contra imaginum calumniatores orationes tres* [*Imag.*] II, 12, pp. 102-104). Also, it is not surprising that, in the third treatise against the iconoclasts, John connects the defence of the veneration of the icons with a passage from the New Testament (Matthew 22:17-21) that had been extensively used for the justification of the secular authorities and the obedience of the Christians to them: 'And in the Gospels the Lord Himself answered those who questioned and tested Him saying, "Is it lawful to pay taxes to Caesar?" He said to them, "Show me the money for the tax," and they brought Him a coin. And Jesus said to them, "Whose likeness and inscription is this?" They said, "Caesar's." Then He said to them, "Render

between the immanent and the transcendent in Byzantine society.[37] In such a context, the view that John Damascene's writings are addressed only to the monastic public of his era is shown to be erroneous.[38]

Interestingly, the victory of iconophiles and the unambiguous sanction of the veneration of icons within the Church were not accompanied by a correspondent change in Byzantine society. While the veneration of icons re-established the relation between the visible and the invisible, the immanent and the transcendent according to the Christian tradition, Byzantine society preferred a more secular way of existence. The testimony of Michael Psellos, the most representative thinker of the eleventh century who mapped an essential transition in Byzantine society is very interesting. Michael Psellos, in his *Chronographia*,[39] clearly indicates that the Byzantine Empire was not a religious state but rather a secular imperium.[40]

Even though the veneration of icons prevailed, the societal orientation that was implied by it did not survive because of the transition of Byzantine society from the Dark Ages and the disruption of the old social links towards an individualised model of life. The veneration of icons was a type of worship with strong societal characteristics, as the icons were available to all believers and they were considered as a common mean

therefore to Caesar the things that are Caesar's, and to God the things that are God's." Since the coin bears Caesar's likeness, it is united to Caesar's person and you must give it back to him. Likewise, the icon of Christ is part of Him, and you must give it what is due' (Imag. III, 11, pp. 122-23).

37. The consideration of the intervention of Leo III as a reaction to the power claims on the part of the monks was another aspect of the ideological conflicts within Byzantine society (Phidas, *Ἐκκλησιαστικὴ ἱστορία II*, pp. 84-90). The aim of this study is not the systematic consideration of the causes of iconoclasm and the assessment of the different propositions in the field but rather the identification of the grounds upon which the eventual veneration of icons was characterised as a 'triumph of Orthodoxy'. John Damascene defends the possibility of depicting the incarnate God and, consequently, the presence of God within the *cosmos*. The reality of the incarnation of God and its implications for human life is in the very meaning of Orthodoxy. John's teaching in the *Three Treatises against Those Who Attack the Icons* is but the Orthodox view regarding the limits of the relationship, and the analogies, between the immanent and the transcendent.
38. Studer, 'Jean Damascène ou de Damas (St)', *Dictionnaire de spiritualité* (DS) VIII, p. 455.
39. Michael Psellos' *Imperatori de Bisanzio (Chronografia)* is considered to be the most popular work of Byzantine historiography. It consists of a number of colourful portraits of individuals such as emperors (Chron. I, 1-37) and princesses (Chron. VI, 1-75) who dominated the life of the Empire during the tenth and eleventh centuries. Through these descriptions one learns about very interesting elements that characterised Byzantine life at that time.
40. Kaldellis, *The Argument of Psellos' Chronographia*, pp. 77-80.

towards the development of a relationship with God. It is not accidental that the veneration of icons was supported principally by the monks who lived in the monasteries organised as coenobitic houses or *koinobia* following the monastic tradition of St Pachomius and St Basil the Great.[41] On the contrary, it is after the seventh century that communal life in the villages turned to an individualised life consisting of isolated families. At that time, the *koinobion* was seen as an odd social group bound by organic links and its existence within Byzantine society as a contradiction to the new social order in Byzantium. Within this context, the argument of the iconoclastic emperor, Constantine V, that participation in Holy Communion – participation with highly individualistic nuance – is sufficient for salvation is easily comprehended.[42]

Indeed, the new social order in Byzantium, the social order during the ninth and the tenth centuries, was principally secular and individualistic. Symeon the New Theologian[43] lived at the end of the tenth and the beginning of the eleventh century. He is known as a representative of mystical theology and the teaching of the way towards a personal or individual experience of God.[44] This shows not only that Symeon was part of the cultural characteristics of his era but also that his teaching could be taken as representative of Christian individualism.

Despite the long-standing belief that Symeon did not deal with the cultural and spiritual interests of his time,[45] it is this author's contention that his thought was not detached from the dominant ideology of the society in which he lived. Moreover, he was critical to the development of an alternative approach to the dominant ideology. Symeon's engagement in the life of Constantinople is easily justified by looking at his constant involvement with the centre of Byzantine society and his position vis-à-vis

41. Phidas, *Droit Canon*, pp. 166-75.
42. Kazhdan and Epstein, *Change in Byzantine Culture in the Eleventh and Twelfth Centuries*, pp. 1-13.
43. For a thorough discussion of the debate around the traditional name of Symeon as 'New Theologian', see Krivocheine, 'The Writings of St Symeon the New Theologian', pp. 315-27.
44. Though he does not make any precise reference to the 'prayer of the mind' or the distinction between 'essence' and 'energy' in God as St Gregory Palamas (1296-1359) did, he understands Christianity as a personal communion with and experience of God (Meyendorff, *Byzantine Theology*, p. 74).
45. Alfeyev, *St Symeon the New Theologian and Orthodox Tradition*, pp. 10-11. A gifted man like Symeon who lived in a monastery situated in Constantinople – a place that was not only the capital of the eastern Roman Empire but also the most important city in terms of contemporary theological and philosophical discussions – could not be unaware of or uninterested in what was taking place outside his monastery and what was affecting the life of churchmen.

ecclesiastical practices in his era. He was taken by his father at a young age to Constantinople to be educated and to be placed in the emperor's service. Though it appears that he did not receive any higher education, he lived in the capital of the empire for more than fifteen years, and some of the time within the Senate as *spatharocubicularios.*[46] In other words, Symeon grew up, was educated and lived at the centre of political and cultural developments in the Byzantine Empire. In addition, Symeon's contact with current ideology did not cease after he became a monk, given that both the monastery of Studios where he was tonsured and the monastery of St Mamas, where he was professed, ordained priest and elected abbot, were located in Constantinople. As an abbot of the monastery of St Mamas, he would regularly receive visits from lay people,[47] following a long-standing monastic tradition according to which 'monks were closely knit into the fabric of Byzantine life'.[48] The fact that Symeon's *Catecheses* survived in versions addressed to laymen and not only to monks[49] is an additional argument in favour of the assumption that Symeon was, in a way, an active participant in the contemporary historical and cultural life of Byzantium and against the theory that Symeon was simply an ivory-towered monastic writer and theologian.[50]

46. Life, 2-9. The term comes from the Greek word σπαθάριος (literally 'sword-bearer') which means dignity and refers to those imperial *spatharioi* who belong to the corps of the *koubikoularioi* (*The Oxford Dictionary of Byzantium* [ODB] III, pp. 1935-36) whose function, among others, was to escort the emperor (ODB II, p. 1154).
47. Ware, 'The Mystery of God and Man in St Symeon the New Theologian', p. 229. The location of the monastery of St Mamas in Constantinople reinforces even further the belief that Symeon was at the centre of the life of the city. There are two traditions regarding its whereabouts. The first tradition locates the monastery in the southwestern section of Constantinople near the gate of Xylokerkos (ODB II, p. 1287) and, therefore, well inside the city (Janin, *La géographie ecclésiastique de l'empire byzantin*, pp. 318-19), whereas the second tradition places it in the district of St Mamas, which included a harbour that by the terms of the treaties of 911 and 945 was assigned as the compulsory dwelling place of the visiting Russian merchants (Phidas, 'Μονὴ ἁγίου Μάμαντος', *Encyclopaedia Papyros Larousse Britannica* [EPLB] 40, p. 176). Obviously, both traditions justify the assumption that Symeon lived in a very active area of Constantinople that made him, in a way, part of the life of the city.
48. Hussey, *The Orthodox Church in the Byzantine Empire*, p. 349.
49. Krivocheine points out that these versions were designed by Nicetas Stethatos and not by Symeon, (Krivocheine, *Sources Chrétiennes* [SC] 96, pp. 169-74). Nevertheless, the design of these versions make sense because Symeon 'was a well-known abbot and spiritual father in Constantinople, and through his works he exerted incalculable influence on later generations' (*The Cambridge Medieval History IV: The Byzantine Empire Part II* [CMH], p. 199).
50. For the adoption of such a theory, see Alfeyev, *St Symeon the New Theologian*

On the other hand, the connection that is made between Symeon and individualism should not be linked to his characterisation as one of the representatives of the kind of monastic individualism that preaches an individual road to salvation and considers an occupation with the monastic community or other monks as spiritual destruction.[51] On the contrary, it is connected with his presence in a society where the emphasis on the individual is a point of reference in ideological discussions. Michael Psellos, a contemporary of Symeon, in his *Chronography*, a work that exemplifies the importance of individual creation, expresses the ideological climate of that era. In addition, Symeon's era is considered as the beginning of modernity, in the sense that the revitalisation of the *polis*, along with the emergence of the bourgeoisie and the development of trade are the first indications of a process that resulted in the modern state and the transition from self-governance to autonomy and the declaration of freedom and human rights.[52] Constantinople, the city in which Symeon lived, resembled the big cities during the revival of the *polis* in the West.[53] The individualistic environment of his time is also visible in the practice of providence as well as in the system of *charistike*. The former was the seizure of imperial-owned land by individuals, who would take the income from the land in return for military service, whereas the latter was a public programme sponsored by the emperor and the ecclesiastical hierarchy for the private management of religious institutions.[54]

---

and Orthodox Tradition, p. 11, and Gouillard, 'Syméon le Nouveau Théologien', *Dictionnaire de Théologie Catholique* [DTC] XIV, p. 2948. Similarly, Fountoulis thinks that Symeon did not deal with the relation between God and history or with issues related to the world outside the monasteries (Fountoulis, Λειτουργικὰ Θέματα Α, p. 103). Obviously, all these cases show an underestimation of the unavoidable historical designation of human life, even of the lives of the Sts. Johannes Koder, who was one of the editors of the *Hymnes* of Symeon in the series *Sources Chrétiennes*, adopts the opposite stance (as is also done in this book), although he uses completely different arguments when he talks about the dominant presence of political verses in the *Hymnes* – because of Symeon's association with Court circles in Constantinople and the fact that the event is not directed towards the monks of St Mamas but towards all those people (laymen, monks and priests) who are ready to understand and not to misinterpret (Koder, 'Γιατί ο Συμεών ο Νέος Θεολόγος έγραφε τους ύμνους του', pp. 813-18).

51. Kazhdan and Epstein, *Change in Byzantine Culture in the Eleventh and Twelfth Centuries*, pp. 148-51.
52. Cipolla, *Before the Industrial Revolution*, pp. 142-45.
53. Pirenne, *Les villes du moyen âge*, pp. 76-77.
54. *Byzantine Monastic Foundations Documents* (BMFD) I, pp. xxviii-49. Given the relationships of Psellos within the cultural environment of the eleventh

In short, John Damascene can be considered an astonishing interpreter and a representative of both the first period and the beginning of the second period of Christian theology, which has been influenced by his thought up to modern times.[55] Damascene was primarily occupied with the designation of the proper relationship between the immanent and the transcendent by dealing with how far the divine is allowed to impinge on the human world. He also lived in a cultural environment that was implicitly oriented towards the centrality of the human being in human history and into which he tried to introduce an enduring spirit of an Orthodox kind of humanism.[56] Symeon experienced the flourishing of humanism that led to modernity and attempted to found a Christian form of individualism as a prophetic reaction to the changes of his era. In other words, the selection of John Damascene and Symeon the New Theologian allows us to delineate Christian thought during a period which eventually resulted in the revitalisation of the 'modern' *polis* [57] and from which the roots of modern society and thought may be traced.

III. The Synthesis

The critical evaluation of modern society, as well as the presentation of a Christian alternative with regard to the issue of euthanasia based on the theological inquiry of this book, is the final step of the whole work. This is achieved by bringing together the ideological principles of modern society and Christian theology and by looking at the possible interplay between the two. This interplay coincides with the ongoing task of the Church to elucidate Christian understanding of the relation between the immanent and the transcendent in and for every era. This book aims to accomplish such a task, for it constitutes an attempt to make the proper transition from the theological tradition of the Church Fathers to contemporary society with a view to discussing the issues surrounding euthanasia.

The privilege of the Christian tradition is that it examines that very 'world' (i.e. the inner world of every human being), where moral decisions are actually made, namely the anthropological parameters of moral decisions, and this offers some interesting insights into current bioethical debates. It highlights the invisible and hidden – either consciously or

century in Constantinople, his designation as a notable *charistikarios* (BMFD II, p. 449) is quite interesting.

55. Karmiris, 'Ἡ δογματική διδασκαλία τοῦ Ἰωάννου Δαμασκηνοῦ', p. 3.
56. Matsoukas, 'Εἰσαγωγή', p. 9, and Duffy, 'Hellenic Philosophy in Byzantium and the Lonely Mission of Michael Psellos', p. 145.
57. Karayiannopoulos, *Ἡ Μεσαιωνική δυτική Εὐρώπη*, pp. 109-11.

unconsciously – sides of the moral issues, and therefore enriches the various arguments in the field with a view to more convincing and more thought-out moral processing. The seriousness of bioethical issues deserves such careful consideration.

Thus, this book seeks to demonstrate the positive consequences of including a religious tradition in a debate that has been characterised as secular by elaborating a Christian form of individualism, given that the issues surrounding euthanasia constitute the after-effects of individualist and autonomous human being. Therefore, the designation of the fundamentals of Christian individualism is presented in contrast to modern individualism. What then emerges is a reshaping of the rationale that dominates the current debate in bioethics regarding the deliberate administration of death. As a consequence, the whole context within which euthanasia has appeared as an issue with a societal interest is challenged and redefined. In other words, this book ends with the provision of the necessary tools towards not only a Christian but also a secular 'treatment' of bioethical issues, such as euthanasia, tools that are sensitive to the Christian tradition as well as the concerns of modern society.

IV. Outline of the Book

This book, even though it belongs to the discipline of Christian ethics, is characterised by the inclusion not only of theological, but also philosophical, sociological and historical arguments. Such an interdisciplinary approach contributes to a better understanding of the ethical issue under discussion and consequently to a more profound analysis and an elaboration of more finely developed arguments. For a preview of this book as a whole, a brief presentation of its outline is necessary.

This book is divided into three parts. The first and second chapters constitute the first part. The first chapter contains a thorough-going analysis of bioethics as a discipline and delineates the necessary basis upon which all bioethical issues must be understood. More particularly, first the polemical and subjective character of bioethics is defined, and the way in which it is oriented towards power claims over those expressing a different reality is revealed. What follows is an exposure of the disguised power claims of bioethics by demonstrating the close link between bioethics and the just war theory, and by identifying the common ground shared by traditionally opposed bioethical approaches, such as, principlism and utilitarianism. The implications of such a reality are elaborated in chapter two by focussing on a specific bioethical issue, namely euthanasia. In this chapter, the power claims of bioethics are particularised in the efforts towards the 'creation' of a 'new' human being, efforts that are fully justified on the part of theories of human existence that are interested in their sovereignty in the public arena. These efforts clearly imply an orientation towards a supposed objectivity and a universalisation based on the possibility of a common morality among the moral agents, a morality that at least in part underestimates the so-called 'particular' moralities. Throughout the first part, the authority of such a kind of morality is challenged and the prospect of including particular moralities in the current debate on bioethical issues is instigated.

Chapters three and four comprise the second part of the book and present a particular morality that is based on moral arguments that are rooted in the patristic tradition. The selection of John Damascene and Symeon the New Theologian gives a different slant on issues surrounding euthanasia compared to secular bioethics. The theological arguments of the two Fathers are developed along the lines of establishing a Christian form of anthropology and thus of a content-rich morality.[58] Issues such as the character of human existence, our free will, suffering and death are discussed. This discussion lays the foundations for a different kind of moral argumentation regarding euthanasia and lays out the necessary grounds for a substantial critique of arguments used by either the proponents or opponents of euthanasia. These arguments are briefly mentioned in this part.

In the third part the theological arguments on issues surrounding euthanasia are fully explained and placed within contemporary society and in relation to individualism, the view of human existence that predominates in this era. Taking into account the basic components of secular bioethical thinking as presented in the first part, as well as the centrality of individualism to the emergence of the issues surrounding euthanasia, this book applies theological arguments that link from the Scriptures and the patristic tradition to the current debate via the elaboration of the fundamentals of a kind of Christian individualism. On these grounds, the presentation of moral arguments surrounding issues relevant to euthanasia may represent a substantial contribution to the current debate of euthanasia.

58. To the best of my knowledge, the first attempt to discuss a modern bioethical issue, such as, in vitro fertilisation, from the viewpoint of Orthodox theology was undertaken as early as 1958. This was a fascinating paper by Metropolitan Konstantinidis, who presented a Christian ethical discussion of the issue in an interesting way (Konstantinidis, 'Τεχνητὴ γονιμοποίησης καὶ θεολογία', pp. 212-30).

Part One

Power Claims over Human Life and the 'Creation' of a 'New' Human Being

Most of the works in the field of bioethics praise their own sufficient and valuable results in order to designate the role of medicine in the medical context, a role that is secured through the creation of lists of principles and rules and the designation of procedures. Besides this approach, there are other works that emphasise various parameters such as good communication between the moral agents involved (physicians, patients and relatives) or the adoption of laws that protect the integrity of those agents. In the first part of this book we argue that all these works converge in one direction. In modern medicine, as in other aspects of human society, subjective views are imposed on human persons through disguised power claims over human life. The implications of these subjective views on human life are very important once they are oriented towards the 'creation' of a 'new' human being. Since bioethics touches upon human existence itself, a systematic identification of the character of bioethics and its role in modern societies is necessary. What follows is not an attempt to discard bioethics as a field related to ethical issues in the medical context, but rather a critique of bioethics with the view to describing its future role, according to which it should take into account not only its own limitations but also the possible contribution of the 'particular' moralities. This is attempted through, on one hand, taking a diachronic view of human existence with regard to the character of sovereign bioethics in modern society and, on the other, revealing the implications of such an approach in the discussion of a particular bioethical issue, namely euthanasia.

Chapter 1
Bioethics and Power Claims on Human Life

Introduction

Amidst the remarkable progress of medical technology, bioethics has emerged with a view to the establishment of an ethical framework appropriate to coping with newly-emerging ethical issues. From the beginning, this new field has devoted all of its efforts to the proper anticipation of moral issues, created by the immoderate power of medicine in the medical context.

Jonas was one of the first philosophers to discuss the new world that technological progress had created along with the technological orientation of modern societies. He described the manner in which the 'deification' of technology and the consequent exercising of the power of scientific knowledge over nature had resulted in self-destructive outcomes for human beings, such as the ecological crisis. Since, in our times, the survival of human beings is at stake, Jonas proposes the exercise of the ethic of responsibility as a restraining force over the excessive power of technological knowledge.[1]

While Jonas examined the catalytic role of technology in human life, Foucault discussed more specifically the changes in the medical context. By raising the issue of the institutionalisation of disease and the patient due to the development of modern medicine over the last centuries, Foucault explained how excessive power had been placed in the hands of

1. Jonas, *The Imperative of Responsibility*, pp. 140-42.

the physician as the result of the removal of power from the hands of the patients and their relatives.[2] He also went further, highlighting both this sovereign kind of power, as administered within the complex technical and administrative structure of hospitals and health authorities, and the bio-power that is operated through the control exercised by medicine to powerfully manipulate the human body.

Undoubtedly, all these efforts towards revealing the power claims of modern medicine and its offspring, bioethics, over human life, enable one to make a substantial contribution to understanding the current reality in the medical context. However, this is not sufficient if the decisive role that bioethics plays, the field devoted to the protection of man by medical power, is ignored. This book, and this chapter, in particular, attempts to transfer our interest from the power of medicine to the power of bioethics over human life, arguing that there is a continuous struggle for power claims over human life by all relevant theories. Like all theories that want to claim sovereignty over human life, bioethics is proven to be polemical by nature.

The first part of this chapter sets out the common ground that all theories relevant to human existence throughout the centuries, including bioethics, share. On one hand, the belief in the possibility of a common morality is challenged and, on the other, the subjective character of bioethics is identified. The second part of this chapter presents a number of arguments that show explicitly the polemical character of bioethics and that demonstrate practices that are oriented towards disguising its polemical quality. This camouflage is necessary for bioethics to secure societal approval. In short, the first chapter of this book gives a description of the character of sovereign bioethics based on a synchronic view of human existence.

I. The Polemical Character of Bioethics: Subjectivity and Power Claims

1. The Challenge of Common Morality

In the 1960s, bioethics joined the range of types of ethical discourse as a discipline that deals with moral issues relevant to medical practice and that would strive to secure the respect of the academic community. Bioethics has gained high popularity both in academic fields (philosophy, medicine, law, sociology and theology) and in social domains (governmental bodies, social and religious institutions, the public

2. Foucault, *The Birth of the Clinic*, pp. 16-20.

debates and the mass media). From principlism to virtue theories and from contractualism to casuistry and liberalism, all theories in bioethics purport to cope sufficiently with the issues raised in the medical context such as those of life, suffering[3] and death. Indeed, bioethics in the modern world seems to enjoy the status of a religion that governs human life in its most fundamental aspects,[4] even though it is presented as a field that secures its claims to objectively justified ethical practices at the expense of ethical reflections that are based on 'particular' moralities. However, what is the truth of this assumption?

a) The Subjective Character of Decisions

Bioethics consists of a number of different theories, each of which claims a universal character, a character that justly pleads for objectivity on the basis of the designation of the most appropriate principles and rules or of a given common morality. If so, the question remains as to whether all or some of these theories are entitled to contend for such a universality over and applicability to human life. The recently introduced common morality project may serve as a paradigmatic case for exploring the character of bioethical theories. The project of common morality has been chosen as an example of the character of the various bioethical theories for two reasons. First, it represents a general tendency of ethics in a variety of domains such as political philosophy[5] and, second, it is implied in all bioethical approaches, since each one of them claims that it is sufficient to meet the needs of all moral agents involved.

---

3. The term 'suffering' in this book includes all those elements in the life of a patient that are viewed as negative experiences, and entails not only the pain that derives from the disease of the body and the feeling of approaching death, but also the sorrow that is related to non-physical aspects of human existence, such as a difficult patch in personal relationships (e.g. the introduction of a patient into the medical context is quite often accompanied by the removal of the patient from his real life, in which, among other things, he has a variety of personal relationships and common activities with others).
4. As early as 1970, Arendt foresaw that intellectuals would constitute a new, and by virtue revolutionary, class that would be interested in power and authority (Arendt, *On Violence*, pp. 72-73). In our case, we may infer that her description could apply to all those who are active in bioethics and who represent academic disciplines such as philosophy, the law, sociology and theology.
5. The common morality project in bioethics is not a trend that can be identified only within the context of modern medicine. It is also evident in political philosophy and the development of an ethics that is attempting to confront the fragmentation of the modern world. See, for example, Walzer, *Thick and Thin*, where Walzer supports, among other concepts, the idea of the ethical minimum for the justification of dynamic actions in international relationships (pp. 63-83).

A comprehensive definition of common morality reveals a characteristic vagueness. Veatch states, 'The core idea of a common morality is that all humans – at least all morally serious humans – have a pretheoretical awareness of certain moral norms.'[6] Inevitably, this definition raises a number of questions regarding the person who is entitled to identify who these 'morally serious humans' are or regarding the designation of 'certain moral norms', as well as the criteria upon which the 'morally serious humans' and the 'certain moral norms' are determined. What lies behind the scenes is revealed through applying Kondylis' descriptive theory of decision.

The basic assumption of DTD is that the finite subject cannot grasp the objective world, but rather shapes his own world and more precisely his own worldview by choosing from the existing one (the 'preliminary world') elements that interest him. This is the procedure of decision that takes place through a rude or gentle violence of the 'preliminary world'. If the objective world is defined by the totality of all the 'preliminary worlds' and of all the worldviews that arise from each decision, then the decision of a subject can only be subjective. Similarly, since the subject is unable to apprehend objective reality and since the empirical finding justifies the presence of many, more or less different, decisions and worldviews, the outcome of the decision procedure of the subject is always subjective.

Once the subject has established a specific worldview, henceforward, reality is evaluated according to the subject's criteria and rational tools. It is through these criteria and tools that the subject decides what is interesting and what is important to his own worldview. The attribution of an interesting and important character to certain elements is enforced by the denial of their subjective character and at the same time the adoption of an objective character for them. As such, the worldview of a particular subject turns out to enjoy 'objectivity' which, in its turn, safeguards the justification of a particular decision.[7] In the same way, the questions that are raised with regard to the vagueness of the definition of common morality and, particularly, the inevitably subjective character of any decision regarding the fulfilment of the requirements of such a definition, is an indication that the project of common morality that is oriented towards its universal establishment is always subject to a particular worldview, even though it attempts to conceal this self-evident truth. Consequently, even such a project of common morality is subjective by definition.

---

6. Veatch, 'Is There a Common Morality?', p. 189.
7. Kondylis, *Macht und Entscheidung*, pp. 14-17.

b) The Distinction between the Worldview Decision and the Choice among Alternative Solutions

The proponents of common morality may oppose the position stated immediately above by saying that: 'Universality is located in common morality and non-universality in other parts of the moral life, which parts are called "particular moralities ".'[8] This response implies a distinction between universality and these 'particular moralities'. However, such a distinction makes no sense once its vagueness is demonstrated. What is hidden in this distinction is what really counts.

According to Kondylis, there is always a conscious or unconscious confusion of what actually happens when we take a decision. The generally accepted position is that we choose among alternative solutions that safeguard our self-confidence and self-control, and that our identity functions as a weight measure. However, this position is a delusion, as the consideration of the links between the worldview decision, identity and self-preservation of the subject explicitly shows.

Without getting into a detailed discussion, DTD not only explains how the worldview, identity and decision are interwoven, but it also justifies the parallel birth of the worldview and the identity in question. Interestingly, the history of the human being is the history of the decision, that continuously moves towards the establishment of a worldview and the delineation of the identity of the human being. This procedure is not static but dynamic, and it is always accompanied by important or unimportant decisions.

In such a context, the worldview decision is considered a presupposition for the choice among alternative solutions. This happens as the subject makes choices by presuming a particular worldview. It is at the centre of this worldview that alternative solutions rival each other. It is difficult to distinguish between these alternative solutions and the dynamic procedure of a decision that results in the creation of a worldview and an identity. In fact, the alternative solutions, on the one hand, constitute segmental decisions upon which, in the service of self-preservation, the history of the subject is reflected partially or totally. On the other hand, they preserve the way of thinking and the desires implicit in the worldview decision in such a way that the coherence and the orientation of the subject on the basis of his worldview are safeguarded.[9]

Therefore, the distinction between worldview and segmental decisions indicates that the distinction between 'universality' and 'particular moralities' in bioethics is elusive, since both parts of this distinction belong to the category of segmental decisions that are based on and connected with

8. Beauchamp, 'A Defense of the Common Morality', p. 259.
9. Kondylis, *Macht und Entscheidung*, pp. 22-28.

the worldview of the subject(s). Before deciding what is universal and what is not, another, more fundamental, decision must be taken. This fundamental decision is related to the very identity of the decision-maker and as such is linked to the ground upon which the segmental decisions are taken. In other words, any approach to universality such as the project of common morality is not convincing once it ignores or hides what really matters, that is what really designates the supposed universalistic or particular norms.

c) The Oneness of Theory and Practice

The proponents of the substantiality of common morality may argue that, while the subject(s) of the various decisions have their own worldview, their decisions could not but share in the common universal ground or 'a pretheoretical awareness of certain moral norms'.[10] Obviously, such an argument implies a clear division between the theory, namely the worldview, and the practice, namely the segmental decisions that are taken by the subject(s). However, this division is another erroneous belief and cannot be substantiated by DTD.

Kondylis says that what we have identified here as the fundamental decision is characterised by the complete existential participation of the subject, which indicates the complete presence of the multidimensional impulse of the subject for his self-preservation along with his unconsciousness, consciousness and rationality. This complete existential participation of the subject reveals that any distinction between the cognitive and the volitional elements, or between the intellect and volition, is not legitimate regarding the interpretation of human decisions.

More particularly, as has been said above, the subject, through the action or procedure of decision, wants to secure his self-preservation. This volition is fulfilled by means of the framing of a worldview through the selection of those elements of the world available to the subject. This procedure, that presupposes a distinction or a judgement of what is interesting to the subject, is in fact the starting point towards the understanding of the subject. This understanding is none other than the interweaving of the subject with the object, where the latter is submitted to the former (another indication of the subjective character of decision), a kind of submission that is based on specific criteria, upon which the volition is particularised for the self-preservation of the subject. Thus, the understanding and the volition are fused in the worldview decision, a fusion that is perfectly exemplified in the dependence between the worldview decision and segmental decisions. Such dependence justifies the oneness of theory and practice.

10. Beauchamp, 'A Defense of the Common Morality', pp. 260-61.

The oneness of theory and practice is a very important aspect of the character of decision-making, since it rejects the fallacious dualism of keeping the action independent from the theory and the worldview of the subject. Through the discussion of the relationship and the fusion between understanding and volition, Kondylis aims to reject not only normative and axiological principles but also the anthropological and gnoseo-theoretical remnants of metaphysics and modernity. This view contradicts classical metaphysics, according to which pure knowledge reaches its apogee in pure and real being, and it also contradicts modernity, which gives priority to ontology and searches for relations between knowledge and volition.[11]

Thus, it is self-evident that theories of human existence, such as the project of common morality, which strive to prove their objectivity and to generalise their implications, are founded on an artificial distinction, namely the distinction between the worldview (i.e. theory) and the segmental decisions (i.e. practice or actions) of the moral agents.

2. The Character of Bioethics: Polemical by Nature

The subjectivity of all theories and, therefore, of bioethics is better justified through the identification of their profound character that is proved to be polemical by nature. This point of view is further elaborated and disproves the well-established impression that bioethics is a quest towards the application of ethics in the medical context with a view to meeting the needs, protecting the rights and respecting the personalities of the agents involved without any self-interested incentive.

a) From Self-preservation to the Broadening of Power: the Friend/Enemy Schema

A decision (the action or the procedure of abruption and breakaway from which an ideology has arisen) is taken through the dynamic impulse for self-preservation that gives to the subject making the decision a particular orientation, provided a worldview has already been framed and the

11. Kondylis, *Macht und Entscheidung*, pp. 28-33. See, also, Kondylis, *Das Politische und der Mensch*, pp. 453-65, and particularly pp. 464-65, where he justifies the fusion between thinking and volition with reference to Aristotle. Kondylis reminds the reader that, when Aristotle talks in *Nicomachean Ethics* about intention, that is the intent of someone who does something based on a choice that he has made among many possibilities open to him, he defines this selection or intention as a 'desiderative reason' (ὀρεκτικὸς νοῦς) or 'ratiocinative desire' (ὄρεξις διανοητική) (Aristotle, *Nicomachean Ethics*, 1139a 31-33, 1139b 4-5).

subject has taken up a particular position within that worldview. Once such a procedure is accomplished, the subject feels powerful. While the desire for self-preservation and its successful accomplishment betrays the presence of power claims on the part of the subject, the support of this desire upon the basis of the worldview that predominates in society secures the broadening of the power of this subject.

In particular, a worldview is supposed to be in agreement with the workings of the world and not directed against it; otherwise, this worldview could not stand as a sufficient basis for the self-preservation of the subject of a decision. Thus, since self-preservation, which is a dynamic procedure, is connected with power claims, and since the subject wants to safeguard his position against antagonistic factors, self-preservation is presented as being the continuous broadening of the power of the subject. Consequently, linking the worldview decision with the self-preservation of the subject results in the fusion of decision and power claims.

If, according to DTD, a decision is synonymous with power claims, then it always has to be directed against the 'enemy', namely the antagonistic factors in question. Such factors may include those of an inorganic or organic nature, a collective or individual threat, a foreigner, neighbour, brother or even elements of the innermost ego to the extent that all these constitute disadvantages for the self-preservation of the subject. What is remarkable is that the various faces of the 'enemy' are not considered something outside the worldview of the subject. On the contrary, they occupy a specific place in the worldview of the subject, either consciously or unconsciously. In other words, since the worldview is based upon specific power claims, it is also continuously addressed at particular enemies.[12]

Kondylis introduces the dipole schema of friend/enemy as something fundamental to understanding the framing and sovereignty of the different worldviews in the history of humankind.[13] At this point, it should be kept in mind that Kondylis, in his descriptive theory of decision, does not refer only to individual subjects. In fact, he refers to three kinds of subjects of decisions: the genus, the group (in its different social and historical forms) and the individual, even though he does not detect any great differences between groups and individuals as subjects of decision.[14] As a consequence, the schema of friend/enemy must not only

12. Kondylis, *Macht und Entscheidung*, pp. 33-37.
13. Though Kondylis borrows this schema from Schmitt (in *Political Theology*), who applied it to political theories, he applies it more broadly to all cases in the development of human civilisation.
14. Kondylis, *Macht und Entscheidung*, pp. 40-45.

be applied to the understanding of human existence on an interpersonal level but also in a broader sense, such as within social groups or society as a whole.

The application of this schema regarding the description of bioethics on a non-normative and non-axiological basis shows that bioethics, as a secular discipline that wants to shape human life in the medical context, has to be considered as polemical by nature. The self-preservation of bioethics passes inescapably through its power claims over human life. This accusation is not in fact an accusation, as long as it refers to all the available worldviews, and it may not be convincing since it is not ostensibly derived from a completely theoretical model. Therefore, further justification is necessary.

b) The Polemical Character of Decision: Its Disguise and Objectification

Any objection regarding the polemical character of bioethics can only be sustained if, and only if, bioethics as a field refers to the establishment of norms that serve the public and limit any self-interested incentives. In such a case, there is a strong possibility of there being objectified norms and not norms with a profound subjective character.

In an excellent description, Kondylis argues that efforts towards objectifying the character of a subject's decision presuppose the strength of the subject's support for self-preservation. The belief in the objectivity of a decision is an existential necessity, since it instils in the subject the certainty that his orientation is consistent with reality, and that he possesses the criteria to judge what is objective and what is not. Such a procedure can only be understood through an analysis of the subject's efforts at self-preservation and to broaden his power.[15]

The survival of a particular form of societal life depends upon its ability to guarantee the collective, as well as the individual, security of the majority of the members of a society. Since the decision of the subject is aimed at his self-preservation and the broadening of his power, and evidently presuppose an individualistic orientation, such a decision and its power claims must adhere to normative principles that are considered necessary for the survival of a particular civilisation. Through this procedure the power claims permeate the normative and general principles that have been established for the limitation of power claims. In other words, what we find are disguised power claims, which allege to be normative principles and not subjective and self-interested, high-handed acts.

15. Ibid., pp. 48-49.

Once subjective and self-interested incentives are eliminated, the prospect of objective and universal claims begins to be created. This prospect has two main consequences.

First, the transition from self-preservation and power claims to the ideal and normative level is very crucial for the subject who is making the decision. This transition ensures, on one hand, the belief in a particular meaning of life, which is necessary for presenting a particular decision as the one most appropriate for the majority of the members of a social group, and, on the other, it ensures that respect is secured for those elements related to the self-preservation of the subject through both the idealisation and the limitation of those elements. For example, murder, though prohibited, may become a 'just case'. As a consequence, the subject's decision is objectified. The objectification of such a decision is successful to the extent that the decision – in fact, a violation of objective reality by its subject – is disguised.[16]

Second, normative principles as disguises of those things related to self-preservation, such as power claims and the broadening of the subject's power, introduce the problem of interpreting the content of these principles. Thus, the centre of interest is shifted and efforts are directed at the dominance of a particular interpretation and, consequently, the dominance of a particular interpreter. These efforts are successfully realised through a hierarchy that is designated within the subject's worldview, where the placement of the 'enemies' (antagonistic beliefs, arguments, etc.) is strictly allocated. The specific interpreter establishes such an allocation by making the distinctions of immanent /transcendent (the transcendent is always unreachable by the 'enemies' because it represents the absolute orientation of a particular worldview) and the distinction of Being (*Sein*)/ Appearance (*Schein*) (the presence of the 'enemies' is always attributed to 'Appearance' and as such their power to challenge those that represent Being – indisputable reality – is eliminated). These hierarchies aim at defeating 'enemies' through the dominance of the subject as interpreter of normative principles. In such a case, the objectification of a decision becomes the monopoly of interpretation.[17]

Therefore, it is not surprising that all theories in bioethics pretend that they are, on the one hand, consistent with the norms, principles and values of modern society (at either an individual or societal level) and, on the other hand, supply the appropriate safety valves that prohibit any misuse or overstepping of generally accepted norms and principles in modern society, by claiming for themselves the authority to interpret

16. Ibid., pp. 49-59.
17. Ibid., pp. 61-70.

their content objectively. Such an allegation against bioethics clearly shows the manner in which particular historical circumstances (i.e. the characteristics of modern society) can be used as a means towards the process of disguising the power claims of all theories in bioethics. Thus, the connection between a decision and specific historical conditions results in a kind of objectivity that can be considered as a basis for consent among different subjects. For example, Engelhardt, one of the most influential scholars in bioethics, in his book *The Foundations of Bioethics*, supports the idea that, due to the particular circumstances (the particular historical situation), the principle of autonomy, that presupposes the free consent of the agents involved in the medical context, is the only principle that seems to be compatible with modern (liberal) society. This idea clearly implies that the particular historical situation should play the leading role in the establishment of universally respected principles and norms, and therefore, in the sovereignty of a particular worldview.

On the contrary, according to DTD, the specific historical situation shapes the decision but in a different way. A historical situation circumscribes a decision in the sense that it designates the particular circumstances through which the decision of the subject obtains power claims in favour of his friends and against his enemies. Therefore, despite the connection between historical circumstance and decision, the decision cannot have any objective character. Similarly, since the subjective character of the decision never changes, the normative principles that arise in a particular historical situation cannot claim universal adherence due to the subjective character of their origin. The inescapably subjective character of normative principles is apparent in the empirical reality that different theories of normative principles exist.[18]

c) The Importance of the Distinction between Structure and Content: All Theories are Polemical

The above argument could raise a number of objections by the proponents of all theories in bioethics. Any agreement with it could lead to the loss of their power claims and would result in their defeat. A further application of DTD may shed more light on the character of decision.

According to DTD, even though all worldviews (social, political or ethical theories, or religious) have a different content, they all share the same framework of concepts or the same structure. Regardless of their derivation – from either metaphysics, atheistic humanism, or postmodern common morality and ideology – the actual difference

18. Ibid., pp. 37-38.

between them pertains only to their different content. The long-standing belief in the profound divergence between the normative and axiological system is upheld when the fundamental distinction between structure and content is ignored.

Disregarding this distinction in this way is not accidental. On the contrary, the confusion made between structure and content throughout human civilisation, even today, is intentional. Acknowledging a common structure between the different worldviews coincides with acknowledging a common ground of initiation. This coincidence results in the self-revelation of the polemical character of all worldviews. The fact that the subjects of every decision have power claims over their 'enemies', results in the affirmation of the profound subjective character of all decisions. Obviously, such an acknowledgement diminishes those efforts towards objectifying a decision, and consequently towards ensuring its dominance in the public arena.[19]

Understanding the distinction between structure and content is very important and becomes clearer by looking at the priority of the former over the latter in the decision-making process. In particular, according to DTD, a decision is presented as the end result of any conscious or unconscious process that has always been characterised by the efforts of the subject(s) making the decision at securing permanent axes of orientation and safeguards – such efforts are considered part of the common structure shared by all theories. Both orientation and safeguards are provided through the connection of the relevant actions with either a meaningful life, belief in God, prosperity of human beings or particular inclinations and desires that the subject making a decision considers universal and natural. Moreover, the provision of orientation and safeguards is counted as the particular content that is adopted by a particular theory. Though this placement of the subject seems to correspond to the agreement of his actions with his specific worldview, this subject may be, at the same time, subordinated to the sovereignty of a different worldview that is more powerful.[20] Despite the fact that the character of a decision is subjective, there is a quest for safeguards that may lead the subject, consciously or unconsciously and to a different extent in each case, to his submission to alien worldviews for the sake of making the transition from a subjective to an objective decision. Thus, while the content may alter, the quest towards a permanent point of orientation and safeguards, namely the structure, remains always the same.

19. Ibid., pp. 66-68.
20. Ibid., pp. 43-45.

An important example of this kind of subordination is described by Hauerwas who, when he discusses the emergence of medical ethics as a messianic dawn for philosophers and theologians, points out that: '"Religious ethicists" could turn to medicine using the same terms as the philosophers and be rewarded for how useful their analysis was, even though their theological presuppositions were not brought into play.'[21] This example illustrates quite neatly, on one hand, how a departure like the 'turn to medicine' may be beneficial for the subjects in that they are then placed in the 'world' that predominates at that moment at the price of rejecting their own presuppositions. On the other hand, it illustrates how a structure that is oriented towards safeguarding respect and authority for one or other worldviews is the same, though the content of the worldviews may be different. Those who choose to turn towards, or better subordinate themselves, to a more powerful worldview are convinced that they do not have to abolish their own worldviews, given that the preservation of their own worldview is *sine qua non* a precondition for their self-preservation and polemical orientation.

To sum up, the application of the descriptive theory of decision to bioethics has shown, first, the absence of any objectivity or common norms or principles and, second, that all theories in bioethics are polemical in character, which means that they fight for self-preservation and sovereignty by exerting power claims on each other. As a consequence, there are self-interested incentives in all theories of secular bioethics and there is also a power struggle among them. Therefore, the assumption that bioethics secures objectively justified ethical practices, as opposed to an ethical reflection that is based on a 'particular' morality, is by no means warranted.

II. The Exposure of the Disguised Power Claims of Bioethics along with Their Subjective Character

As DTD has shown, all theories in the history of human beings throughout the centuries have been characterised by power claims that were necessary for the self-preservation of their subjects and the eventual sovereignty of one over the other. The previous section has revealed the polemical character of all theories in the history of humankind. The disclosure of the disguised power claims of all theories, and particularly those of bioethics, along with their subjective character, follows. This is made through, first, a brief history of the emergence of bioethics; second,

21. Hauerwas, *Suffering Presence*, p. 5.

the presentation of the necessary presuppositions for power claims over human life by bioethics; third, the establishment of the relationship between bioethics and the just war theory (a theory that justifies waging war and the power claims of one nation over another); and, finally, the discussion of the implications of the power struggle over life, suffering and death within bioethics.

1. From Medicine to Bio-politics: Why Bioethics Does Not Deserve Its Name

What makes bioethics extremely important is its involvement with absolute questions, with matters of life and death and, consequently, with human nature itself. Even the name bioethics – the term *bio* comes from the Greek word βίος that means life – implies a discipline that claims authority over the establishment of the ethics of life. If bioethics claims responsibility over the ethics of life, then it has to include issues that cover the whole spectrum of life and not only parts of it. Otherwise, bioethics cannot justify its name. This observation has been, intentionally or unintentionally, forgotten. To gain a better understanding of the character of bioethics, a brief historical overview is provided.

Medicine, as a profession that has always dealt with matters surrounding life and death, has always been accompanied by so-called medical ethics that traditionally had the responsibility of defining and determining not only the responsibilities of physicians towards their patients but also the relationship between physician and patient. Medical ethics, by exploiting the techniques and theories of moral philosophy, has always been a respected discipline dedicated to the study of ethical questions in the medical context.[22]

In the 1960s, the continuous increase in medical and technological power, along with an increasing interest in the rights of patients[23] and rising fears about the possibility of profound changes not only in medicine but also in human nature, revealed the restrictive nature and inappropriateness of medical ethics in dealing with such a wide range of interests and concerns.[24] This led to the coining of a new term and a new field that comprised a series of different disciplines, those of moral philosophy, medicine and health science, theology, sociology and law.

22. *The Oxford Companion to Philosophy* (OCP), p. 544.
23. Gillon, 'Persistent Vegetative State, Withdrawal of Artificial Nutrition and Hydration, and the Patient's "Best Interests"', pp. 75-76.
24. Engelhardt's preface in Potter's *Global Bioethics*. See also Clouser, 'Bioethics', pp. 54-55.

Potter's articles, such as 'Bioethics, the Science of Survival' and 'Biocybernetics and Survival', introduced bioethics as a new discipline that would deal not only with the moral issues relevant to medicine in the world of advanced technology but also with the main issues pertinent to the survival of humans. Despite Potter's understanding of bioethics as a discipline oriented towards the survival of human beings,[25] the current use of the term betrays a choice that, on one hand, confines bioethics strictly to the medical context (for Jonsen, the 'Birth of Bioethics' is fulfilled dealing with subjects such as 'death and dying, human experimentation, genetic engineering, reproductive technology, and organ transplantation'[26]) and, on the other hand, barely widens the horizon of traditional 'medical ethics' to meet the new challenges in medicine, for the 'new challenges' are limited simply to the 'problems of truthfulness, privacy, justice, communal responsibilities and the like'.[27] The result is that bioethics is limited to a context designated by technologically advanced medicine and the moral issues that are created by it.

Bioethics, by claiming authority over moral issues in the medical context, claims power over human life, and particularly over those aspects that are shaped by modern medicine, such as suffering and disease. Despite the importance of technological power in modern medicine and its influence on healing, other aspects of human life are also important for a human being, even in the medical context. However, this self-evident truth is consistently ignored by modern bioethicists, as they prefer to answer the questions that are caused by medical technology without placing much interest in the human condition itself.

The choice by bioethicists to focus only on the tip of the iceberg and deal, for example, with the issue of euthanasia as an issue related to the permissibility of death, and not as an issue dependent on the character of human existence, is not accidental. It need not be pointed out that such a choice designates the orientation of bioethics towards power claims over health policies and practice in the medical context from either a philosophical, legal, sociological or psychological perspective. This orientation is easily betrayed by the underestimation of the decisive role of

25. Potter makes his thought explicit in an interesting presentation, in which he incorporates medical and ecological bioethics into biological knowledge, the knowledge of human value systems, as well as individual, societal and population problems (Potter, *Global Bioethics*, p. 72). In a broader sense, according to Jonsen, Potter, like his fellow scientists who gathered at the conferences of the early 1960s, considers bioethics a description of 'values that should frame human life' (Jonsen, *The Birth of Bioethics*, p. 34).

26. Ibid., p. viii.

27. Beauchamp and Childress, *Principles of Biomedical Ethics*, p. 1.

worldviews (the identification of the character of human nature is always based upon a particular worldview), upon which an ethical decision is taken. In other words, bioethics, instead of being an ethics of human life, becomes bio-politics,[28] since it is occupied with the provision of the appropriate justification of all relevant health policies and practices – the elaboration of bioethics is strongly related to governmental policies on issues related to health and the safeguarding of certain secular principles in the wider society. This transition indicates an attempt towards the implementation of politics, rather than towards the service of human life as the real meaning of bioethics implies.

2. How Does Bioethics Make Its Power Claims over Human Life?

The consideration of bioethics as bio-politics is the first step towards understanding its power claims over human life. However, how does such a bio-politics have power claims over human existence?

First, due to the authority of universities in modern society, bioethics – from its inception – required the necessary academic respect in order to become the successful successor to traditional medical ethics. Based on this reality, bioethics had inevitably to accept the compartmentalisation of knowledge as found in modern universities (and which results in an incomplete understanding of reality) and become part of a community that reflects the moral order of modern society.[29] In other words, bioethics had to pay an important price.

---

28. The term bio-politics is used by Foucault to indicate that in modern society the biological life of man is integrated more and more into the mechanisms and plans of the given authority (see, for example, Foucault, *The History of Sexuality*, pp. 140-43). Here this term is used with the meaning that it acquires when it is placed in the context of Kondylis' thought, which is the fixed (in all eras) practice interpretation of human life that shows power claims through the 'release' of the subjectivity and the contest for a dominant role in the configuration of modern reality at all levels.

29. A very interesting critique of such a reality is made by Hauerwas, who responds to the question of how universities contribute to the corruption of youth (Hauerwas, *Christian Existence Today*, pp. 237-52). Manent is particularly expressive when he describes the unlimited freedom of the scientist to formulate his hypotheses and to draw conclusions: 'He is the absolute sovereign over his province of "facts", which is methodologically exempt from connecting to other facts, which is to say from the whole of the human phenomenon. He is in fact more than exempt – he is formally forbidden even to sketch such a connection, which would constitute an offense against scientific rigor and a lapse into "literature" or "ideology" or even "philosophy"' (Manent, *The City of Man*, p. 111).

Second, as DTD has shown, a theory or a discipline will survive only by occupying a central place in the currently most powerful worldview (in our case, that of secular society) and by being persuasive it can cope with the needs of the majority of the people. A substantial step in this direction is the demarcation of clear lines between those efforts that promote the supposed universality of bioethical theories and those that encourage particularistic convictions. In this context, bioethics chose to draw separating lines from other disciplines and particularly from theology and the so-called 'particular moralities'. Indeed, since bioethics has power claims over human life in the medical context, theology may be considered as one of its opponents. However, the drawing of such lines is not justified once, according to DTD, there is no theory, set of principles or norms that may legitimately claim universality and censure others for sectarian positions. The establishment of any principles, theories or norms cannot be universal by definition. The movement towards dividing realms is what has been used by all worldviews, throughout the centuries of human civilisation, since this practice is the means *sine qua non* by which they may broaden their control over human life. Consciously or unconsciously, the promising new discipline of bioethics, while it suffered, from the very outset, from an incomplete understanding of reality, was, however, oriented towards sovereignty over human life and pretensions of universal applicability.

Third, this orientation towards sovereignty over human life and pretensions of universal applicability implies an internal interdependence. The acknowledgement of the universal applicability of bioethics is possible only through effectively masking its motivations for sovereignty over decision-making regarding human life, and consequently for the 'self-preservation' of bioethics itself. This facade is framed through the adoption of the current values of society and, particularly, through the defence of these values. For example, in a hedonistic society where the fulfilment of individualistic pleasures enjoys high priority, an ethic that serves such an orientation has a high chance of success. On the contrary, ethics that challenge such an orientation seemingly have no future.[30]

It is in this context that the emphasis of most of the bioethical theories on the right of autonomous patients to choose between alternatives according to their own interests and preferences has to be viewed. It is

30. For a systematic presentation of the hedonistic character of modern society and particularly the dominance of individualistic hedonism, see Kondylis, *Der Niedergang der bürgerlichen Denk- und Lebensform*, pp. 169-283.

worth noting that support for the autonomy of the patient and the choice between alternatives is always accompanied by the imposition of a particular worldview. It is not accidental that Beauchamp and Childress, two of the most influential supporters of the application of this principle of autonomy in bioethics, try to justify the general availability of substantial (there being not a complete absence of influence) autonomous choice by giving examples such as the free choice of a house or university.[31] This connection reveals a particular approach as to how the autonomy of a human being is measured. This approach is indicative of a particular worldview, and this worldview undoubtedly shapes the understanding of autonomy in, for example, the medical context where suffering, life and death are anticipated. As DTD states, there is a profound dependence of segmental decisions (the various alternatives) on the respective worldviews.

Such dependence is obvious from the way that these alternatives are presented and the designation of their connotation and particular content with regard to the worldview that rules the medical context. It is for this reason that the dependence of the provision of alternatives on particular worldviews is fiercely denied by those theories that want to endure through broadening their power and disguising their self-interested motives. It is in the context of their efforts towards disguise that one should understand the suspicions of secular bioethics towards theological ethics, which, in contrast, openly declares the foundation, for example, of Christian bioethics on a lucid worldview.

3. Bioethics and Just War Theory: the Justification of Power Claims

The fact that bioethics has power claims over human existence, along with its aim of broadening its power and, consequently, its dominance in the public arena, can be demonstrated even more forcefully through identifying the common ground between bioethics and just war theory.[32] In the following section, it is argued that the character of bioethics could be considered as another form of the just war theory, a theory that is used for justifying the waging of war, namely the justification of causing harm and/or death. This assertion is not recent. As early as 1954, Joseph

31. Beauchamp and Childress, *Principles of Biomedical Ethics*, p. 60.
32. The relationship between medicine and war has also been discussed by Hauerwas. He points out that: 'the essays on medicine are designed to help illumine how the republic that war serves and embodies also resides in the very practices designed to "help" people' (Hauerwas, *Dispatches from the Front*, p. 27).

Fletcher proclaimed that Christians should allow an exception for killing to alleviate suffering near death, given that Christians allow exceptions to the Sixth Commandment for killing in wartime.[33]

Bioethics is presented as a discipline that deals with the moral issues that are raised in the medical context as a result of technological developments in medical practice, and reflects the character of modern society – the ideologies that predominate in western developed societies incline towards priorities and preferences that inescapably shape medicine and vice versa. Because the moral issues that are raised in the medical context are issues relating to human life itself, its destiny and its meaning (the meaning of disease, suffering, death etc.), the power claims of bioethics over human existence concern the most significant parameters of life.

Along the same lines, the just war theory as a means as a means of justifying war is directly connected with human life itself. The waging of war turns one human being against another, causes harm and death, and violates some human values in the name of others. Apparently, like bioethics, the just war theory clearly implies power claims over human life.

The connection between bioethics and the just war theory attempts to show that both share common ground by having power claims over human life. This sharing of common presuppositions is evident in the efforts of those pushing bioethics and the just war theory to present as objective what is fundamentally subjective, and to disguise their aims towards broadening their power and their sovereignty over their 'enemies'.

a) Bioethics and Just War Theory: Two Sides of the Same Coin

Just war theory states that wars are just only when the conditions of *jus ad bellum* (regarding the just recourse to war) and *jus in bello* (regarding the just execution of a war in progress) are fulfilled.[34] This framework of the just war theory presupposes moral absolutism that separates war crimes from just wars. Just like the proponents of bioethical theories and

33. Fletcher, *Morals and Medicine*, pp. 195-96.

34. *Jus ad bellum* requirements for waging war include a public declaration, a proportional just cause, a reasonable prospect of success, its justification as a last resort and a legitimate authority. *Jus in bello* requirements for waging war include deployment of means proportional to the cause only, respect for non-combatants' immunity from attacks and the treatment of prisoners of war as non-combatants (Childress, 'Just-War Criteria', p. 41). For a critique of such dualism that constitutes the very essence of war, see Walzer's *Just and Unjust Wars*, p. 21, where historical war cases such as World War II and the Vietnam War are discussed, in order to expose the problematic character of the division of the moral reality of war into the reasons states have for fighting and the means they adopt.

the proponents of the common morality project, the proponents of the just war theory base most of their arguments on absolute claims – claims that bespeak an objective and universal character.

Baker,[35] in a remarkable paper, reveals the strong links in objectivity and universality between the just war theory and bioethics. She argues that the application of criteria borrowed from just war theory in resolving medical-ethical dilemmas at the bedside is acceptable.[36] She tries to formalise and expand Dyck's process[37] and applies eight criteria of the just war theory[38] to demonstrate the ethical character of making an appendectomy. Baker's main argument is that decision-making in the medical context that is based on just war criteria is appropriate within the context of a pluralistic society, once this basis provides the practitioner and patient with the necessary tools for daily use. Moreover, the application of just war criteria in the medical context is able to stand the tests of universality and generality.

Baker supports her position by identifying similarities between decision-making in the medical and wartime contexts. Her position is that in both medicine and war all those involved cause harm – harm in the form of pain, restriction or invasion – and thus exemptions are established with regard to the duty 'not to harm'. Moreover, by using just war theory criteria, she discovers further connections between the medical and the war context. Among others, the legitimate authority in medicine (the physician and the patient) is analogous to the model of the government (the elected officials and the electorate constitute the legitimate agents in politics); the just cause for medical intervention corresponds to intervention in war; the just intention towards the well-

35. Baker, 'The Application of the Criteria of the Just War Theories in the Resolution of Medical-Ethical Dilemmas at the Bedside', pp. 3-19.
36. Baker's article has been published by the official journal of the National Federation of the Catholic Physicians' Guild. In my view, this is not accidental, because the historical roots of the just war theory trace back to Augustine and because the ethical arguments that are quite often used in both the medical and wartime contexts, such as the doctrine of double effect (which is discussed later in this chapter), also originate in the Catholic tradition and, particularly, the teaching of Aquinas. This is, however, by no means to say that recourse in every case to the arguments of the just war theory as well as the doctrine of double effect is in accordance with Catholic tradition.
37. Dyck, 'Ethics in Medicine', p. 13.
38. Dyck follows the model of just war theory proposed by Childress, whereby legitimate authority, just cause, reasonable hope of success, just intention, due proportion, just means, declaration and last resort are identified as the criteria that have to be fulfilled in order to wage a just war (Childress, 'Just-war Theory', pp. 427-55).

being of the patient in medicine matches the just intention of peace through the waging of a war; and finally, the application of particular medical treatment that affects human life is considered as the last resort in medicine just as war is regarded as the last resort in politics.[39]

Undoubtedly, Baker's contribution to the present discussion is very interesting. However, her approach focusses only on the external and superficial similarities between the just war theory and bioethics. The fact that she applies just war criteria without questioning the theoretical presuppositions that lead to the development of the just war theory prevents her from looking at the profound common ground that both just war theory and bioethics share. Therefore, she can see neither their willingness to seek justification of the application of power over human life, nor their demand for objective recognition, despite the fact that they are subjective *au fond*.

The application of DTD has shown that such absolute claims on the part of bioethics cannot be justified. Likewise, Calhoun, in a noteworthy article, raises the same problem within the just war theory by revealing the inconsistency that is connected with the supposed absolutism. This inconsistency emerges through paying closer attention to the conditions that have to be fulfilled for a war to be considered as just. The cornerstone of Calhoun's thought is that a specific authority, which is considered legitimate, must make the judgement as to which conditions need to be fulfilled. Therefore, the just war framework, though it presupposes moral absolutism, simultaneously implies moral relativism. As such, the interplay between absolutism and relativism in the just war theory results in a meta-ethical paradox. To use Calhoun's words, 'Just war theory paradoxically commences from moral absolutism, while implying that the morality of the killing of innocents is context-dependent, which is precisely the statement of relativism.'[40] What is clearly implied is that the particular authority pleading for the justification of a war is historically determined, temporally limited, and that its leaders are appointed in the conventional manner. Calhoun concludes that, if relativism is true, then any application of the standards of one society beyond its own parameters, as happens when one nation attacks another, is misguided, and therefore there are no moral grounds for waging wars.[41] This conclusion is at root in agreement with the analysis of the character of bioethics through the application of DTD.

---

39. Baker, 'The Application of the Criteria of the Just War Theories in the Resolution of Medical-Ethical Dilemmas at the Bedside', pp. 6-15.
40. Calhoun, 'The Metaethical Paradox of Just War Theory', p. 53.
41. Ibid., p. 55.

In a few words, the basis for both bioethics and the just war theory is that there is a common morality that serves as a common ground towards justifying power claims over issues related to human life, and particularly over the administration of actions that have profound effects on human life (in either a medical or a wartime context). Also, in both cases, justification is necessary due to the voluntary violation of particular ethical standards (e.g. the killing of innocents). Additionally, in both cases what plays the most important role is the specific authority that is presented as being the legitimate authority for taking decisions. Finally, in both cases, any decision that is made is fundamentally subjective, even though presented as objective.

b) Just War Theory, Bioethics and Disguised Attempts at Power Claims

To achieve a more complete overview of the relationship between just war theory and bioethics, it is necessary to look at the criticism of just war theory by so-called pacifists. A glance at the confrontation between the proponents and opponents of the just war theory reveals the common presuppositions of both bioethics and the just war theory. Although this work does not aim to present a systematic discussion of the arguments of either side, some useful lessons for bioethics could be drawn from a brief examination of this moral conflict.

According to just war theory, the waging of war is justified once several criteria are met. The absolute focus on simply fulfilling a series of criteria in order to justify and legitimise causing undesirable harm to human beings implies that care for human life is reduced to the level of politics. As a consequence, the waging of war and the consequent administration of harm and death – which transgresses the threshold of human existence – are considered as part of the particular policy of a nation or of a group of nations. Such policy is justified through the fulfilling of criteria (or principles or norms) and does not deal with, either directly or indirectly, human life itself: the application of just war theory is never explicitly accompanied by the essential content of a particular worldview for the self-evident reason of avoiding the consideration of waging wars as the outcome of a particular culture.

Cahill, when looking at the theological context of just war theory and pacifism, asserts that just war theory is based on the setting of minimal criteria. This is self-evident in those efforts at making compromises between different and antagonistic religious, moral and cultural beliefs with a view to universality. Additionally, just war theory, even though it presumes values like peace or justice, does not offer a substantive view of those values.[42] Obviously, just war theory, as is common practice in bioethics, is characterised by self-limitation in a construction of principles, norms or criteria, and is presented as not being oriented towards a specific worldview. We have already shown that such self-limitation is necessary in order to provide the appropriate ground for the successful broadening of power in solving moral disputes.

Without a doubt, the proponents of just war theory could not accept such an accusation. It is for this reason that just war theorists attempt to re-orient their contradistinction with pacifists by taking into account the fact that focussing on specific criteria or principles is misleading for understanding the character of the just war theory. Unfortunately, even these efforts are subject to the same weaknesses identified above.

Childress, one of the proponents of just war theory, appeals to the human sense of duty in order to retaliate against the accusations of pacifists. He wants not only to defend just war theory but also to present a formal theory, devoid of substantial ethical content or content-less, that would be applicable to pacifism as well. He therefore elaborates the just war criteria in the light of the *prima facie*[43] duty of non-maleficence, the duty not to injure or kill others that the justification of war must override.[44] After grounding the just war criteria in the condition of overriding the *prima facie* obligation not to injure and kill others, Childress concludes that just war theorists and pacifists fail to notice their common starting point, according to which non-violence has moral priority over violence and that violent acts always need justification because they violate the *prima facie* duty not to injure or kill others.[45] He believes that, through the emphasis on the priority of non-violence over violence, common ground between pacifists and their opponents can be established. It is interesting that Childress believes that, by offering a formal theory of just war, a theory that is devoid of any particular content, and by not being aligned to a particular worldview, agreement between the just war theorists and the pacifists can be achieved, given that this does not require material consent.

Among other efforts to reconstruct the just war theory in order to secure a universal applicability, feminist studies offer their own alternatives. For example, Peach, by criticising the intimate dichotomies

42. Cahill, 'Theological Contexts of Just War Theory and Pacifism: A Response to J. Bryan Hehir', p. 261.
43. A *prima facie* duty is a duty that can be overridden if a competing moral consideration should arise. For the notion of *prima facie* duties or principles, see Ross, *The Right and the Good*, pp. 16-47.
44. Childress, 'Just-War Criteria', pp. 41-42.
45. Ibid., p. 53.

of the traditional just war theory, such as the dichotomies between male and female, combatant and non-combatant, soldier and citizen, ally and enemy, state and individual, pleads for a more particularised, contextualised, and individualised approach. Such an approach focusses on the effect of going to war on the lives of particular individuals.[46] Apparently, even Peach and her feminist just war theory stick within the external parameters of the waging of wars by proposing more sensitivity to particular individuals without any appeal to the specific worldview from which such sensitivity may be derived.

It is remarkable that such beliefs that have been developed within the context of the just war theory are also, *mutatis mutandis*, recognisable in the medical context, since they, despite the proposal of particular principles, are based on the systematic purging of all theories of any content. As the application of DTD has pointed out, all theories focus on their principles and responsibilities as regards society, and they exaggerate the differences between them as regards their own, unique, content in order to successfully objectify the subjective character of their decisions.

c) Just War Theory, Bioethics and the Doctrine of Double Effect

The close ties between bioethics and the just war theory is further justified with reference to the doctrine of double effect (DDE). The case of the doctrine of double effect (also called the principle of double effect) holds a central position in understanding the polemical character and power claims of all theories, including just war theory and bioethics. DDE is invoked to explain the permissibility of an action that causes serious harm, such as the death of a human being, as a 'side effect' while some good end is being promoted.

DDE is a doctrine that has been applied with the same frequency in both war and medical contexts. This common use at least shows, though implicitly, the common ground between these contexts.

(i) The Disputes over the Formulation and Interpretation of DDE: The development of DDE can be traced back to Catholic theology and, in particular, to the teaching of Aquina s. However, contemporary philosophers, either proponents or opponents of DDE, tend to provide a rationale independent of Catholic moral theology. This tendency, however, underestimates the survival, even in a non-theological form, of the theoretical presuppositions that gave rise to DDE. Therefore, while there is a kind of agreement as to the conditions that constitute DDE, there is a definite disagreement as to the precise formulation and interpretation of this doctrine. The disagreement about the precise

46. Peach, 'An Alternative to Pacifism? Feminism and Just-War Theory', pp. 152-72.

formulation and interpretation of DDE is not irrelevant to the modern tendency to keep DDE separated from its origins.[47] At this point, a brief history of DDE may shed some light on the issue as a whole.

Among those who articulate and apply DDE, it is a common premise that this dogma has its theoretical roots in the *Summa Theologica* of Thomas Aquinas and, in particular, his attempt to justify killing in self-defence.[48] Though Aquinas' analysis as to whether it is lawful to kill a man in self-defence[49] has attracted a lot of attention, the placing of his analysis in a particular section of *Summa Theologica* has been ignored. Accordingly, it should be remembered that Aquinas' teaching on killing a man in self-defence forms part of a broader consideration of murder, whereby a human being inflicts the greatest iniquity on another human being. Without a doubt, the study of a single paragraph isolated from the whole text from which it is derived, is, at the least, misleading.[50]

In the section devoted to murder, one may notice that Aquinas does not hesitate to justify killing, but this is always in two specific circumstances. In the first instance, the act of killing has to be for reasons of the welfare of community and the consequent preservation of the common good – it refers to the killing of evildoers, that resembles the severing a decayed limb by a physician for the sake of the health of the whole body.[51] In the second instance, the act of killing has to be carried out either by a person who has public authority, which implies that such a person acts for the common good, or by a person who acts in self-defence, which shows that the priority of one's own life rather than of another's is natural.[52] Aquinas has a particular understanding of what is the common good of the community (the Christian community or the Christian State) and it is the preservation of this common good that leads to the killing of

47. Powers shows how different contemporary attempts to defend DDE have not been successful. By scrutinising the rationales proposed by scholars in the field, such as Joseph Boyle, Michael Bratman, Warren Quinn, John Mackie, Thomas Nagel and Charles Fried, he concludes that they have failed to resolve either the deeper theological issues surrounding DDE or its disputed application in cases involving death in medicine (Powers, 'Contemporary Defences of the Doctrine of Double Effect', pp. 341-56).
48. See, for example, Boyle, 'Toward Understanding the Principle of Double Effect', pp. 10-11, and Berkman, 'How Important is the Doctrine of Double Effect for Moral Theology? Contextualizing the Controversy', pp. 95-97.
49. St Thomas Aquinas, *Summa Theologica*, SS, Q. 64, 7.
50. The article in the *Summa Theologica* that discusses the lawfulness of killing a man in self-defence is one of the eight articles that deal with the lawfulness of killing in a variety of forms (ibid., SS, Q. 64, in the introduction).
51. Ibid., SS, Q. 64, 3.
52. Ibid., SS, Q. 64, 7.

those who are opposed to it.[53] It is in this context that Aquinas attempts to develop some criteria that may justify the administration of death and which later resulted in the elaboration of DDE.

(ii)The Justification of Killing and DDE: It is not accidental that the fundamental presumptions that stand behind the justification of killing in particular circumstances connected with a kind of common morality ('common good' for Aquinas) and with the authorisation of subject(s) ('public authority' and 'self-defender' for Aquinas) coincide with the analysis of the descriptive theory of decision, according to which a worldview can have power claims once the absolute defeat of its opponents is achieved. Undoubtedly, the acceptance of killing is crucial, since it opens the way towards the administration of death in specific circumstances. Therefore, it is not surprising that DDE has been used in the context of both war and medicine. In the former, it was used for the justification of waging wars, and as consequence of administering harm and death, whereas in the latter, it was used for the justification of administering death in abortion and euthanasia. Interestingly enough, though DDE is primarily related to a justified administration of death, almost all studies on DDE are oriented towards its consistency as regards the distinction between the intended and foreseeable effects of an action.[54] The evaluation of DDE and its criteria in the light of the substantiality of this distinction for the justification of killing follows immediately below.

Regardless of the differences in the formulation of these criteria by contemporary proponents of the dogma,[55] there is a basic agreement on the conditions that should be met for an act to be judged morally permissible.[56] The first condition refers to the agent who must act to reach

53. There is substantial disagreement as to whether Aquinas actually justifies killing in self-defence or whether he gives enough weight to the mandate to care for one's own life and well-being (Berkman, 'How Important is the Doctrine of Double Effect for Moral Theology? Contextualizing the Controversy', pp. 95-97). Here, the emphasis is placed on the general framework that resulted in the development of the doctrine of double effect and not on the provision of an analysis of Aquinas' thought and the exact limits that he places on the justification of actions.

54. See for example, Quinn, 'Actions, Intentions, and Consequences: The Doctrine of Double Effect', pp. 335-47.

55. Marquis discusses four different versions of DDE that aim, unsuccessfully, to bypass any problems of inconsistency that older versions had (Marquis, 'Four Versions of Double Effect', pp. 516-42).

56. Although many scholars in the field have proposed their own versions of DDE, the formulation that is proposed by Powers in his 'Contemporary Defences of the Doctrine of Double Effect' has been selected because of its explicitness of the presuppositions of DDE. An almost identical description of the four condition of DDE is found in NCE.

some good end or purpose, or at least some morally neutral end. The second condition refers to the agent's lack of intention to harm innocent people, although he may foresee it as a consequence. The third condition refers to the agent's unintentional harm to others as a means to reach a good end or purpose, even though he may foresee it as a side effect. The final condition refers to the proportional relationship between the intended good end and the foreseen harmful effect. Obviously, the main idea found in these criteria is that of the intention ('an act of the will, presupposing the act whereby the reason orders something to the end'),[57] given that moral actions take their character from their end (from what is intended), even though other unintended effects may result.[58] Then, what are the implications of these criteria for the consideration of human existence?

First of all, what derives from the criteria of DDE is the focus on the morality of an act and not on human behaviour as a totality. This focus implies that a specific action can be isolated from human life as a totality. The consideration of an act as independent and as a sole activity, without there being any substantial dependency on the subject, and particularly his specific worldview, is quite arbitrary. The descriptive theory of decision detects a very serious confusion between a segmental decision (the choice of a particular action among alternative solutions) and a person's worldview. Interestingly, it is through this confusion that the foundation stone of DDE is laid with a view to the successful objectification of a subjective act, and finally to the justification of an act that leads to death.[59] This 'objectification' disguises the subjective character of an act and at the same time disguises power claims of the subject(s) of an act over human life.

Second, the issue that also derives from the same criteria is the individualisation of the decision of an agent. This introduces a problem, since an agent and his actions should not be considered

57. Aquinas, *Summa Theologica,* FS, Q. 12, 1.

58. Aquinas identifies the end of an action with what is intended by that action. Any other effects that may accompany the intended end are placed among those that are characterised as accidents, namely those that do not belong to the constituent elements of a species, which cannot be regarded as sin (*Summa Theologica,* SS, Q. 43, 3).

59. The 'objectification' of an act is quite often connected with absolute presuppositions. Traditionally, the DDE theorists are absolutists, despite the divergence among them (Cavanaugh, 'Double Effect and the Ethical Significance of Distinct Volitional States', pp. 139-40). Others maintain that behind the application of DDE stands the absolute character of Catholic morality (Boyle, 'Who Is Entitled to Double Effect', pp. 486-88).

as divided from the rest of those human beings who constitute the interpersonal interactions in a small group of people, i.e. a family, hospital, community, or a whole society. Every agent is a member of a small or a large community and is always dependent on a particular worldview. Therefore, his morality has to be viewed within a broader picture than that of the close-knit picture of DDE.[60] It is definitely an issue that DDE may consider someone who enjoys absolute autonomy as an agent, and independence like the autonomy and independence of God.[61] In this context, DDE as a doctrine that is able to give man the authority to administer death (when the appropriate criteria are fulfilled) is absolutely consistent, and man is somehow conferred with the 'divine' power that makes him eligible to have power claims over human life.[62] Once more the descriptive theory of decision is proven to be true, given that the denial that human existence is founded on a particular worldview and, consequently, on a particular understanding of human life ensures the presence of the necessary implications towards a disguised exercising of power over human life.

Third, what emerges through the DDE criteria is that the permission or acceptance (or lawfulness for Aquinas) of an action that leads to death is counted as a particular mental element of a human being, a mental element that is viewed in isolation from his other mental states. By considering intention as an efficient and necessary condition of permitting killing, the moral character of human behaviour is at least oversimplified once it ignores the complexity of human personality. The primacy of intention in the morality of human acts sets up a human being spoiled by his substantial elements such as his sentiments, passions and unconscious inclinations. All these reveal the subjective and problematic character of intention with respect to its use as a crucial criterion. In other words, before discussing whether a specific effect of

60. The view of the moral agent as a being that is separated from the rest of humankind, even from his most intimate partners, has been criticised by many authors whose interests range from Christian theology to feminist philosophy.

61. The relationship between autonomy and DDE is discussed by Bole, though without implications as to the possibility of an absolute autonomy on the part of human beings (Bole, 'The Theoretical Tenability of the Doctrine of Double Effect', pp. 470-72).

62. Boyle points out, based on the Catholic tradition regarding the problem of evil, that God does not intentionally bring sin but only accepts it as a side effect. In this context, it is implied that man, like God, can do the same by being in a position to distinguish clearly what is intended and what comes out as a side effect (Boyle, 'Who Is Entitled to Double Effect', p. 493).

an action can be considered as either intended or a foreseeable effect based on the DDE criteria, the sufficiency of the DDE rationale for the justification of death administration has to be examined. Otherwise, any relevant analysis turns a blind eye towards the eligibility of such dogma.

To sum up, the establishment of the common ground that bioethics and just war theory share makes it evident that bioethics has power claims over human existence with a view to the broadening of its power and dominance over its 'enemies'. All these are feasible through the efforts for the objectification of what is subjective by definition, based on content-less ethics. This practice is clearly evident even among competitive bioethical theories.

4. Bioethics and the Power Struggle over Life, Suffering and Death – When Principlism and Utilitarianism Do Not Imply Any Difference

The elaboration of any theory in bioethics is an expression of the submission of its power claims to normative principles (where 'normative principles' include all the principles, norms, values, virtues, commandments etc. as well as their relationships that are proposed as sufficient ethical ground for taking decisions) over human existence. This is to be completely expected, since those who assert power claims know that they have to control their unconscious and non-rational inclinations by respecting the law and institutions in order to achieve their disguised practice.[63] The submission to normative principles of two of the bioethical theories that are traditionally considered to be opponents, namely principlism and utilitarianism, is very expressive of the common ground that they share regarding their structure as theories of human existence.

a) The Imperative of Autonomy: Principlism and the Focus on Procedural Issues

The majority of bioethicists focus their discussion on the importance of principles and rules to issues relevant in the medical context. The most important principles that have surfaced through this trend are those of

63. It is widely accepted that power claims and ethics are heterogeneous as they represent what is 'bad' and 'good', respectively. This is an idealistic rather than a realistic interpretation. Undoubtedly, power claims do not necessarily lead to an uncontrollable exercise of power (Kondylis, *Macht und Entscheidung*, pp. 73-74).

autonomy, beneficence and justice. Though others support additional principles[64] or re-baptise them,[65] the interpretation of the principles of autonomy, beneficence and justice as well as their interrelationships are central to the issues surrounding decisions on euthanasia. The specific interest of this research in such decisions leads primarily to the examination of the principle of autonomy.

The tradition of so-called principlism emerged at the same time as the initial appearance of bioethical issues, with Beauchamp and Childress' *Principles of Biomedical Ethics*[66] giving it systematic endorsement. In fact, these two eminent bioethicists have chosen to concentrate not on the elaboration of a content-rich account of autonomy, but rather to raise the importance of respect for autonomy, apparently with a view to universality. This is quite evident when they consider liberty (independence from controlling influences) and agency (capacity for intentional action) and not a content-rich autonomy as the essential conditions to all theories of autonomy. Thus, human behaviour is not considered as the result of a particular understanding of autonomy that comes from a particular worldview. On the contrary, what matters is the focus on the 'autonomy as a choice'.[67] Consequently, the disengagement of 'autonomy as a choice' from any content and from any dependence on a variety of inescapable influences, such as the character of the subject of the autonomy itself or the historical circumstances in which he lives, is necessary. Otherwise, a systematic account of the sources and the nature of these influences is required.[68] In this context, it is

64. For example, Beauchamp and Childress include as the fourth principle that of non-maleficence (*Principles of Biomedical Ethics*, pp. 113-64). Battin adds dignity, which includes 'autonomy, self-determination and responsibility for one's acts . . . self-awareness and cognizance of one's condition and acts, together with their probable consequences' (Battin, *The Least Worst Death*, p. 282).

65. Engelhardt refers to the principle of autonomy as the 'principle of permission' in order to emphasise the authority of the moral agents in the medical context (Engelhardt, *The Foundations of Bioethics*, pp. 102-21).

66. The first edition of Beauchamp and Childress' *Principles of Biomedical Ethics* was published in 1979, while the fifth edition, to which the quotations cited in this work correspond, came out in 2001.

67. Beauchamp and Childress, *Principles of Biomedical Ethics*, p. 58.

68. Though a systematic account of what stands behind the idea of 'autonomy as choice' is not attempted, arbitrary presumptions are made. For example, Beauchamp and Childress call the agents of 'autonomy as choice' 'normal choosers'. The 'normal choosers' are those who act intentionally by exhibiting various degrees of understanding and control of influences (ibid., p. 59). Beauchamp and Childress use the term 'normal chooser' in contrast to the 'ideal chooser', or those who control first-order desires or preferences through

not surprising that the interpretation of the principle of autonomy can range from it being a choice, a right[69] or a negative/positive obligation[70] to a *prima facie* principle.[71]

In other words, Beauchamp and Childress, on the one hand, avoid the absolution of autonomy in decision-making in medicine since such absolution has been considered weak in establishing arguments in bioethics. On the other hand, they suggest rather a procedural use of autonomy by not proceeding to any profound account of human autonomy, since such an account entails the risk of revealing elements of a particular worldview and of losing the flavour of universality towards which principlism is oriented. Notably, though alternative approaches to autonomy have been proposed in bioethical discussions, the focus of interest remains, more or less, on the procedural treatment of human life in the medical context.

The testimony of Engelhardt, the bioethicist who laid the foundations of principlism in bioethics,[72] though he later rejected the idea that

---

second-order desires or preferences (Dworkin, *The Theory and Practice of Autonomy*, pp. 3-81). However, the attribution of the characteristic 'normal' or 'ideal' cannot be legitimised without explicit definitions of 'normal' or 'ideal' along with the designation of the context in which such definitions make sense.

69. The respect for autonomy is the acceptance of all decision-making rights that enable people to act autonomously. On the contrary, disrespect for autonomy implies attitudes and actions that not only ignore but also insult or demean the rights to autonomy of others (Beauchamp and Childress, *Principles of Biomedical Ethics*, p. 63).

70. As a negative obligation, an autonomous action should be not subjected to controlling constraints by other(s) and should foster autonomous decision-making (ibid., p. 64). However, the assertion that the idea of negative obligation derives from Kant's use of autonomy, and his imperative towards the respect of persons as ends in themselves, cannot be justified if Kant's autonomy is viewed on the basis of the 'kingdom of ends' – that is the union of different rational beings in a system governed by common law and in which the relationships between rational beings are characterised by their treatment as ends and means (Kant, *Groundwork of the Metaphysic of Morals*, pp. 100-01).

71. Beauchamp and Childress, *Principles of Biomedical Ethics*, pp. 63-64.

72. Jonsen, presenting the history of the Belmont Report (the report that assigned authority to principlism), comments that two of the three principles chosen for the published version of the report (National Commission for the Protection of Human Subjects of Biomedical and Behavioral Research, *The Belmont Report*, Appendix, Vol. 1) had been derived from an Engelhardt paper that proposed, among other things, 'respect for persons as free moral agents' and 'concern to support the best interests of human subjects in research' (Jonsen, *The Birth of Bioethics*, pp. 99-104). The former was termed 'the principle of respect for persons' (later it was re-baptised as the principle of respect for autonomy) and the latter as the principle of beneficence.

principles can serve as a panacea in bioethical issues,[73] is very interesting. Engelhardt does not see any way out of this vicious circle. He argues that the Enlightenment project, with its roots in natural law and the philosophical assumption regarding the capacities of reason, has failed to establish a content-rich secular bioethics. As a consequence, the only means available to resolve controversies between individuals and societies is a 'libertarian character of morality',[74] according to which the emphasis must be placed upon the individual and his or her authority to establish social structures, while at the same time moral choices can only be justified by the permission of those individuals involved. Engelhardt re-baptizes 'the principle of autonomy' as the 'principle of permission' to better indicate that secular moral authority is derived from the permission of those involved in a common undertaking.[75]

To sum up, both principlism and the libertarian account of morality propose procedural decision-making in the medical context (the taking of so-called segmental decisions according to DTD) and establish a worldview according to which human life, suffering and death are simply parameters for the sufficient accomplishment of the decision-making procedure, rather than being considered substantial and content-rich criteria. Such procedure results in the re-orientation of human life from a substantial to a procedural view of life. This re-orientation not only undervalues the human being as a whole being, but also challenges (by its power claims) the appropriateness of any other account of the character of human existence that may put the priority of the procedural understanding of human life at risk. In a pluralistic society, principlism ensures, through following a number of abstract principles, its societal role as well as the continuous expansion of its power in terms of the sovereignty of its worldview over human life.

73. He characterises his contribution to the salience of principles as one of the sins of his youth and, as such, he confesses it (Engelhardt, *The Foundations of Christian Bioethics*, p. 66).

74. Engelhardt, *The Foundation of Bioethics*, pp. x-xi.

75. Ibid., p. xi, and Engelhardt, 'The Many Faces of Autonomy', pp. 293-96. Even though Engelhardt acknowledges that not only the respect for autonomy but also the respect for human beings is necessary, he proceeds to a rather abstract definition of the character of a person that includes: self-consciousness (the ability to reflect on oneself), rationality (the need to be rational), moral sense (the capacity to understand the concepts of worthiness of blame and praise) and freedom (the capability of giving permission) (Engelhardt, *The Foundation of Bioethics*, p. 139). See also Engelhardt, 'Respect for Life and the Foundations of Bioethics', pp. 30-33.

b) The Imperative of Consciousness: a Utilitarian Approach

Those bioethicists who were previously mentioned deny any link with the provocative work of Peter Singer in the field of bioethics. Utilitarian at root, Singer lays the foundations of bioethics in the rewriting of the Commandments[76] upon which traditional ethics had been based. Even though he prefers the term 'Commandment' over 'principle', a preference that may indicate an absolutism regarding the relevant directives, Singer shares common ground with the proponents of principlism.

In Singer's ethical theory, principles like autonomy allot a pivotal place to the imperative of consciousness. Just as respect for the autonomy of a moral agent is a prerequisite for making choices, for permitting or for consenting, likewise consciousness is the prerequisite for having forward-looking desires that extend beyond periods of sleep or temporary unconsciousness (i.e. a desire to have children or to get out of painful or distressing situations)[77] or for having conscious preferences for continued life and enjoyable experiences.[78] Obviously, the capacity to make choices of principlism becomes in Singer's theory the capacity to have preferences and desires. Nevertheless, at root they are interested in the same things.

Singer wants to challenge the human-centred view of traditional ethics which, according to him, has been influenced not only by religion (man was created by God according to His own image) and the ancient philosophers such as Aristotle (everything exists for a particular purpose; what is less rational must serve what is more rational), but also by modern philosophers such as Descartes (the possession of an immortal soul makes a human rational and thoughtful) and Kant (since humans are rational, self-conscious and autonomous beings, they must be respected as ends in themselves).[79] Singer fails to notice that, in the medical context, the human-centred view of ethics is also successfully challenged by theories such as principlism once the successful management of current ethical dilemmas becomes the centre of interest. What Singer tries to

76. Singer's use of the capital 'C' for Commandments has been followed.
77. Singer, *Practical Ethics*, p. 127.
78. Singer, *Rethinking Life and Death*, p. 191.
79. Ibid., pp. 167-68. Singer considers the origin of the human-centred view of traditional ethics mainly in Genesis and, in particular, in the creation of man by God according to His own image and the subsequent sovereignty of man over the whole creation. He also believes that the exceptional position that humans enjoy was further enforced under Christianity and its assertion that only humans have immortal souls (pp. 165-66). However, the assumption that the Genesis narrative leads to the foundation of a human-centred view of ethics is by no means justified, at least with regard to the Christian tradition that is elaborated in this book and that is discussed in its second part.

accomplish is already a fact which he fails to notice. In the era of mass democracy, not man, but the satisfaction of his desires, his choices, his preferences and his needs for pleasure, are the elements that are believed to be important in ethics.

The boldness to found, from the point of view of the foundation of ethics, the responses to ethical dilemmas on general principles or orders is evident Singer's pretext, for he does not hesitate to refer to the concept of 'person', a term that refers both to existentialism in terms of philosophy – existence precedes substance and as a result the person is the most fundamental of all perceptions of what is valuable and what is not as regards the human constitution (i.e. consciousness),[80] and to modern theological literature – the development of a theological anthropology with reference to an understanding of what a person is through his relation to God, others, the self and the world.[81] As a result, Singer, in starting with the Lockean definition of person, according to which 'a thinking intelligent being has reason and reflection and can consider itself as itself, the same thinking thing, in different times and places',[82] concludes that there is always a borderline between a human being and a living body. Once this borderline is crossed, then the maintenance of the physiological processes in the body is not possible. In fact, the whole discussion no longer refers to a human being but only to a single body.[83] The important question here is where this borderline is drawn and when it is crossed. Undoubtedly, for Singer, this borderline is crossed once the loss of consciousness and the ability to choose have been irreversibly lost.[84] If these conditions are fulfilled, then death can be administered without a feeling of guilt.[85]

80. See, for example, Kierkegaard, *Repetition.*
81. See, for example, Zizioulas, *Being as Communion.*
82. Locke, *An Essay Concerning Human Understanding*, Book II, ch. 9, 29.
83. This position does not constitute the expression of an extreme utilitarian approach towards bioethical dilemmas as the opponents of Peter Singer want to believe. Giorgio Agamben detects the fundamental bio-political structure of modernity in the decision about the merit (or the demerit) of life as such. As a result, the birth of euthanasia is a modern event and is characterised by man's obligation to 'separate in someone else the life from the *bios* and to isolate in him a kind of naked life, a life that can be killed' (Agamben, *Homo Sacer*, p. 142).
84. Singer, *Rethinking Life and Death*, pp. 191-92.
85. Singer does not hesitate to say that patients without consciousness are mere biological existences and, consequently, that their life does not have the same value as that of the rest of humankind. Thus, he suggests the rewriting of the first old Commandment, 'Treat all human life as of equal worth', with a new Commandment, 'Consciousness is essential if continued life is to be worth having', by arguing that it must be recognised that the worth of human life varies (ibid. pp. 190-92).

In short, whether speaking either of autonomy or consciousness, principles or commandments, the convergence point of both principlism and Singer's utilitarianism is the praise of choice as the most crucial parameter in ethical dilemmas and, consequently, of the 'deification' of the subject as long as he or she is self-conscious. If the descriptive theory of decision is right, then, either explicitly or implicitly, we find an 'objective' character of the corresponding subjective worldviews along with their power claims over human existence – Singer's Commandments are presented as general, common rules like the Ten Commandments, whereas principlism is presented as content-less and, therefore, as a universally applicable ethical approach.

III. Concluding Remarks

All theoretical approaches in bioethics, like all theories relevant to human existence, have been shown to be subjective and polemical by definition. The application of the descriptive theory of decision (DTD) has demonstrated that even the most powerful theories in bioethics share common ground, which is the disguised subjectivity of their respective assertions in order to claim power over human life by their being presented as objective and universally applicable.

The most fundamental argument that supports the subjective character of any decision is that all moral agents always act according to their own worldview and not according to abstract principles. This argument is based on two assumptions. First, though each moral agent has the tendency to pretend that the character of his own worldview is objective, his decisions are subjective. Second, though there is a distinction between the worldview of a moral agent and his choices, such a choice is inescapably dependent on his own worldview and, thus, there can be no clear-cut separation among them. It is for this reason that DTD supports the argument that the choice among alternatives is based on the fundamental decision of each moral agent (his worldview) and that it is called segmental decision. The dependence of any segmental decision on the particular worldview of a moral agent is further supported by the oneness of theory and practice that challenges both metaphysics and ontology. Thus, any assertion that common rules or principles, and finally a common morality, for all human beings are possible is at least naive.

The application of DTD in the process of the identification of the character of bioethics reveals another inherent characteristic of this discipline, which is the striving for self-preservation among competitive worldviews; one can easily conclude that each worldview has its own 'enemies'. Consequently, the moral agents of a particular worldview have to fight their 'enemies' (the other competitive worldviews) for their self-preservation. Inescapably, the character of each worldview, and consequently that of bioethics, is polemical by definition.

As indicated by its name, bioethics is a field devoted to the development of ethics relevant to human life. However, dealing with human life is not a simple task, since a number of parameters, such as the character of human existence and the character of the era in which given persons live, must be taken into account. Unfortunately, bioethics, through the ages, instead of being the ethics of life, was transferred to the politics of life (bio-politics). This has resulted from the array of interests of bioethics, which includes suffering and the coming of death in the medical context, though isolated from human existence as a whole. As a consequence, bioethics has been aligned with the priorities of governmental health policies, which focus on the control of medical technology over the body. Thus, bioethics is self-limited and, consequently, has violated the actual content of its name.

The choice of bioethics to become in a way bio-politics has some important implications. Bioethics, as an academic discipline, is therefore subject to the compartmentalisation of knowledge and to an incomplete understanding of reality, for it draws separating lines between its academic evolution and the development of the so-called particular moralities, such as the morality of the Christian Church. These dividing lines have been necessary to assert power claims and, consequently, to rule over human life, an orientation that had to be masked. This is achieved through the adoption of current social values, such as the priority of the fulfilment of individualistic pleasures. Therefore, bioethics is presented as being objective and universal, though such assertion, according to DTD, cannot be justified, as has been demonstrated. In fact, while bioethics denies any relation to the particular moralities, it eventually expresses its own, very particular, morality.

The fact that bioethics has power claims over human life, for it deals with life, suffering and death in the medical context, provides a parallel between this and another theory that also has power claims over human life through an 'objective' justification to cause harm and death. This is the just war theory. This parallelism contributes to a better understanding of the character of bioethics. Both bioethics and the just war theory represent a tendency to create a list of principles or criteria to abide by, and not a content-rich account of human life. This practice, though it claims to be objective, is always subject to the personal interpretation of each moral agent involved in each particular case. Despite the endeavours of bioethics and the just war theory to assert objectivity and, consequently, to justify their power claims over human life, both fall into an inescapable subjectivity. This claim is obvious in the use of the doctrine of double effect by both bioethics and the just war theory.

The subjectivity upon which DDE was developed and is currently used is easily betrayed in those different formulations that have been proposed. Moreover, this doctrine focusses on the morality of an act, which it considers independent from any particular worldview of the moral agent. Thus, DDE, on the one hand, considers an ethical decision isolated from the whole life of the moral agent and, on the other, pretends that human persons enjoy a kind of independence that only God (whose intentions and decisions are not biased) has, and that such independence is not based on any self-interested or subjective incentives. In other words, the framework of DDE explicitly shows that, although bioethics and the just war theory are fundamentally subjective, they are oriented towards power claims over human life.

The common ground that is shared between bioethics and the just war theory is also identifiable synchronically and particularly among bioethical theories that are traditionally considered to be opposed to each other. Principlism and Singer's utilitarianism, even though they have different content, share the same structure of thought regarding the drawing up of a list of principles or Commandments. This designation reveals that both theories try to present as objective what is, by definition, subjective. They therefore attempt, through the application of a list of principles and Commandments, to impose particular worldviews on the meaning and destiny of human life. This attempt breaks down any distinction between so-called common morality and the 'particular' moralities once all theories of human existence are shown to be profoundly 'particular'. In addition, the focus on content-less principles, that is accompanied by the ignorance of the fundamental nature of the character of human existence, leads to a shift from a human-centred to a principle-centred view of ethics. The implications of such a transition on the human being are discussed in the chapter that follows.

Chapter 2
Bioethics, Euthanasia and the 'Creation' of a 'New' Human Being

Introduction

Anyone who wants to have power claims over human life has to be in a position to play the role of the Creator of human life.[1] To do so, he must be presented as a competent and legitimate authority. Bioethics in its various theoretical forms, despite its limited spectrum by nature (it is subjective, self-interested and therefore 'particular') and by choice (the focus on bio-politics), shapes or tries to shape human life in modern times.

The application of the descriptive theory of decision has shown that all theories, including the theory of bioethics, have a dual character. On the one hand, they are subjective and polemical by nature and, on the other, they are presented as being objective and authoritative by having power claims on human life. This dual character results in the following paradox. While bioethics claims that it aims to resolve moral disputes in the medical context, as a result of the impressive development of medical

1. The position that sovereign bioethics signals the 'creation' of a 'new man' does not happen in isolation from the characteristics of our civilisation. This is something that has arisen in this book. It is not accidental that such a tendency or practice has been detected elsewhere, although in a different framework: in the political philosophy of Pierre Manent, who notes, when speaking about the ideologies of Europeans after World War II, that: 'It was their ideologies of course that assured them that everything was possible and nothing was forbidden, that man could be remade or a "new man" be made' (Manent, *A World beyond Politics?*, p. 83).

technology and the application of excessive medical power over human existence, at the same time, it claims power over human life, namely it acts as an authority that resembles the authority of the Creator. Not surprisingly, those bioethicists who insist that their theories respect the cultural and religious diversity in modern societies reject such accusations.

The substantiation of the power and authority of bioethics over human life is achieved by looking at the character of the proposed decisions on issues surrounding euthanasia. This examination provides a synchronic view of euthanasia, which in turn reveals that the 'creation' of a 'new' human being leads to a human being compatible with the character of bioethics.[2]

While decisions on euthanasia constitute only a part of the decisions which bioethics deals with, they hold a position of a particular interest. The end of human life in the medical context along with the suffering and the corruption of the living human nature raise issues that touch human life itself. Since suffering and corruption are interwoven with human life from its very beginning, the issues surrounding such decisions do not refer only to the medical context but have implications for the daily life of human beings. Therefore, the selection of euthanasia as a paradigmatic case in this work may serve towards a further disclosure of the power claims of bioethics over human life and particularly the shaping of a 'new' human being.

The first part of this chapter reveals the manner in which the character of bioethics results in a human being 'stripped' of those characteristics traditionally considered as constituent aspects of his nature. A human being created on the basis of content-less principle and procedures is a human being highly fragmented, once the necessary backbone is missing. The second part of this chapter incorporates the remarkable efforts being made to reconstruct such a fragmented human being. Despite the remarkable contribution of these efforts in creating a morality that takes into account the character of human existence, they cannot escape their inclusion in the descriptive power of the descriptive theory of decision.

2. The idea that bioethics wants to play the role of Creator is different from the argument against euthanasia according to which man wants 'to play God'. While the latter signifies the objection to man's attempt to take the role of God in the administration of death – the administration of death on behalf of God sounds strange since God cannot be the cause of death (despite the presence of evil and, consequently, the problem of evil that results in the most powerful objection of traditional theism, Christianity considers God as omnipotent, omniscient and perfectly good), the former designates a more profound influence on man.

I. The Gradual 'Creation' of a 'New' Human Being

Before commenting in particular on the way that bioethics shapes human life, it is necessary to provide a concise overview of the history of the reshaping of the human being in the medical context during the last centuries. The 'creation' of a 'new' human being by bioethics is not something that is rooted only in recent developments in medical technology and in the raising of a number of moral issues within the medical context. On the contrary, it starts as early as the beginning of the progress of medicine over the last three centuries. This development was brought about within broader advances in human thought.

Foucault's work explains how the ability of man to map his own body with the precision of mathematics had profound implications for medicine. This ability, by revealing both the 'space' of the organism and the time of disease, enables us to grasp the truth of life and the nature of illness, or better, it provides an unsupersedable model, prescribed by nature.[3] In this context, death becomes the point from which corpses are opened up, and as such man is able to see and know empirically the human body and its finitude.[4] From this time onwards, medicine requires power claims on human life once it is proved able to, first, penetrate the adytum of human nature through the elaboration of pathological anatomy and, second, that it is based on the only legitimate procedure in the sciences, which is the empirical justification of truth. Thus, the body turns out to become an object of the empirical view of science, namely an object whose destiny is shaped by medicine, the scientific discipline that has power claims over it. Such medicine becomes engaged in the philosophical discussion on human nature.[5]

The development of pathological anatomy was accompanied by another important turning point in the treatment of the patient and disease. In fact, this turning point is a presupposition for the elaboration of pathological anatomy. This fundamental change is characterised by a progressive distancing of medicine from the individual perception, family assistance and home care, that resulted in the clinical

---

3. Foucault, *The Birth of the Clinic*, pp. 124-46.
4. Ibid., p. 144.
5. Ibid., pp. 196-99. Foucault criticises the claim for the objectivity of modern medicine by stating that medicine is shaped by the particular historical context and the social and cultural attitudes in which it developed. What actually happens is something like the use of language, that is undoubtedly designated by the constraints of each historical period. Similarly, medical knowledge is a subjective form of knowledge.

institutionalisation of disease.[6] The institutionalisation of disease shaped the profile of medicine in the twentieth century. Vovelle, focussing on the treatment of death in the last century,[7] refers to the hospitalisation and the medicalisation of death, whereas Ariès, in his *Essais sur l'histoire de la mort en occident*, describes the same reality as the medicalisation of the concept that people have of life.

According to Vovelle, the crucial point regarding the time of death, despite the ongoing debate, has irrevocably passed into the hands of physicians. In fact, Vovelle distinguishes the situation that was predominant until the 1950s and 1960s from that of the following decades. While both situations share the same ground (the hospitalisation and medicalisation of human life and death), the efforts of society for the exclusion of death and the dead from ordinary life characterise the former period, whereas the rediscovering of death as an issue that deserves attention and discussion marks the latter. The rediscovery of the question of death in the last decades is not a paradox. It is during the last decades that the development of medical technology and the consequent unprecedented power of medicine and of its representatives gave rise to a substantial critique regarding the limits of medicine.[8] In such a context, the development of this critique is not surprising, but rather to be expected, since the growth of power of specific agents spontaneously results in the reaction and criticism of those upon which such power is applied. This reaction is often substantiated through the claiming of, on the part of the patient, the right to die or the right to a dignified death. Nevertheless, even though patients or their relatives authorise physicians to administer death, the patients definitely do not shape the context.

In the same vein, Ariès gives attention to the displacement of the process of death from the patient's home to the hospital, where death becomes a technical case – death comes when care stops. Consequently, the displacement of this process is accompanied by the transferral of power from the patient and his family to the physician. The physician exercises this power alone as the absolute master in the medical context and deprives the patient of his death, in the sense that he designates the procedure of how death comes about. Due to progress in medical developments, this power seems more important because of the prolongation of life and the postponement of death. Rather, the physician decides when death should come in most cases. Again, there

6. Ibid., pp. 3-21.
7. Vovelle, *La mort et l'occident de 1300 à nos jours*, pp. 673-761.
8. Ibid., pp. 748-50.

is a dispute as to whether the physician or the patients are entitled to decide on this matter.[9] However, such a dispute ignores the importance of who designates the context of the decision-making.

In short, during the last century, and particularly during the last decades, there has been a significant change not only in the status of medicine as a science but also in the hierarchy of the agents involved in the treatment of a disease (i.e. physician, patient, family). Despite the critical assessment of the role of medicine and the growth of bioethics, the displacement of the power of the agents involved into hospitals implies that the ruler of the 'game' is the physician once the 'game' takes place where he, by definition, is sovereign. On the other hand, the critical change in the status of medicine signifies that medicine has embarked on an anthropological quest that begins at the point when corpses are opened up and results in a perception of man that starts and ends with his body. Thus, the physician, as a representative of the power of modern medicine over human life, deals only with the life of the body and, as a consequence, the 'end-of-life' decisions that are taken in the medical context become 'end-of-body' decisions.[10] In such a context, man is, in a way, 'recreated' once he is considered mainly a body that has to be treated properly, particularly towards its end. Let us now discuss a series of characteristics that are identified in the current bioethical discussion and that are implicitly oriented towards this 're-creation'.

1. The Human Being as a Moral Agent Who Accomplishes Procedures

A real creator is a creator who assigns the limits of the 'world' over which he wants to have power claims. In the medical context, bioethics assigns the limits of the discussion on issues surrounding euthanasia through the application of particular definitions. While the provision of definitions is necessary for methodological reasons, it also determines the character of

9. Ariès, *Essais sur l'histoire de la mort en occident*, pp. 61-76 and 167-212.

10. The point that 'end-of-life' decisions, such as euthanasia, become 'end-of-body' decisions clarifies the fact that bioethics, in dealing with the issues surrounding the administration of death in the medical context, has, at least in a significant part, chosen to focus only on the 'end' of the human body. Medicine, strictly speaking, can only deal with the human body. However, there is a significant difference between, for example, the treatment of the body as a machine and the treatment of the body as the constituent part of a human being – the latter implies consideration of the relationships that exist between this part and other constituent parts of humanity, as well as the relationships that the patient may have with other human beings.

the discussion around euthanasia. Since the decisions on euthanasia are related to the issues of life, suffering and death in the medical context, the proposed definitions have implications for what human life is or, better, how human life must be seen.

To start with, all definitions that are relevant to euthanasia focus on either how (with or without consent, by administering a lethal injection or by withdrawing or withholding a life-sustaining treatment) or by whom (the patient, the physician or a relative) death takes place in the medical context. Such a focus prioritises the procedural character of these definitions as well as the categorisation of the decisions surrounding euthanasia. For the best depiction of the different cases in the medical context, a series of distinctions and categorisations are provided here.

One of the two main criteria for the distinction of the different forms of the administration of death is the person who administers death. When a physician administers death by means of a direct act (i.e. by lethal injection), then the occurrence is called euthanasia. When death results after the administration of a particular dose of drugs prescribed by a physician, the incident is called physician-assisted suicide. Both practices result in death. What changes in each case is the moral agent who executes a professionally (i.e. by the physician) designed assignment. Obviously, what matters is the designation of the moral agents involved and, therefore, of the procedural character of the administration of death.

The second main criterion refers to the means by which decisions about euthanasia are reached. Two such practices can be identified. The first is the presence of the consent of the patient and the second is the manner by which these decisions are arrived at.

The conferral of consent by the patient leads to a further categorisation that includes voluntary euthanasia (when it is carried out at the request of a competent patient), non-voluntary euthanasia (when it is carried out on a patient who is not in a position to make a choice and has never previously expressed his choice) and involuntary euthanasia (when it is carried out on a patient, though competent, without his consent).[11] However, there is an intrinsic vagueness in this categorisation that gives rise to a series of questions. Who decides, and according to which criteria, whether, when and under which circumstances a patient is or is not competent to give consent to die? Apparently, such questions set up the problem of the subjectivity of the different moral agents involved in the taking of these decisions.

The manner by which decisions on euthanasia are made, leads to another categorisation and to two other kinds of administration of

11. Kushe, 'Euthanasia', pp. 295-96.

death. The first is active or positive euthanasia, which is carried out through the injection of lethal drugs. The second is passive or negative euthanasia, which is administered through withdrawing or withholding a life sustaining treatment. What underpins this distinction is quite an old agreement (or disagreement) on whether there is a moral difference between an act and the omission of an act in medical practice, or between killing and letting someone die,[12] and whether such differentiation makes sense when not only the result but also the intentions are the same.[13] Once more, the definitions that are used for euthanasia suffer from vagueness and subjectivity.

If what really matters in decisions on euthanasia is included in the definitions that are presented above, then the administration of death in the medical context considers man to be diminished 'by definition'. Even though decisions on euthanasia affect the life, suffering and death of human beings, which are the most extreme realities in human experience, these realities do not play a role in the definitions regarding euthanasia drawn up by modern medicine. In such a consideration, a person (either a physician, patient, relative or a surrogate) is viewed as merely an agent whose role has to be defined and controlled, for example, through the presence of the appropriate consent or the justifiable intention, for the accomplishment of a specific procedure. However, this is not the only concern. What is really worrying is that such a consideration is not based on a definite moral account, and as a consequence results in a profound vagueness.[14] By applying the descriptive theory of decision, one may argue that the choice of vague definitions is better understood if this is viewed as a way to secure the power claims of subjective moral accounts.

This particular designation of the context of decisions on euthanasia is neither an accidental nor a non-rational choice. On the contrary, it is in deep agreement with the mores of modern society and the established imperative of 'procedure'. Kondylis argues that, due to the pluralistic

12. A detailed discussion of this controversial issue is provided in a collection of papers entitled *Killing and Letting Die*, edited by Steinbock and Norcross.

13. There is a long tradition of raising the importance of intention in medical practice. It is the rationale of double effect that is actually derived from the judgement of the physician's intention. The doctrine of double effect, along with its meaning and weight, has already been discussed in chapter one.

14. Kushe, though he accepts that there are profound differences between the various definitions of decisions on euthanasia, notes: 'Whether or not these differences are morally relevant, and if so on what grounds, is a debate that is still continuing' (Kushe, 'Euthanasia', p. 301). For Kushe, the absence of a definite moral account that would offer the grounds for the clear designation of any morally relevant differences is evident.

character of postmodern society, the 'legitimacy' of a decision has to pass through a procedure without reference to any system of values. In the same vein, the truth does not have any content. It is rather the outcome of consent through a procedure.[15] Focussing on the procedure prevents the consideration of issues such as the meaning of suffering in human life that may result in the disclosure of the disguised polemical character of the procedure (who is entitled to carry out the procedure, how the procedure must be accomplished etc.). However, the assumption that by focussing on procedures, as well as by 'stripping' man of important elements in his own life (the discussion of which follows immediately below), a status quo may be secured has not been successfully established. This assumption cannot exclude the implicit power claims over human life once the character of life and death are designated by applying a particular worldview such as the procedural consideration of human life.

Generally speaking, the whole discussion in bioethics is geared towards a particular perspective, according to which man is, among others, a moral agent who is oriented towards accomplishing procedures. This view constitutes the first fundamental 'stripping' of man of the substantiality of his own existence (where 'existence' means something more than the accomplishment of a procedure). These procedures are intentionally 'stripped' of any meaningful framework (where 'meaningful' is the consideration of a system of values, virtues or anything that may give an ethical orientation to the moral agents involved). It is in such a context that the foundation of a systematic fragmentation of human life is accomplished.

2. The Procedures Need Principles: Man's 'Imprisonment' in His Autonomy

What emerges spontaneously when the discussion turns to issues surrounding euthanasia is the autonomy of the moral agents involved. While, for a long time, the autonomy of the subject has been the anchor of modern ethics, its application in bioethics reveals such a divergence that it leads to confusion and vagueness.[16] Taking into account that the

15. Kondylis, *Der Niedergang der bürgerlichen Denk- und Lebensform*, pp. 221-23.
16. The autonomy of the subject in the medical context figures in such diverse texts as the medical codes of medical associations (for example, the declarations of the World Medical Association) and documents that express particular theological traditions, such as 'The Declaration of the Basic Principles of Bioethics Based on the Orthodox Tradition' of the Interparliamentary Assembly on Orthodoxy at a conference in Bucharest, 2002.

vagueness of a principle or of a norm is always an efficient weapon for power claims, the focus on the autonomy of the subject and his centrality in bioethical discussions are by no means mere offsprings of modern ethics. Rather, it is a means by which humans are shaped.

a) The Illusion of Kant's Autonomy in Bioethics

The representatives of bioethics claim that their theories, as well as their arguments, can be traced back to the teaching of the eminent moral philosophers of the modern age in order to ensure their own appropriate prestige in the public arena. This is evident regarding the centrality of the subject along with the imperative of one's own autonomy, which was substantiated by Kant in the most radical way.

Kant's contribution to moral philosophy has long been recognised and characterised as a substantial break from the dominant tradition that existed before him, which was natural law. Natural law was a moral law that was seen as imposed by God or an external authority. Man's only obligation was to obey this law under threats of punishment in case of disobedience. Kant established a new way of thinking in morality. He actually proposed a diametrically opposed interpretation.

Kant argues that the designation of what morality consists of cannot be successfully accomplished if a law is imposed on man externally (this imposition implies a necessity of acting from a certain interest and as such cannot serve as a moral law). On the contrary, when man is considered as a subject 'only to laws which are made by himself and yet are universal', a moral law can be established.[17] The imposition of a framework of morality on man externally is considered as heteronomy (it comes from the Greek word ἑτερονομία [*eteronomia*], which is composed of the Greek words ἕτερος [*eteros*], that denotes something different from one's own being, and νόμος [*nomos*], that is the equivalent for the English word 'law'), whereas the designation of one's moral laws by oneself is called autonomy (which comes from the Greek word αὐτονομία [*autonomia*], a compound word that is composed of the Greek words αὐτός [*autos*] that signifies the particular being [ὁ ἴδιος],[18] and νόμος [law]). For Kant the notion of autonomy is the supreme principle of morality.

In particular, autonomy is connected with the will of all rational beings. The autonomy of the will is 'the property the will has of being a law to itself (independently of every property belonging to the objects of volition)',[19] that is the power of will to legislate itself and to choose

17. Kant, *Groundwork of the Metaphysic of Morals*, p. 100.
18. Andriotis, *Ἐτυμολογικὸ λεξικὸ τῆς κοινῆς νεοελληνικῆς*, p. 44.
19. Kant, *Groundwork of the Metaphysic of Morals*, p. 108.

maxims (subjective principles of a volition)[20] for itself, independently of any desires of any nature. Moreover, Kant considers the autonomy of the will as the capacity to choose maxims that can give universal laws.[21] In other words, autonomy identifies the moral imperatives of the moral agent's own freely and rationally adopted moral policy. As a result, the moral agent and his autonomy become the centre of morality and, at the same time, the legislator and the subject of the moral laws.[22]

Although moral philosophy, as well as its application in bioethics, cannot be understood without taking into account Kant and his philosophical tradition, the Kantian roots of bioethics are questionable. For example, principlism and its focus on the centrality of the subject and on principles like respect for the autonomy of the subject, while it seems to share some common ground with Kant, is characterised by a superficial similarity. The so-called 'respect for the autonomy' of the subject does not entail an autonomy that gives universal laws. Rather, it is an imperative towards the self-determination of each human being.

Along the same lines, libertarian approaches in bioethics, such as Engelhardt's approach that traces back to Nozick and his account on individualism, do not justify a profound relation to Kant. While Nozick's theory is based on Kant's view that rational beings are 'ends in themselves', and as such each rational being must always treat others or be treated by others never simply as a means but always as an end, it goes further and establishes an individualistic perspective of humanity. Nozick does so by putting 'deontological' or 'side' constraints to reveal the inviolability

20. According to Kant, 'A *maxim* is a subjective principle of action and must be distinguished from an *objective principle* – namely, a practical law. The former contains a practical rule determined by reason in accordance with the conditions of the subject (often his ignorance or again his inclination): it is thus a principle on which the subject *acts*. A law, on the other hand, is an objective principle valid for every rational being; and it is a principle on which he *ought to act* – that is, an imperative' (ibid., p. 88).

21. The determination of the will according to universal laws is an obligation that is demanded by the categorical imperative. The categorical imperative 'would be one which represented an action as objectively necessary in itself apart from its relation to a further end' (ibid., p. 82). It is the categorical imperative that tests maxims by prescribing an experiment in which one wonders whether one could consistently will one's maxim as a universal law.

22. The notion of the heteronomy of the will stands at the very opposite of the notion of autonomy once the will 'seeks the law that is to determine it *anywhere else* than in the fitness of its maxims for its own making of universal laws' (ibid., p. 108). As a consequence, it is not the will that gives the law but the object to which the will is related. This mode of action is distinguished from autonomy since the law under which an action arises has not been designated by the rational being.

of other persons, and concludes that 'others may not be used in the specific ways the side constraints exclude'.[23] For Nozick, the fundamental principle of a modern society should be the acknowledgement of the existence of distinct individuals who are treated as resources for others, since there is no social entity that can justify the sacrifice of someone else for its own good.[24] Therefore, though Nozick starts out from Kant, his actual conclusions have little in common with the Kantian understanding of the autonomy of the subject or of an autonomy merged with the quest towards universal laws. Accordingly, the libertarian approach of Engelhardt, who considers the autonomy of the patient as the imperative of giving permission, is a far cry from Kant's perception of autonomy. Once the patient, as a moral agent, is considered merely an agent who gives permission, then the patient is nothing else than a being who is designated by others (those who administer particular actions towards him), even though he retains the right of consent by giving permission for a particular action to be carried out.

Tauber summarises the outcome of adopting a supposedly Kantian account of autonomy in bioethics. He criticises the Kantian roots of the notion of autonomy and talks about the loss of Kantian autonomy in bioethics. This loss has resulted in the understanding of autonomy as self-governance.[25] Obviously, the understanding of autonomy as self-governance does not share substantial ground with the Kantian notion of autonomy.

The choice of bioethics not to closely follow a particular tradition such as the ethical tradition of Kant is not accidental, since bioethics aims to shape our understanding of what a human being is. The application of DTD in this context also bears out this conclusion.

While Kant's moral philosophy remains a particular theory that was worked out in a particular historical context and was always based on a particular worldview, modern bioethicists use the cardinal principle that accompanies such a philosophical tradition with a view to the securing of their 'objectivity' and their power claims over human beings in the medical context. By doing so, they ignore the strong interdependence

23. Nozick, *Anarchy, State, Utopia*, p. 32.
24. Nozick's theory encourages the establishment of a libertarian individualistic society. He proposes that, from a political philosopher's point of view, a minimal, as opposed to an extensive, state can be justified. In fact, he stresses the importance of each person having individual rights, being treated by the state with respect for his rights, choosing his ends, defining the conception of himself and cooperating voluntarily with other individuals.
25. Tauber, 'Historical and Philosophical Reflections on Patient Autonomy', pp. 307-309.

between theory and practice, where theory is always defined by the specific worldview of their subjects, given that the principle of autonomy can be easily identified with numerous terms and in extremely diverse contents – as many different moral accounts as the number of the moral agents involved.[26] More clearly, bioethics, as a creature of a particular historical context and as a field that wants to serve man in a particular way (i.e. the accomplishment of procedures in the medical context on the basis, among others, of the principle of autonomy), is the tradition that shapes the relevant context, and not Kant and his moral philosophy.[27] In other words, even though bioethical theories have aimed at being grounded on respectable philosophical theories, the practice in the medical context corresponds to modern society and its values and priorities as well as to the particular worldview of the moral agents involved.

b) The Transition from the Human Being to the Autonomic Being

The illusion of Kant's autonomy in bioethics, and particularly the understanding of autonomy as self-governance and self-determination on the basis of an individualistic consideration of human existence, reveals the ways through which the particular character of bioethics shapes the human being of the modern age.

For example, McKenny points out that what is morally important in the issue of physician-assisted suicide is the self-determination of the patient along with the procedural safeguards and restrictions, such as the requirement that the patient be in a terminal condition. Such self-determination coincides with the expansion of the reign of human choice over the body. Since the aim of bioethics is oriented towards serving what McKenny calls 'the Baconian project' – the unquestioned commitment to the technological control of the body for the sake of eliminating human misery and necessity– moral convictions about the place of illness and

---

26. Engelhardt, 'The Many Faces of Autonomy', pp. 283-85.

27. It is in this context that Shuman criticises Pellegrino and Thomasma's *A Philosophical Basis of Medical Practice*. According to Shuman, Pellegrino and Thomasma, to distinguish between the 'good' of the patient, as subjectively defined by the patient as an autonomous being, and the good of medicine, that is objective as it is based on the ontology of the patient's living body that is determined by science, is simply to reproduce the problematic distinction between fact and values. What Shuman says is that any serious approach in bioethics is by no means without theoretical presuppositions (values) upon which specific practices (facts) are shaped (Shuman, *The Body of Compassion*, pp. 67-71). The importance of the interdependence between theory and practice has been elaborated through the application of the descriptive theory of decision in bioethics in chapter one of this book.

health in a morally worthy life are being replaced by moral convictions about relief from suffering and the expansion of choice.[28] If so, the choice of bioethics to see decisions on euthanasia from the self-determination point of view restrains the human being once human life and death are presented as dependent on a single parameter, namely the expansion of choice as part of a larger effort to control death. It is worth noting that the orientation towards self-determination, the expansion of choice and the control over death results in a fallacious reality.

McKenny states that, even though its proponents do not admit it, the permissibility of physician-assisted suicide is based upon two assumptions. The first assumption is the physician's ability to control death, and the second is attribution by medicine of this control to the patient.[29] Thus, the consideration of any decisions on euthanasia merely on the basis of self-determination results in a fallacy, not only because it gives the impression of man's control over death, despite the fact that death comes unavoidably, but also because a human being who suffers must prioritise the control over suffering and death despite the fact that suffering is considered a meaningless element in human life. Once autonomy is identified with self-determination, then, inescapably, man is placed within a fallacious reality that ignores what man and human life really stand for.

In such a context, efforts towards the refinement of the application of autonomy in bioethics have been developed. A vivid example is provided by feminist scholars who, among others, have set up the reconsideration of autonomy as a decisive principle in decisions on euthanasia, through the establishment of a relational framework that may include not only family relationships within the family, but other social connections as well. This line of thinking rejects the dominant individualistic concept and favours an autonomy that is understood relationally, by accepting the significance of an interdependence of the moral agents involved.[30] In the same vein, a wider interpretation of the autonomy of the patient is also provided. This time autonomy is interpreted not in the context of an ideology of control but rather in the context of a specific community. Therefore, the autonomy of a human being is expressed through his relationship with others and understood in terms of its social character.[31]

---

28. McKenny, *To Relieve the Human Condition*, pp. 7-24.
29. Ibid., pp. 25-32.
30. Donchin, 'Autonomy, Interdependence, and Assisted Suicide: Respecting Boundaries/Crossing Lines', pp. 201-204, and Little, 'Assisted Suicide, Suffering and the Meaning of a Life', pp. 292-95.
31. Fuchs, Lalive d'Epinay, Michel, Scherer and Stettler , 'La notion d'autonomie: une reformulation interdisciplinaire', pp. 178-79.

Consequently, autonomy with societal characteristics may limit the excessive emphasis on the individuality of the patient. However, even a relational understanding of autonomy does not break out from the vicious circle where content-less autonomy is at the centre of issues that touch human existence. Such a form of autonomy still remains the cornerstone that predefines the whole issue of these decisions, even though it is viewed on a societal level. The absence of a content-rich morality that would give some meaning to the exercising of autonomy in the medical context weakens the authority of such efforts.

Every person in good will could accept that autonomy, at least in the sense of the self-governance of a human being, plays a significant role in modern society. Similarly, someone could agree that the autonomy of the subject, respect for the autonomy of the subject or the right of the subject to make his own choices are important parameters in decision-making in the medical context and, in particular, for the issues surrounding euthanasia. However, there is an important difference between these positions and bioethics attributing the central role vis-à-vis these decisions to autonomy, which implies that autonomy is the most essential element of the human person. Needless to say, sovereign bioethics does not support such a view.

In short, the exceptional position that autonomy occupies within bioethical thought is safeguarded through the assumption that all human beings are autonomous beings by nature and, therefore, regardless of any particular consideration of morality. It is also assumed that each moral agent can keep his worldview separated from the application of the principle of autonomy and, therefore, that a content-less account of autonomy makes sense. If the bioethical debate on euthanasia is one that is oriented towards the justification of a particular decision regarding the life, suffering and death of human beings, and if this discussion primarily and predominantly revolves around a content-less notion of autonomy, then the human being, for whom and by whom this discussion is elaborated, is considered an autonomous being. To be more precise, the most appropriate predicate of such a being should be 'autonomy' rather than 'human', once 'human' as predicative of a specific being is no longer indicative of a content other than that of autonomy. In other words, though the 'objective' foundation of morality on the popular principle of autonomy is attempted, the result is not the safeguarding of the wholeness of a human being once he is 'stripped' of the most essential elements of his existence. Even when the relational character of human existence is taken into account, it is made on the basis of a human being who is basically autonomous.

3. Division and 'Undifferentiation' within Human Existence

The absence of a content-rich consideration of human existence, along with the focus on particular principles, inescapably results in the vision of a fragmented human being, once the human being's own existence is no longer at the centre of interest. Neither the wholeness nor the fundamentals of human existence are considered of central importance. In such a context, the confusion regarding the inwardness of humanity, i.e. the presence of a profound division or the absence of differentiation among the elements that constitute the inwardness of humanity, is not surprising.

Traditionally, the division of man into two fundamentally different constituent parts (this takes various forms, such as soul-body, mind-matter, mind-body, will-body, consciousness-unconsciousness etc.) is called dualism, whereas the absence of any differentiation between them is called materialism. As a matter of fact, materialism consists of a cluster of theories that understand the absence of separateness between, for example, mind and matter differently. What is clear in both dualism and materialism and their constant confrontation is the need for balance.

a) Dualistic and Materialistic Views of Human Existence

The philosophical roots of dualism go back to the ancient Greek philosophers such as Plato, Aristotle and the Epicureans. The modern interpretation of dualism derives from Descartes' philosophical system. Descartes' famous assertion '*cogito, ergo sum*' ('I think, therefore I am') supports the idea that the mind, the soul or the spirit (the non-material element), and the body or matter (the material element) are entirely distinct things.[32] Descartes categorises all things into those that think (*res cogitans*) and those that are extended things – they have an extent (*res extensa*). He asserts that, 'my essence consists in this alone: I am a thing that thinks', whereas he is certain that he can exist without his body since it is considered as an extended thing distinct from his essence.[33] The main idea of dualism that results in a division within man is, either explicitly or implicitly, extremely present in bioethics.

The common belief in bioethics is that the body is a distinct part, upon which the sovereignty of human will is applied. As a consequence, the

32. Descartes, by making the existence of a human being dependent on the capacity of thinking, points out that nobody 'can ever bring it about that I am nothing so long as I shall think that I am something . . . the statement "I am, I exist" is necessarily true every time it is uttered by me or conceived by mind' (Descartes, *Meditations on First Philosophy*, p. 17).

33. Ibid., p. 49.

human will and desires are alienated from the body. Shuman says that the body is considered a passive machine and points out that in modern medicine the body is not an aspect of personal agency and identity. Obviously, behind such a belief there is a strong connection between the dualism of Descartes and the modern tendency towards the principle of autonomy. He notes: 'The modern tendency to privilege individual autonomy as a moral principle *sine qua non* is at least partly connected to a dualist assertion that the body is passive and inert and thus obedient to the self-legislating will.'[34] Given the centrality of autonomy as a norm or a principle in bioethics, and particularly in the discussions that deal with the issues surrounding decisions on euthanasia, dualism sheds some light on the foundation of such discussions.

The sovereignty of dualism is not limited to a conceptual division within man. On the contrary, it shapes the understanding of human life once man is divorced from the real life of ordinary experience. McKenny says that, in treating the body as a machine, the lived body of ordinary experience is set aside. Since medicine is shaped by the development of technology, the issue is not the affirmation of the moral significance of the body but rather the expansion of choice and the elimination of suffering for the sake of the so-called Baconian project.[35] As a result, man, in the medical context, loses his own life and is placed in a new world where what matters is the body as machine. Therefore, dualism not only influences the way that modern medicine treats patients but it also divides human life into two irreconcilable parts – the body and the 'rest' of human existence. It can be in no doubt that modern medicine and its ethical offspring intrude into life and shape our vision of what it is to be human.

The body as a machine that is alienated from the human will (or soul, or mind) reminds one of Ryle's characterisation of dualism as the dogma of 'the Ghost in the machine', according to which the mind is the ghostly counterpart of the body.[36] Ryle represents one of the critics of Descartes' dualism, which is a critique from a materialistic point of view. He, at the very opposite pole to dualism, argues that there are only physical objects and physical happenings, such as instances of human behaviour. The distinction between mind and matter (or body) does not make sense once the mental processes are sort of an abbreviation for talks about kinds of behaviour and, therefore, the mind is not behind the behaviour of the body but a part of a physical behaviour. Thus, Ryle, while critical

34. Shuman, *The Body of Compassion*, p. 15.
35. McKenny, *To Relieve the Human Condition*, pp. 198-99.
36. Ryle, *The Concept of Mind*, pp. 11-18.

of the dualistic tradition of Descartes, presents a refined behaviourism[37] that, inescapably, signifies the transition to the opposite extreme that limits man to the observable aspect of human life.

b) Dualism and Materialism: Two Sides of the Same Coin

Interestingly, both dualism and materialism, at least in bioethics, seem to be two sides of the same coin. Either by separating mind (or will, or soul) from matter (or body), or by denying any differentiation between them, the result is the same. For example, man, in the context of decisions on euthanasia, is considered as a being who is 'stripped' either of his bodily life (the treatment of the body as a passive machine, rather than as a substantial element of a human being, coincides with the dualistic perspective of human life) or of his discernible mental state (the treatment of man as merely the sum of behaviours coincides with the materialistic perspective of human life). The case of Peter Singer is a very characteristic example of how fundamentally different ethical approaches share common ground. He, while utilitarian, supports both a dualistic and a materialistic view of life. In fact, he does not see a clear-cut distinction between dualism and materialism and bases the dualistic aspects of his theory upon a materialistic approach to bioethics.

The dualistic character of Singer's bioethical approach, where a human being and a human body are presented as distinct entities, has been discussed in detail in chapter one. In what follows only the materialistic aspect of Singer's bioethical approach will be discussed.

Singer, just like every proponent of the naturalistic point of view, a point of view that has a profoundly materialistic character, supports a concept of life according to which 'life can be meaningful even if there is neither God nor soul and that certain ways of living in a purely physical world can be sufficient for meaning in life'.[38] In other words, the

37. Ryle's refined behaviourism is not the only materialistic theory. Armstrong supports a purely physicalist theory by trying to interpret the mental processes in man as part of the central nervous system. He believes that even the consciousness of man's own states of mind can be identified with purely physical states of the central mental system. Within such an interpretation, the inner mental states become material states and, as a consequence, man is a physico-chemical reality (Armstrong, *A Materialist Theory of Mind*, pp. 54-72). Others go a bit further by arguing that human mental life is similar to the life of a machine (Putman, *Mind, Language and Reality*, pp. 291-303). Even though there are significant differences among all these approaches, they all share a common ground, according to which even the non-material aspects of human nature are treated in a materialistic way.

38. Metz, 'Recent Work on the Meaning of Life', p. 792.

naturalistic view considers life as simply a biological phenomenon of a higher order than the natural processes in the inorganic world.[39] In this context, the values of human life are equated with the life of animals, which represents a challenge to the human-centred view of ethics. Singer's purpose is to indicate that human beings do not deserve any more special respect than other beings and to reject the idea that human beings are the result of a special creation or are infinitely more precious. He characteristically states that, due to the evolutionary history of human beings, 'the possibility of human and chimpanzee interbreeding cannot be ruled out'.[40] In other words, Singer considers human existence as the sum of behaviours, a consideration that implies neither a meaningful nor a substantial differentiation, such as between mind and body within man.

Generally speaking, Singer challenges the uniqueness of the human being by following a materialistic point of view while, at the same time, elaborating specific arguments on issues surrounding euthanasia based on a dualistic point of view. In other words, both traditions that deal with the mind-body problem are not in a position to establish equilibrium. In addition, they result in either a divided or an 'undifferentiated' human being. In any case, human existence is 'stripped' of either an internal union or meaning. As a result, it is not surprising that a confusion between humans and animals is possible. The absence of a content-rich consideration of human existence regarding its inwardness is more than tangible.

4. The Division among Human Beings and the Fallacy of Reaching Agreement or Consent

The implications of discarding a human-centred view of ethics are not only limited to the inwardness of human existence. They are also evident in the outwardness of human existence, namely the relational character of human life. Such an example is evident in the relationships between the moral agents involved in the medical context where the decision-making and its procedural character must be controlled in order to reach a desired result that is synonymous with the successful accomplishment of procedures. The two sovereign ideas for reaching consent or agreement are justice and communication.

39. Heyd, 'The Meaning of Life and the Right to Voluntary Euthanasia', p. 169.

40. Singer, *Rethinking Life and Death*, p. 180. Singer concludes that the old Commandment, 'Treat all human life as always more precious than any human life', must be rewritten as a new Commandment 'Do not discriminate on the basis of the species' (ibid., pp. 201-06).

a) Man as Contractor – the Fallacy of Objectified Consent

One of the most influential traditions in bioethics is the tradition of contractualism that raises the importance of so-called informed consent. Informed consent is a controlled and objective approval that serves the administration of a particular medical intervention such as the administration of death in euthanasia. The profound character of informed consent can be elicited from the context into which it was born.

It has already been argued that modern society – where mass democracy rules as the most appropriate way to achieve social symbiosis – is characterised, among other things, by the rise of individualism. Due to the realm of individualism, the truth is synonymous to consent.[41] In this context, what is important is establishing a system that may preserve the individuality of the moral agents and at the same time secure the attainment of consent between individuals.[42] The application of this rationale in the medical context has resulted in the elaboration of informed consent as a practice that provides a controlled procedure towards achieving consent between the moral agents involved (the physician(s), the patient, the relatives, the wider society). While informed consent is encountered in the medical context, its philosophical roots hark back to Locke, Rousseau and Kant and the elaboration of contractualism. The modern representatives of these philosophical traditions highlight different aspects of desired consent. Among others, the cases of John Rawls and Jürgen Habermas reveal the origins of the foundations of modern contractualism and their insufficiency.

Rawls tries to combine the importance of society with an interpretation of the Kantian insistence on autonomy. He proposes the idea of justice that can only be achieved through something like a social contract, in which men autonomously agree on how the basic institutions of society must be structured in order to be just. Rawls starts from the Kantian notion of the 'kingdom of ends'[43] and tries to present his moral theory on the autonomy of the subject and the categorical imperative in a social perspective. He believes that the only way towards this direction

41. Kondylis, *Der Niedergang der bürgerlichen Denk- und Lebensform*, pp. 221-23.
42. 'The empire of consent spreads, the process of individualization intensifies, and thus the authority of the communities of different orders in which human beings hitherto found the meaning of their life – the nation, the family, the church – declines more and more each day' (Manent, *A World beyond Politics?*, p. 116).
43. The kingdom of ends, though only an ideal, is a kingdom where a systematic union of rational beings arises under common objective laws. Since these laws are oriented towards the relation of rational beings towards one another as ends and means, the kingdom can be called the kingdom of ends (Kant, *Groundwork of the Metaphysic of Morals*, p. 101).

is the connection between autonomy and objectivity, along with its dependence on a theory of justice. This is substantiated through the original position – 'a hypothetical situation characterised as to lead to a certain conception of justice'.[44] The original position is a thought experiment, which considers that people, as 'rational contractors' (free and equal beings respecting one another)[45] and separated by a 'veil of ignorance' from the knowledge of their particular status as human beings (social position, wealth, skills etc.), may accept the same set of principles. This set of principles, defined by the original position, corresponds to a specific consideration of justice. In other words, free and equal human beings in a well-ordained society act autonomously based on principles that have been consented to and as such these principles are objective and lead to the same judgement in particular cases.[46]

Without doubt, the aim of Rawls' theory of justice is to provide an empirical alternative to Kant's morality and to establish a realistic framework for objectified contracts between the moral agents in a society. However, the use of words such as 'well-ordained society', 'free' and 'equal' beings, as well as the hypothetical basis of the foundations of the original position, show at least how far from the real world such considerations are. For example, given that the medical context is a 'society' where the moral agents involved (physicians and patients) have an entirely different status – the patient is a human being who suffers from an incurable disease in an institutionalised context, where the desired consent is inevitably influenced by the worldview of those who designate the character of the medical context, namely the physicians, who as a consequence have power claims on the procedure towards the attainment of consent – the outcome of the contact between these moral agents is a biased form of consent.

b) Man as Communicator – the Fallacy of Reaching Agreement

A theory of justice cannot secure an objective-informed consent once it is founded on disputable presuppositions such as the equality of those involved in a procedure towards obtaining consent or forming a contract. Therefore, other elements of human existence such as the communication

44. Rawls, *A Theory of Justice*, p. 11.
45. Along with Kant, who argues that rational beings are 'ends in themselves', Rawls proposes a concept of moral equality, according to which each person matters and matters equally, and that each person is entitled to equal consideration impartially. This impartiality is the basis for the justification of rights in Rawls' theory (ibid., pp. 160-68).
46. Ibid., pp. 392-96.

action based on rationality have been proposed. Like Rawls, Habermas, influenced by Kant's tradition and the principle of universalisation,[47] elaborates a theory of justifying human actions on rationality. The basis of Habermas' model is the assumption that all subjects involved in all social actions are oriented towards either the attainment of a successful outcome (of an end) or the reaching of an understanding ('The agents involved are coordinated not through egocentric calculations of success but through acts of reaching understanding').[48] Reaching an understanding is considered a process of reaching an agreement between speaking and acting subjects in such a way that the agreement is not imposed but is a result of a free choice.

The core element of Habermas' theory is the presupposition that agreed consent can be based on reason. He believes that the main prerequisite of a possible agreement is that both the speaker and the listener understand a linguistic expression in the same way. However, the vagueness of such an assertion in the medical context is easily betrayed with reference to only one of the three conditions that according to Habermas have to be fulfilled by the communicative intention of the speaker. This condition is the truthful expression of the beliefs, intentions, feelings and desires of the speaker.[49] Without a doubt, such a condition is out of place in the medical context (not least in all social contexts according to the descriptive theory of decision) since it accounts for abstract and subjective considerations.

However, it is within such a context that contractual theories in bioethics have been developed. A representative example, namely a 'triple contract' theory, is presented in Veatch's *A Theory of Medical Ethics.* Veatch sees, through informed consent in the medical context, a social contract between the physician and the patient parallel to those of social policy (the contract between society and each human being) and of health

47. Kant's influence on Habermas is evident in the efforts of the latter to dress his theory with the authority of a universal law. Habermas supports the idea that the communication action incorporates the principle of universalisation. He also states that understanding as a process for the acceptance of the norms of an action, which hypothetically ought to be adopted, corresponds to the acknowledgement of the principle of universalisation (Habermas, *Moral Consciousness and Communicative Action*, p. 92). For a critique of the universalistic foundation of Habermas' *The Theory of Communicative Action*, see Habermas, *Die Zukunft der menschlichen Natur*.
48. Habermas, *The Theory of Communicative Action I*, pp. 285-86.
49. The other two conditions are the rightness of the speaker's speech in respect to a given context and the truthfulness of his statement as justified with reference to its presuppositions.

policy (the contract of medicine as a profession with the members of a society along with prescriptions of principles and rules). He, like Rawls and Habermas, is interested in the autonomy of the subject as well as the subject's orientation towards an objectified consent. His philosophical presuppositions are essential for the assessment of his theory. Indeed, without hesitation, Veatch rejects any metaphysical grounding of morality and seeks an epistemological foundation for secular universality by denying both a theory of value (a theory that provides an account of what is good) and a virtue theory. On the contrary, he proposes 'the theory of principles of right action'. Even though he acknowledges that there is no general agreement on the precise list of principles, he defends his theory by saying that there is a kind of convergence or an agreement when these principles are applied to all people (despite their divergence in terms of their nationality, race, or religion).[50] While he justifies, for example, a place for autonomy in the social contract of a community or of a 'social contract theory' in bioethics, he does not provide a precise meaning for autonomy. Similarly, he neither focusses on the situation of the patients (the medical context designates, in a way, the autonomy of the patients) nor on the character of human beings (each human being has his own personal worldview that always shapes his life) as moral agents who are involved in the social contract. Thus, Veatch seems not only to follow the general accepted practice of 'do not touch' the ground upon which any contract between human beings is formed, but also to ignore the fact that, by placing man in a contract theory, a theory that focusses on the attainment of consent, one contributes to the further 'stripping' of man of the most substantial elements of his own life.

To sum up, the treatment of man as communicator or contractor towards the forming of a contract or acquiring of consent shows that priority is not given to the moral agents themselves (their tradition, character or values) but rather to principles for the sake of a social life grounded upon a social contract or an agreement. While the profound desire of such contract theories is the escape of man from his own individuality and the serving of society for better efficiency (whatever that means), these efforts provide nothing more than the unhindered accomplishment of procedures. The transition from the autonomy of the subject to the creation of a social contract is an unjustified, long leap, since it ignores the real life of the moral agents involved by simply applying abstract definitions of communication and justice.

50. Veatch, 'The Foundations of Bioethics', pp. 212-17. Veatch, almost two decades after the initial publication of his theory, has not altered the core of his theory, though he acknowledges that its difficulties are still present.

5. The Establishment of a Rights-based Human Existence

A relational human life that is based on the notion of justice and proper communication between human beings culminates in the establishment of a rights-based human existence. Thus, the emergence of bioethics as a discipline that coincided with the emergence of human rights is not accidental. The notion of a right is based on what human beings have in common, on their common needs and capacities, which are more important than their differences.

However, the notion of rights is by no means definite. For example, so-called human rights are rights that must be respected because they exist in all human beings. History has shown that such an assertion is problematic. In practice, even the most developed western countries deny that human rights are universal and based on our shared nature. Even though all human beings are supposed to be equal in all circumstances, the truth is that this equality is always framed and limited by national standards. Such an example might include employment laws that separate the inhabitants of a country between the indigenous population and foreigners.[51]

Bioethics is framed by the rationale of the fallacy of universal respect for human rights, and therefore faces a number of inevitable questions. In particular, there is not an *a priori* agreed response to the questions of who deserves a right, since there is no agreement on the content or the object of a right. For some, the criterion of someone possessing a particular right is the capacity to suffer;[52] for others, it is the ability to possess reason or having personal interests;[53] and for others, it is the ability to desire that to which one has a right.[54] In addition, there is no agreement on the possible response to the questions of how the rights are justified. For example, Mill grounds rights on utility,[55] since a utilitarian justification cannot give priority to rights. On the contrary, Rawls justifies rights by prioritising them in contrast to utilitarianism.[56] Another inevitable question is related to the identification of those rights that are inalienable. Although there are fundamental rights, such as the right to life and the right to freedom, that are easily applied in the case of the elimination of slavery, their direct application in the desire of a patient who requests his own death is considered problematic.

51. Kondylis, *Ἀπὸ τὸν 20ᵒ στὸν 21ᵒ αἰώνα*, pp. 61-67.
52. Loewy, 'The Role of Suffering and Community in Clinical Ethics', p. 86.
53. Gillon, 'Persistent Vegetative State, Withdrawal of Artificial Nutrition and Hydration, and the Patient's "Best Interests"', pp. 75-76.
54. Singer, *Writings on an Ethical Life*, p. 195.
55. Mill, *On Liberty and Utilitarianism*, p. 14.
56. Rawls, *A Theory of Justice*, pp. 30-33.

It is not an overstatement to say that current bioethical discussion has designated a rights-based human existence in the medical context. This does not only mean that decisions on euthanasia are taken in the courts[57] but it also means that traditional rights, such as the right to life, justifies a right, where the object stands at the very opposite of what was supposed to be traditionally respected, namely the right to die.[58] Though human life and death are mutually exclusive (death comes when life ends), the legalistic approach towards such decisions considers both as two sides of the same coin or two sides of human existence. Once such a view is legitimised, then the passage from the right to suicide to the right towards the administration of death to a patient through the assistance of the physician is very easy, since the imperative of rights must always be preserved (the elaboration of arguments that may justify the inclusion of the physician as a representative of the medical profession in the administration of death for the sake of rights is not very difficult in a society where individualistic morality is based on these rights).[59]

Interestingly, the recent efforts towards the establishment of the right to die are not the last step in a procedure towards a rights-based human existence; rather, recent discussions reveal a transition from the right to die to the duty[60] or the obligation to die.[61] The oxymoron is that, through the establishment of a duty or an obligation to die, the right to die is placed within the realm of the moral character and integrity of the patient and is justified through objectively true moral principles 'under which each of us ought to choose death over life'.[62] In other words, through the endless legalistic argumentation, another 'imprisonment' of the patient is attempted, where a rights-based human existence also has to think about the basis of imposed 'universal' and 'objectified' rules and principles. Obviously, such a shaping of human existence is only possible when life and death are 'stripped' of any meaningful context

57. See, for example, US vs Salerno, 481, US 739, 745 (1987) and Cruzan vs Director, Missouri Dept of Health, 497, US 261 (1990).

58. For a criticism of such a right, see Kass, *Life, Liberty and the Defence of Dignity*, pp. 201-29.

59. For example, Rachels argues that, once suicide is morally permissible, so is assisted suicide (Rachels, *The End of Life*, p. 86). For a critique of Rachels' argument, see Gunderson, 'A Right to Suicide Does Not Entail a Right to Assisted Death', pp. 51-54.

60. Corlett, 'Is There a Moral Duty to Die?', pp. 41-56.

61. Loewy and Loewy, '*Lebensunwertes Leben* and the Obligation to Die: Does the Obligation to Die Rest on a Misunderstanding of Community?', pp. 26-27.

62. Corlett, 'Is There a Moral Duty to Die?', p. 56.

such as the ordinary life of the patient, namely a content-rich human life that involves, among others, personal relationships, values, virtues and membership of a community.

As a general conclusion in relation to the efforts towards the 'stripping' of a human being of the essential aspects of his own life in the medical context, one could notice that, despite widespread assertions in bioethics that the enforcement of a particular anthropology is not attempted in current bioethical discussions, the previous analysis has shown the contrary. If the descriptive theory of decision is correct in saying that the enforcement of a particular anthropology is but the imposition of the particular worldview of the subject(s) of a decision (who is as such subjective by definition) – an enforcement that is oriented towards the securing of its power claims on human life – then, through the identification of those characteristics of human existence that matter in the medical context, the practice of modern medicine and of bioethics towards the misappropriation of the role of creator and the 'creation' of a 'new' human being is no longer disguised. A human being 'stripped' of his own ordinary life is a fragmented human being. Thus, the reconstruction of such a human being is imperative.

II. Efforts Towards Reconstructing the Fragmented Human Being

The previous analysis has shown that the choice of bioethics to be based on content-less ethics regarding human existence has resulted in a fragmented human being who searches for his foundation in the fulfilment of procedures and the establishment of rights through consent and agreement. In fact, human existence, along with the particular moralities, are excluded from the bioethical debate because of the fear of the violation of the supposed universality of the relevant moral account of human actions in the medical context.[63] Therefore, it is not surprising that throughout the last decades a limited number of scholars have tried to develop theories towards the reconstruction of such a fragmented human being. Despite the partiality and the unavoidable subjectivity of these efforts, since they cannot escape the implications of the descriptive theory of decision, it is essential to refer to them as they represent a

63. Manent comes to the same conclusion when he comments on the political message of the wars of the twentieth century: 'we nonetheless do not cease to hesitate between the particular political bodies that are the nations, whose particularity the past wars have rendered unworthy, and a universal idea of humanity that we do not know how to concretize' (Manent, *A World beyond Politics*, p. 85).

willingness towards the preservation of the human being and against his exclusion from the centre of the ethical debates, as well as against his vulnerability, in terms of unimpeded power claims over him by self-appointed creators. Interestingly, these efforts are based on philosophical traditions that are not popular in modern times.

1. Revising the Idea of Nature: an Anthropology of Metaphysics

Many believe that modern biomedicine has abandoned any ontological and teleological account of humanity.[64] This abandonment was a prerequisite of the quest for a common and objectified morality, pure and stripped of any anthropology or any content-rich interpretation of human existence. Despite its illusive character, such a belief is widely accepted and applied. It is in this context that the contribution of Hans Jonas[65] to bioethics has to be interpreted. Jonas bases his theory on ontological grounds and in terms of a metaphysical quest.

Jonas, by explicitly denouncing extreme autonomy in man and by supporting an interpretation of freedom in each human being that recognises the importance of the environment and the rest of the world, elaborates a philosophy of organism according to which a human being, as an organism, has chosen to follow the route towards an organic identity that is simply an exchange with the environment. Jonas borrows from science the term 'metabolism' in order to express the continuity of the exchange with the environment (he uses the German term '*Stoffwechsel*' which means 'the exchange of matter'). Once living beings, such as human beings, are in a procedure of continuous exchange with matter, they are never identified with the sum of the materials at a specific time. Therefore, while living beings are always free from their material essence, they, at the same time, are subject to the necessity of the continuous exchange with matter. Otherwise, they cannot exist. For

64. Shuman, *The Body of Compassion*, p. 28.
65. The Jewish-German philosopher Hans Jonas is considered as 'the first philosopher of eminence to arrive in on medical ethics' (Jonsen, *The Birth of Bioethics*, p. 77). In most of his writings of this period, Jonas clarifies his intention to establish a new ethic based on a teaching that would say what is good. An interesting collection of articles that presents his main thoughts for a philosophy of life or organism is available in Hans Jonas' *Philosophische Untersuchungen und Metaphysische Vermutungen* (for the rest of this work, PUMV). Jonas provides a good example of how the philosophy of modernity has turned to bioethical issues by combining different philosophical traditions in order to touch the roots of these issues.

Jonas, the interdependence between the freedom of using the world and the necessity for this use is an indication that life is always under the threat of its negation.[66] Jonas concludes that there is an ontological necessity upon which any living being, including humans, lives and acts. Therefore, any ethic for the future has to be based on ontology and the metaphysical belief that the being proclaims not only what a living being is but also the obligations towards it. The outcome of this foundation of ethics is the imperative of responsibility. Jonas argues that the capability of humans to take responsibility is based on their ontological ability to choose among alternative possibilities for action with knowledge and volition, and argues that this responsibility is adjunctive to freedom. Hence, the two ontological poles of the freedom of human beings and the value of being gave birth to the ethical principle of responsibility as a moderator between them.[67]

Hans Jonas, along with the elaboration of a philosophy of organism, offers the most comprehensive critique of both dualism and materialism in the bioethical context. He highlights the importance of the human being and elaborates an ethic for the future based on the condemnation of both Descartes' dualism and materialism.[68]

For Jonas, the partiality of idealism and materialism with respect to integral reality, cannot solve the problem of 'the existence of a living life in an unfeeling world of matter which in death triumps over it'.

In particular, he believes that dualism has failed to conceive of the insoluble of inwardness (spirit/mind/soul) and outwardness (matter/nature/body) in a living organism (the psychophysical unity which the organism exhibits).[69] As Kass testifies, for Jonas, materialism has ignored 'the inward dimension of all that lives, and therefore failed to understand the difference between the nonliving and the living'.[70]

Jonas chooses three external characteristics of man in order to justify the transgression of materialism. First, man makes tools that are not governed by any organic action or biological planning and, thus, he is able to fulfil the necessity for contact with matter that is a natural bodily

66. Jonas, PUMV, pp. 82-86.

67. Ibid., pp. 129-33.

68. Jonas sees a very strong connection between dualism and materialism. He says that dualism 'is the vehicle of the movement which carried the mind of man from the vitalistic monism of early times to the materialistic monism of our own as to its unpremeditated, even paradoxical result; and it is difficult to imagine how the one could have reached from the other without this gigantic "detour"' (Jonas, *The Phenomenon of Life*, p. 12).

69. Ibid., pp. 17-19.

70. Kass, 'Appreciating the Phenomenon of Life', p. 3.

necessity.[71] Second, man creates images and through them manipulates and changes the content of the perception, as well as creating new forms of objects apart from those of the material world. Third, man is the only being who constructs tombs and therefore he is conscious of his mortality, is able to reflect upon life and death, react to direct visual evidence and raise his thought to the invisible by placing the tool and the image at his service.[72] Thus, Jonas forms an anthropology that is based on the inevitable metaphysical quest.[73] Jonas believes that this is the only way for 'the ethics of the future' since, nowadays, there is an obvious supremacy on the part of those who command the tools due to the dominance of the technological and physical sciences over human life.[74] Even though, in his time, metaphysics was not very popular, Jonas believes that 'the ethics of the future' must be based on metaphysics, since only metaphysics can say why man must continue to exist, why his disappearance is prohibited and how man must exist.[75] Since technological advances 'hurt' the ultimate issues of human being, such as the meaning of *bonum humanum*, the meaning of life and death, the dignity of the person, and the integrity of the image of man (in religious language, the image of God), man needs metaphysics in order to undertake the responsibility against any distortion of his future.[76]

In short, Jonas proposes an anthropology that considers the relationship between human beings and the world as fundamental for human identity. Through this anthropology he lays down the foundation for an ethics based on ontology and metaphysics that challenges modern society and its indifference to questions relevant to the essence of the human being. According to Jonas:

> Ontology as the ground of ethics was the original tenet of philosophy. Their divorce, which is the divorce of the 'objective' and 'subjective' realms, is the modern destiny. Their reunion can be affected, if at all, only from the 'objective' end, that is to say, through a revision of the idea of nature.[77]

---

71. Jonas, PUMV, pp. 37-39.
72. Ibid., pp. 39-49.
73. As Jonas states, 'Out of the tombs arose the pristine metaphysics in the shape of myth and religion. That all is life and that all life is mortal is the basic contradiction it strives to resolve. It meets the profound challenge; and to save the sum of things, death had somehow to be denied' (Jonas, *The Phenomenon of Life*, pp. 8-9).
74. Jonas, PUMV, p. 49.
75. Ibid., p. 136.
76. Ibid., pp. 143-46.
77. Jonas, *The Phenomenon of Life*, p. 283.

For Jonas, the revision of the idea of nature could result in crossing the divide between the objective and the subjective realms, and therefore in a kind of objectivity that respects all subjects. However, since the objective end designates this transgression, it is obvious that such a transgression implies a distance between the moral agents and the end towards which they have to be oriented. This shows that even Jonas's metaphysics is subject to the descriptive analysis of the descriptive theory of decision.

2. The Importance of the Other: a Relational Framework of Ethics

In Levinas the issues regarding the division, as well as the breaching of the division between the objective and subjective realms through a revision of the ideal of nature, is transferred to the relationship between the subject and the Other in the pursuit of a relational account of morality. For those who are interested in the invention of a tie-rod that may reconstruct the fragmented vision of humanity, the contribution of Immanuel Levinas to modern ethics is of great importance.

Levinas' thought starts from the assertion that war is a constant possibility as well as a reality that suspends morality. The suspension of morality happens due to the concept of totality that dominates Western philosophy and forces individuals to play roles incompatible with their commitments since they 'are reduced to being bearers of forces that command them unbeknown to themselves'. In this context, human beings are inescapably subject to self-destructiveness, once within such totality there is not something exterior to which a distance would be kept in order to escape war given that 'every war employs arms that turn against those who wield them'. Any reference to the meaning of individuals outside such a context becomes impossible.[78] For Levinas, the only way towards the elimination of war is the replacement of the concept of totality with the concept of infinity, along with the establishment of exteriority. Therefore, in contrast to the individualistic perception of a human being in liberal societies, Levinas asserts that ethics 'beyond visions and certitudes, delineates the structure of exteriority as such' and, as such, the interest in the subject is expanded to include exterior parameters as well.[79] Indeed, the aim of Levinas is the elaboration of a form of subjectivity, which, through an eschatological lens, becomes objectivity once it welcomes the infinitude, the Other, as hospitality.[80]

78. Levinas, *Totality and Infinity*, pp. 21-22.
79. Ibid., p. 304.
80. Ibid., pp. 25-27 and 220-23.

The cornerstone of Levinas's ethics is 'to be for the Other'. 'Being-for-the-other' is a relationship that subordinates neither the I to the Other nor the Other to the I. Exteriority and I are not antagonists. On the contrary, the face of the Other 'signifies the philosophical priority of the existent over Being,[81] an exteriority that does not call for power or possession, an exteriority that is not reducible, as with Plato, to the interiority of memory, and yet maintains the I who welcomes it'.[82] While 'being-for-the-other' does not imply any transcendence of the one over the other, this way of existence results neither in a kind of contract nor implies an undifferentiated relationship; it rather places the importance on a relationship that is designated by the opening of the subject to the face of the Other in such a way that 'in existing for another I exist otherwise than in existing for me'. This kind of relationship is 'the essence of morality itself'.[83] Thus, Levinas states a relational way of existence that is qualified once existence ceases to be oriented towards the Self and turns towards the Other. Such an orientation is the being interpellated by the Other. To be more precise, the being as an I, as an individual, is defined by his responsiveness to the Other.[84]

Obviously, the way that Levinas views human existence represents a challenge to individualism and to the autonomy of the subject in a self-determinative perception of humanity. Levinas proposes an ethic where the relationship between each human being with the other(s) or Other (the religious presuppositions of Levinas should not be forgotten) is crucial and decisive in all cases. Therefore, the application of Levinas's ethics to bioethics in order to accentuate the relational character of the relationship between the patient and the physician is not a surprise.

Given that the Other designates the Self, or, in other words, the Self is freely designated by the Other, Tauber points out that the patient, by respecting his autonomy, frames the physician's response based on his commitment to cure. Therefore, the patient ceases to be an Other but he rather becomes both the healer and the sufferer as a 'singular unit' through a dialectical relation.[85] Without a doubt, this dialectical relation

81. Levinas criticises the ontology of Heidegger, who affirms the priority of Being over existent and consequently the priority of ontology over metaphysics, which subordinates the relationship with the Other person to the relationship with the Being. He points out that ontology presupposes metaphysics and as such the relationship with the Other precedes any ontology (ibid., pp. 45-48).
82. Ibid., p. 51.
83. Ibid., p. 261.
84. Levinas, 'Dialogue with Emmanuel Levinas', pp. 13-33.
85. Tauber, 'From the Self to the Other: Building a Philosophy of Medicine', p. 179.

does not imply that either the patient or the physician have the authority to impose definitions, for since the Self is defined by the Other, likewise, the Other is defined by the Self, given that the Other is also a Self.[86] For Tauber, such reciprocity in the relationship between the patient and the physician in the medical context has to be the task of medical ethics 'where each (physician or patient) is scrutinized as a *relational* Self'.[87]

Apart from Levinas' contribution to breaching the division among human beings through the re-orientation of the relationship between the physician and the patient, his ethical approach is also related to breaching the division within human existence. Given that the relationship between the I and the Other has a constituent character for a human being, Levinas discards any dualism in human life. He does so by identifying life with a body ('Life is a body'). This identification is based on the assumption that, just as life can be viewed either in its self-sufficiency – the living body (*corps propre*) – or as a crossroads of different forces – the interaction body-effect, likewise, 'to be a body' can be considered either as to be a master of oneself (*se tenir*) or to 'be-in-the-other'. Though life continuously affirms that the inversion of the body-master into the body-slave is always possible, just like the transition from health to sickness, life as a body that experiences both independence (to be a master of oneself) and dependence ('be-in-the-other') does not imply a kind of slavery once 'to be-in-the-other', that is, 'to be encumbered by one's body', results in happiness. If so, any dualism between the lived body and the physical body does not exist.[88]

In the same vein but in the medical context, Fuchs, influenced by the phenomenology of Levinas, adopts a system of ontology, according to which the suffering patient is a living human before the physician and not a pure consciousness or a pure will. Fuchs states that the physician cannot overcome this reality by merely referring to compassion and respect by stating that one should have compassion and respect for the suffering person.[89] Recognising an embodied being in the face of the other, Fuchs 'implies a moral obligation not to destroy her body, not to kill her . . . the killing of his (her) organism is *per se* directed against him

86. Ibid., p. 182.
87. Ibid., p. 184.
88. Levinas, *Totality and Infinity*, pp. 164-65.
89. Fuchs notes that 'once the principle of eliminating suffering by killing the sufferer is acknowledged, then there is no reasonable argument left against the extension of euthanasia to *non-terminal*, unrelievable suffering (e.g. severe depression) and to patients *incapable to give consent* (non-voluntary euthanasia)' (T. Fuchs, 'The Notion of "Killing": Causality, Intention and Motivation in Active and Passive Euthanasia', p. 252.

as a person'.[90] In other words, any action against the living body is against the psychophysical union that constitutes the person and which is the basis of all medical actions. Fuchs argues that the physician deals with an inseparable unity of 'body' and 'soul', a unity of outward and inward, which constitute the so-called 'person in his bodily integrity'.

Taking into account the remarkable contribution of Levinas to the restoration of the vision of the fragmented human being in the medical context, one may argue that his philosophical foundations could be adopted as an appropriate alternative to bioethics. In applying the descriptive theory of decision to the philosophical framework of Levinas, the question that is raised is whether the relational framework of Levinas could overcome the subjectivity and the temptation for power claims over human life.

Levinas presents the infinity, the Other, as the alternative to the totality of beings, where power, war and killing sovereign. He notes that, though the Other precedes any initiatives the Self may take, he exhibits infinite resistance to committing a murder. Such resistance introduces an absolutely other relation once 'the resistance of what has no resistance' paralyses the power of the Self.[91] Therefore, the power (*pouvoir*) to kill becomes a kind of powerlessness (*impuissance*).[92] However, while Levinas challenges the reality of totality, where the first event of the encounter is war, by saying that the face of the Other threatens the eventuality of struggle, he acknowledges that resistance to murder is not real but ethical, and concludes inescapably that: 'War presupposes peace, the antecedent and non-allergic presence of the Other.' Despite the powerlessness of the Self due to the presence of the Other, war, killing and power exist as realities. Apparently, the transcendental character of the Other keeps a distance from the Self, and, as a consequence, verifies the descriptive theory of decision and places it among the rest of the theories that have power claims over human life. Waldenfels argues that, while Levinas refers to a nearness between the Self and Other, such a nearness that originates in otherness includes not only the distance between the Self and the Other but also a distance that is continuously increasing.[93] Tauber's efforts to present Levinas's relational framework of morality as an alternative to an autonomy-centred view of ethics,

90. Ibid., p. 250.
91. Levinas, *Totality and Infinity*, pp. 197-201.
92. Waldenfels, 'Levinas and the Face of the Other', pp. 63-81.
93. Ibid., p. 74. The distance between the Self and the Other becomes even clearer in *Otherwise than Being*, a later work of Levinas (Levinas, *Otherwise than Being or Beyond Essence*, pp. 81-97).

just like the alternative of Nietzsche, are not convincing. Tauber argues that in Levinas the Self is substantiated through his relationship to the Other, whereas in Nietzsche the Self has to strive alone, and asserts that through Levinas the Self is released from his powers, whereas through Nietzsche the Self is a will aimed at securing power claims. However, in the process Tauber ignores the self-evident truth that the emphasis on the relationship between the moral agents, even in the context of Levinas' thought, cannot serve as a panacea to the manipulations that derive from the objectified worldviews, given that the distance between the Self and the Other remains even in such a context.

3. Morality in a Narrated or To-be-narrated Quest

Given that both an anthropology of metaphysics and a relational framework of ethics are connected with either an objective end or the absence of a realistic proximity between the moral agents involved in a particular context, one may wonder what could be a convincing alternative?

MacIntyre believes that such an alternative is provided through the reemergence of virtue ethics and of narrative. In such a case, the fragmented moral agents are placed in a context where they enjoy not only a meaningful system of anthropology but also meaningful relationships. It is interesting that MacIntyre makes his own contrast with Nietzsche.

MacIntyre, in his work *After Virtue*, argues that the human being in modern society has two alternatives. The first one is to follow Nietzsche's tradition that coincides with liberal individualism. The second alternative is to follow the tradition of Aristotle, according to which morality has to be viewed in the context of virtue ethics and of narrative. MacIntyre points out that, while Nietzsche's *The Will to Power* shows that modern morality is encumbered with pseudo-concepts that aim to disguise the will to power and claim an objectivity that is falsely considered as rationally sustained, his 'great man' is also a pseudo-concept that cannot become an alternative to the conceptual scheme of liberal individualistic society. Rather, however, the 'great man' is 'one more representative moment in its internal unfolding'. Thus, Nietzsche's theory, despite the criticism against modernity that it entails, is unwillingly aligned with modernity and, particularly, with its 'deification' of individualism. As a result, MacIntyre proposes the restatement of the Aristotelian tradition.[94]

MacIntyre's main objection is that in the modern society one does not participate in shared activities and is isolated from the community

94. MacIntyre, *After Virtue*, p. 259.

in which one was raised. This results in 'the great man' and his own self-sufficient moral authority. However, man is a story-telling animal who has a moral starting point as this is specified by his own story or his own tradition. Therefore, what is important is not man's authorship but rather 'what story or stories do I find myself a part of'. Only in this way may someone understand his interaction with others. MacIntyre provides an example of how stories designate what human beings learn about the world that surrounds them.

> It is through hearing stories about wicked step-mothers, lost children, good but misguided kings, wolves that suckle twin boys, youngest sons who receive no inheritance but must make their own way in the world and eldest sons who waste their inheritance on riotous living and go into exile to live with the swine, that children learn or mislearn both what a child and what a parent is, what the cast of characters may be in the drama into which they have been born and what the ways of the world are. Deprive children of stories and you leave them unscripted, anxious stutterers in their actions as in their world.[95]

It is in this context that MacIntyre criticises the empiricists, the analytical philosophers and the existentialists, who view man in terms of psychological states and events, in terms of the connection between them or in terms of Leibniz's law for a strict identity (either all the properties of the last heir belong to the claimant or the claimant is not the heir). MacIntyre believes that these approaches fail to see what stands behind a human action, which is the concept of a story from which a character (the roles into which man has been drafted) is generated.[96]

Without a doubt, MacIntyre's priority is not to challenge current philosophical traditions for the sake of the particularity of the personal history of the moral agents. On the contrary, by demonstrating the insufficiency of these philosophical traditions that claim objectivity and universality, he wants to provide an alternative. This alternative, while it begins from the particularity of the personal history (or narrative or tradition) of the moral agents, passes to universality. This transition is based on MacIntyre's perception of virtues that proceeds 'in a narrated

95. Ibid., p. 216.
96. Just like the *Descriptive Theory of Decision*, that emphasises the importance of the 'background' that exists behind human decisions, which is revealed through the distinction between the worldview decisions and the segmental decisions, MacIntyre also talks about the importance of the story that designates the character of a moral agent and consequently the character of a moral action.

or to-be-narrated quest'. Throughout this quest man passes through three different stages. First, by viewing virtues as qualities that allow one to achieve good internal practices, as well as qualities that sustain one in the quest for what is good, man increases his self-knowledge ('What is good for me?'). Second, by bearing in mind that virtues are qualities that contribute to the good of a whole life, he increases his knowledge of the good ('What is the good for man?'). Third, he pursues what is good for every human being within an ongoing social tradition by relating the virtues with this aim. The third stage indicates that, while identity is designated by the membership of particular communities (family, neighbourhood, city or tribe), a person is not obliged either to admit the moral constraints of the particularity of such communities nor simply to abandon or obliterate such particularity. Rather, he has to move forward from such particularity to what the search for the good and the universal consists of.[97] MacIntyre concludes that such a quest is possible only in the context of the Aristotelian tradition, since this tradition is the best example that humans possess that is 'rationally entitled to a high measure of confidence in its epistemological and moral resources'.[98]

MacIntyre's belief that the Aristotelian tradition constitutes the best example of virtues is questionable. Hauerwas and Pinches accuse MacIntyre of choosing a particular moral tradition even though the Christian tradition provides a competitive alternative. Hauerwas and Pinches argue that, while MacIntyre, in considering interpreters of Aristotle's theory of virtues,[99] he proceeds to an essentially Greek understanding of the virtues by ignoring the profound disagreement between Aquinas and Aristotle on this understanding.[100]

Even though the centrality of tradition and virtues may be considered an alternative to other current philosophical approaches, MacIntyre's theory cannot be regarded as universal, since it is based on a subjective interpretation of what tradition and virtues stand for. As a result, MacIntyre's efforts at establishing a moral theory fall within the spectrum of the critical analysis of the descriptive theory of decision that highlights that, despite their subjectivity, all theories want to have power claims over human life, and therefore wish to play the role of the sole legitimised interpreter.

97. Ibid., pp. 218-221.
98. Ibid., p. 277.
99. MacIntyre, *Whose Justice? Which Rationality*, pp. 164-82.
100. Hauerwas and Pinches, *Christians Among the Virtues*, pp. 66-69.

4. Narrative Identity and the Turn towards Self-knowledge

In examining all the attempts at reconstructing the vision of the fragmented human being along with their flaws, it is justifiable to wonder whether it is possible to have a moral approach that could anticipate the diverse questions surrounding bioethics and particularly euthanasia. To attenuate such worries, the promising contribution of Paul Ricoeur is discussed.

Ricoeur believes that the question 'who am I?' is fundamental to philosophy, despite its neglect by modern thought. He places self-knowledge and understanding at the centre of his philosophical interests. Ricoeur's choice signifies a remarkable about-turn in the debate regarding the ethical character of human actions and challenges the popularity of content-less ethics. What makes Ricoeur's contribution to the field much more important is the rationale behind the focus on self-understanding. This rationale consists of two fundamental concepts.

The first is the absence of unmediated self-knowledge. While he focusses on the subject, he is not considered a follower of the Kantian tradition of autonomy once he recognises the opacity of the *cogito*. On the contrary, he asserts that that a subject 'does not know itself directly but only through the signs deposited in memory and imagination by the great literary traditions'.[101] The efforts of Ricoeur to extract man from his own self towards an inclusion of 'other(s)' culminate in his second fundamental concept, namely the narrative unity of a person's life.

According to his second concept, human life is characterised by one's responsiveness or unresponsiveness to others. The responsive self lives in hope that its responsiveness to others can and will bring about a better life for all people, a life in which all participate with and for others.[102] In this context, there is an evident primacy of the other-than-self over the self. Ricoeur prefers to call such a procedure 'narrative identity'. Obviously, he is not interested in the preservation of the Kantian notion of autonomy. Personal identity is a narrative identity, and, therefore, one can make sense of oneself only in and through one's involvement with others. To avoid any misunderstanding, the narrative character of one's identity by no means abolishes the individuality of the moral agent. On the contrary, a dialectic that underestimates neither the individual nor the decisive role of others regarding one's own character as human being is implied.[103]

101. Ricoeur, 'Intellectual Autobiography', p. 16.
102. Ricoeur, *Oneself as Another*, pp. 165-68.
103. Ricoeur, *Le Juste 2*, pp. 85-105.

In other words, Ricoeur's work is marked by a transition from the centrality of human autonomy to the centrality of personal relationships, along with the importance of meaningful stories in the moral orientation of human life. In a way, Ricoeur goes beyond Jonas, Levinas and MacIntyre once he, without recourse to metaphysical paths, establishes the importance of self-knowledge and understanding without the fear of violating the cultural diversity of modern societies, and once he proclaims weaving such self-knowledge into a narrative that incorporates both the self and others. In addition, Ricoeur does not hide the fact that the unity that binds one person to another is based on the common quest for esteem and recognition.[104]

However, is it guaranteed that such a common quest has an aim shared by all moral agents? The answer found in the historical reality is negative. The inclusion of others in the narrative identity of the moral agents by no means secures the absence of conflicting interests that may lead to the absence of power claims between persons, for the self-evident reason that the different worldviews of the moral agents involved do not result in a common worldview. Once the desired esteem and recognition of the moral agents is at stake, the rationale of the imperative of self-preservation continues to rule as sovereign. Though the focus on self-understanding is absolutely necessary to challenge the long-standing accepted morality, this is not sufficient.

5. Which Rationality?

The critique, on the one hand, of the sovereign rationality of contemporary bioethics and, on the other hand, of the promising efforts towards a content-rich consideration of human existence by no means implies the adoption of postmodern rationality.[105] On the contrary, it is the means to introduce the presentation of a Christian rationality that proclaims the necessity of an alternative that would go beyond the antinomies of our ethical system[106] – not through the establishment of an ambiguous common morality but through the coexistence of the 'universal' and the 'particular'.[107]

Contrary to the rationality of modern democracy that seeks 'to construct a rigorous moral and political doctrine without inquiring into the nature, essence or substance of man, and even by rejecting

104. Ricoeur, 'Nature and Freedom', pp. 29-37.
105. MacIntyre's *Whose Justice? Which Rationality* inspires the title of this section.
106. Nagel, 'War and Massacre', p. 143.
107. Changeux and Ricoeur, *What Makes Us Think?*, pp. 272-79.

any affirmation regarding human essence as presumptuous or idle',[108] this book presupposes a rationality that emerges from a particular consideration of human life and consequently of human existence. Such rationality goes beyond a narratively shaped theology and a robust theological metaphysic, as well as beyond their contradiction that is included in modern ethical or religious relativism.[109] Such rationality brings together not only the Trinitarian God and man in Christ but also invalidates the alienation of the human being from his own substantial elements as an existence. This is achieved through the provision of a content-rich response to the question of self-knowledge; a question that from the standpoint of Christian ethics requires an answer, and failure to produce an adequate answer to it is evidence of a defective method of enquiry.[110]

Such an endeavour, on the part of the Christian ethics presented in this work, takes its inspiration from the patristic tradition. This selection allows a smooth passage to be effected from the rationality of modern reality to an alternative rationality. This happens for a specific reason. The theology of the Church Fathers is developed, in large degree, around two axes – individuality (hypostasis as it is called by the Greek Fathers) and the free will, a term that is also used by Pierre Manent to describe the modern reality.

More particularly, Manent, following and developing the thought of de Tocqueville, asserts that modernity, in contrast to democracy in antiquity, and aristocracy, is characterised by the regime of the human will, a regime that indicates the sovereignty of the personal will. More particularly, what happens today is a distinction and not an equation (the same *potentia*, according to Thomas Aquinas) between the free will, that corresponds to the possibility of choosing, and the will that wills – 'Willing is not exactly choosing; willing is stronger than choosing, since one continues to will after choosing.'[111] In fact, we have the victory of the will over the free will as a natural faculty of man. This victory signifies the emancipation of the human will from nature and therefore 'nature evidently no longer can have value as the comprehensive framework in

108. Manent, *The City of Man*, p. 124.

109. 'The *real* contradiction is between a narrative theology that never quite allows itself to claim that the story of God's dealings with us "inscribes" in time the character of the eternal God, and a metaphysic that divorces behavior from the manifestations of God on the grounds that the divine nature is not truly bestowed or participated in the world' (Williams, 'Afterword', pp. 497-98).

110. MacIntyre, 'What Has Christianity to Say to the Moral Philosopher', pp. 18-25.

111. Manent, *The City of Man*, p. 158.

which one dwells and interprets human beings'.[112] The act of the will is identified with the social contract and becomes the principle and the source of modern democracy.[113] Such a sovereign will is separated from the contents of life once there is not a common good but rather 'the common denominator and condition for the possibility of all the goods that individuals can desire: the preservation of life and integrity of its members'.[114] As Manent concludes, the pursuit of moral perfection for the moderns is not 'the victory of the higher part of human nature over the lower part' but rather it 'is a matter of the victory of law, or will, or liberty, over nature as such, both lofty and base, and thus also over free will as a natural faculty of man'.[115] From the point of view of political philosophy, the triumph of the will signifies the separation between the state and society, while from an ethical point of view such evolution signals the alienation between people and between each human being and his or her own nature.

If the above short description highlights particular characteristics of the dominant rationality in modern reality that are useful for the study of practical ethics, then the recourse to the patristic tradition will prove valuable for a particular reason: a central thread of the patristic tradition is the study of human individuality in relation to human nature and in reference to the operation of the human will. It must be noted here that from early on the Church Fathers had foreseen the importance of the will in the understanding not only of Jesus Christ but also of man, by making fine distinctions in the multivalence of the term 'will' and by associating these with both individuality-hypostasis and human nature. In the Christian tradition the dilemma of freedom or dependence on nature does not exist. This consideration of rationality is elaborated in the part two of this book.

III. Concluding Remarks

The political, cultural and religious diversity that characterises modern societies raises the question of establishing a common morality that could serve as a common ground of moral agents with diverse personal backgrounds in order to achieve an 'objective' evaluation in order to deal with moral issues, such as those surrounding euthanasia. As shown in the previous chapter, such an endeavour is fallacious, but necessary for

112. Ibid., p. 161.
113. Ibid., p. 163.
114. Ibid., p. 171.
115. Ibid., p. 182.

the disguised power claims over human life, and could only lead to the 'creation' of a 'new' human being, a human being who is fragmented – a human being who suffers from the absence of the constituent elements of his own existence regarding the moral account of his own life – and therefore who is 'stripped' of the fundamentals of his very being.

This 'stripping' of the human being is in principle evident in the framing of the whole discussion of the issues related to decisions on euthanasia through the imposition of particular definitions. In a society where the truth is nothing else but the outcome of consent through procedures, these definitions would only determine the accomplishment of such procedures. Therefore, the designation of how and by whom decisions on euthanasia are taken becomes central. This designation is not based on a definite moral account and results in general vagueness. Humans become mere moral agents whose choices are controlled to accomplish a vaguely defined procedure.

The accomplishment of such procedures is associated with numerous principles. Among them, the principle that enjoys an exceptional position in the medical context, and particularly in decisions on euthanasia, is the principle of autonomy. Even though linking this principle with the Kantian tradition is attempted, such a connection is rather superficial, since it is stripped of any meaningful account of morality and, therefore, is subject to exploitation and the accommodation of power claims over humans. Additionally, the application of autonomy in the medical context becomes the grounds for an abstract account of the self-determination of the moral agents. Thus, the fallacious orientation towards control over death becomes a priority. Once a vague notion of autonomy becomes almost the most substantive element of humanity, man becomes synonymous with his autonomy and 'stripped' of the constituent elements of his ordinary life. Consequently, this practice leads to the transition from a human to an autonomic being.

The 'stripping' of man from his ordinary life refers not only to his external but also to his internal life. Man loses, on the one hand, his wholeness through the use of dualistic approaches that imply, among other things, that he is a bodiless autonomic being with absolute sovereignty over the body, and that imply, on the other hand, the differentiation of the elements that constitute human nature once they are simply considered as constituents of the bodily aspect of humanity. What then becomes easily discernable is the focus solely on aspects that do not deal with the essentials of the human being, such as those that are identified as being diachronically part of human nature and that were thoroughly discussed in chapter one.

The elaboration of contractualism is another indication of the lack of the human substratum from the ethical debate. Contractualism, an alternative to individualism, attempts to control the autonomic character of human life and results in a procedural account of human life. This procedural aspect of life is accomplished through the establishment of a vague list of principles or rules. Consequently, in the medical context, a social contract or consent presupposes the disconnecting of human persons from their traditions, character or values. Despite the efforts towards an objectified consent, the irrefutable truth is that such attempts deliberately underestimate the influential role of the worldviews of the moral agents involved.

The last indication of a moral orientation that places human existence at the margins is reflected in the emergence of human rights during recent decades and the promotion of a rights-based human existence. This reality has implications in the medical context, where rights such as the right to die go far beyond the more traditional rights such as the right to life. Someone could argue that the boundaries between life and death are no longer clear. This is not coincidental, for rights-based understanding of human existence is founded on principles and notions that do not share any substantial account of morality.

A human being denuded of his own ordinary life and all of his essential elements is a fragmented human being. Therefore, such a human being must be reconstructed. Even though a number of theories that aim in this direction, such as metaphysics, have been developed, all of them have two important failings. The first is the inevitably subjective character of their assertions, like the subjective interpretation of the tradition of virtue ethics. The second is their inability to bridge the objective with the subjective realms, as well as the Self and the Other. Due to this inability, the desired proximity between them is not achieved and, therefore, the application of power claims over human life is unavoidable.

The inclusion of all moral agents involved in a particular context within the same narrative characterises other promising efforts at reconstructing the fragmented human being. Since they are based on the proper self-knowledge and understanding of the moral agents, these endeavours attempt to re-orient the focus towards what really designates the character of moral actions. However, the orientation of such ethics towards the respect for and the acknowledgement of others by no means eliminates the desire for self-preservation and whatever else this desire entails.

What is left after analysing all these theories critically? Is there any way out of such a vicious circle that keeps man, by definition, subject to a tendency for self-preservation through power claims over human existence? Is there a convincing alternative even if metaphysics cannot escape from such subjection?

Given that the current debate on bioethics is framed by a nonsensical distinction between so-called common morality and the 'particular' moralities, discussed in chapter one, as well as by a principle-centred and not a human-centred view of morality that entails a fragmented being, discussed in chapter two, any possible alternative should be free from such ineffective constraints. The following chapters of this book are devoted to the development of such an alternative, which represents a 'particular' rationality that stands in contradistinction to the sovereign rationality found in modern society.

Part Two

The Creation of Man According to the Image of God and the Prospect of Voluntary Death

The first part of this book has provided a descriptive approach to bioethics through the application of Kondylis' descriptive theory of decision. This application has given a description of the character of bioethics through the exposition of the common ground that all theories relevant to human existence share, including bioethics, which is their self-preservation through power claims. The presentation of the character of euthanasia as discussed in modern society followed. Consequently, the anthropological presuppositions of bioethics, which are either consciously or unconsciously kept disguised and result in a vision of a fragmented human being, despite the efforts for the reconstruction of such a being, have been revealed.

The second part of this book is marked by a change in epistemological approach and provides a transition from philosophy to theology. This is a transition towards a normative approach to human existence, an approach that is designated by the elaboration of theological arguments, namely arguments with reference to God. In such a context, even a Christian tradition cannot escape the critique of the descriptive theory of decision. This means that a Christian tradition may also be viewed as a theory of human existence that consequently aims towards its self-preservation and the maintenance of its power claims. However, the anthropological presuppositions of such a Christian tradition must be examined even more closely in order to see whether they match those that designate the fragmented human being of bioethics, and whether they, at least, provide a kind of alternative regarding the commitment to self-preservation and power claims. In other words, the second part represents a switch from a descriptive to a normative approach, and presents theological presuppositions as regards the issues surrounding euthanasia.[1]

Part two presents the theology of John Damascene and Symeon the New Theologian. The theology that derives from the Christian tradition and, in particular, from the patristic tradition, to which the two Fathers belong, is polemical in the sense of St Paul's words: 'For our struggle is not against flesh and blood, but against the rulers, against the powers, against the world rulers of this darkness, against the spiritual forces of evil in the heavens.'[2] Christians quite often confuse the distinction between these two types of struggle. It is for this reason that the discussion of the character of self-preservation within such a tradition is extremely important.

According to the descriptive theory of decision, even Christians are subject to the orientation towards or the inescapable imprisonment within the sovereignty of this world that secures one's own self-preservation. However, the coming of Christ has opened up another possibility for man, that of going beyond one's interest in self-preservation. After the coming of Christ, self-preservation is enlightened and transfigured into self-relinquishment. Therefore, the first priority of Christians is not their mere self-preservation in this world but rather their eternal 'self-preservation'. Can then someone argue that there is a clear-cut distinction between the pursuit of eternal 'self-preservation' within the Christian tradition and self-preservation through sovereignty over the other?

The descriptive theory of decision states that the oneness of theory and practice is fundamentally important for understanding human existence. This is also equally important for the understanding of the Christian tradition on which the theological arguments of this book are based.

1. The inclusion of normative and non-normative approaches regarding human existence enriches this book from a methodological point of view, because it not only entails the involvement of the two major categories on the understanding and examination of moral life, but it also offers the ground for an ancillary relationship between them.

2. Ephesians 6:12. To avoid any misunderstanding, this position neither places Christians outside the life of modern societies nor absolves them from their responsibilities regarding their intervening role. On the contrary, it designates what is important in their 'war' within societies (see, for example, Hays, *The Moral Vision of the New Testament*, pp. 65-66). It is worth noting that John Damascene repeatedly uses this phrase from St Paul in his homilies on the martyrs Barbara and Anastasia (Barb. 2, 17-20; Anast. 29, 11). Obviously, the life and death of the martyrs substantiate, in a way, the polemical character of the Christian life.

However, the voluntary acceptance of particular theological arguments cannot guarantee the corresponding practice once such acceptance does not automatically transgress the fallen state of humanity.

Indeed, the character of human existence cannot justify a clear-cut distinction between the pursuit of 'self-preservation' in eternity within the Christian tradition and the pursuit of self-preservation through sovereignty over the other, since this is not a distinction but rather a continual spiritual endeavour. This is evident in the words of St Paul, 'But I see a different law in my members waging war against the law of my mind and making me captive to the law of sin that is in my members',[3] and in St Peter's denial of Christ that was immediately followed by the recognition of his sin.[4] These examples reveal the character of the Christian life throughout the centuries as it is expressed in every Christian individual or in Christians as a whole, and in members of a community that lives in this world but with constant reference to God and to His Kingdom. A Christian community, being part of this world, is inescapably subject to its constraints. Even though it is subject to such a reality, it must not be passively adapted to contemporary society. On the contrary, the Christian community must criticise the principles of the particular society based on its commitment to a Christian way of life.[5]

The fact that within the Christian tradition self-preservation through power claims over human existence is interwoven with eternal 'self-preservation' transgresses the descriptive power of the descriptive theory of decision, a theory that is strictly limited to the secular aspect of human existence. Such a transgression by no means implies that DTD is not applicable in the case of the Christian tradition that is presented in this book. On the contrary, DTD, as happens with all theories of human existence, reveals the orientation of all persons, including Christians, towards their self-preservation and power claims over others, their supposed enemies. However, within the context of the Christian tradition, this orientation acquires an eschatological prospect, as is clearly indicated by St Paul,[6] and, as a consequence, it is possible that the supposed enemies of human existence would not be identified with a

3. Romans 7:23.
4. Matthew 26:69-75.
5. For such a critique within the contemporary context see in Hauerwas, *Χριστιανισμός και Αμερικανική Πολιτική*, where the introduction (written by the author of this book) discusses the relationship between the Church and State, along with the fear of the institutionalisation of the Church with special reference to the Greek Orthodox Church (pp. 7-33).
6. Ephesians 6:12.

particular human being or a particular group of human beings who are representatives, for example, of a particular theory of human existence. This possibility designates a reality that at least limits the focus on self-preservation and power claims on one another and goes beyond the struggle for power in this world. Christ taught His disciples and through them all people that the rulers of this world, namely those who direct human life in its various aspects, seek absolute dominance over humans and apply absolute authority over them, and that the Christian character stands at the very opposite to the rationale of the world: 'You know that the rulers of the Gentiles lord it over them [κατακυριεύουσιν], and those in high positions use their authority over them [κατεξουσιάζουσιν]. It must not be this way among you! Instead whoever wants to be great among you must be your servant.'[7] It is in this vein that the elaboration of the theological arguments that follows has to be interpreted.

7. Matthew 20:25-26.

Chapter 3
St John Damascene and the Character of Man

Introduction

The aim of this chapter is to elaborate those aspects of Christian anthropology that are, either directly or indirectly, connected with the issues surrounding euthanasia such as the meaning of life and death and the responsibility of man towards life and death. The theological work of John Damascene is taken as a basis for the argumentation. This elaboration is necessary for the proper understanding of the moral character of the decisions taken in the medical context with respect to euthanasia. Given that the character of human life is extremely complex, the whole discussion passes through two axes of interpretation.

The first axis corresponds to the major turning points in the Christian account of human history, that is, the creation of man according to the image of God, the fall of Adam and Eve and the incarnation of the Son of God in Christ. The implications of these changes are very important for the proper understanding of an absolute question such as the coming of death. Following this, a content-rich and meaningful context is established within which substantial moral arguments can be developed.

The second axis of interpretation deals with the significance of the interpersonal character of human life (relationships with one another and with God) and the impact of the internal character of man regarding the coming of death. Despite the contemporary emphasis on the relational character of human life, that is absolutely justified taking into account the centrality of the individual and the emphasis of modern civilisation on the autonomous being, Damascene offers the ground for a balanced discussion that involves both the relational and the individualistic aspects of a human being as they are perfectly exemplified, among others, in the case of the martyrs.

Since this book aims at the discussion of the issues surrounding euthanasia through the elaboration of a specific account of human existence, the choice of the narration of the creation of man in the Old Testament, a narration that connects a fundamental anthropological principle (God created man according to His own image)[1] and the entry of death into human life (God placed him in paradise but warned him that if he ate from the tree of the knowledge of good and evil he would surely die),[2] as a starting point for the elaboration of relevant theological arguments is justified.

For John Damascene, the narration of the creation of man in the Old Testament has a multivalent character.[3] Damascene, in a thorough-paced way, elaborates the concept 'according to the image'. First, people as well as angels were created according to the image of God in terms of the following principles: the rational, the intellectual and the self-determining (κατὰ τὸ λογικὸν καὶ νοερὸν καὶ αὐτεξούσιον), the birth of the word by the intellect and the projection of the spirit and sovereignty (κατὰ τὸ γεννᾶν τὸν νοῦν λὸγον καὶ προβάλλειν πνεῦμα, κατὰ τὸ ἀρχικόν). Second, people have surpassed angels in terms of the unborn (ἀγέννητον) of Adam, the begetting (γεννητόν) of Abel and the procession (ἐκπορευτόν) of Eve. Third, people were given sovereignty by nature (κατὰ τὸ φύσει ἀρχικό), where the body is slave to the soul by nature and is governed by the soul. Fourth, the whole creation is united (κατὰ τὸ συνάγειν πᾶσαν τὴν κτίσιν), since man is the union of the intellectual and the sensible creation (σύνδεσμος γάρ ἐστι νοητῆς καὶ αἰσθητῆς κτίσεως). Finally, Christ, the Son of God, was meant to become according to the image of man (κατ' εἰκόνα, οὗ ἔμελλε γίνεσθαι ὁ υἱὸς τοῦ θεοῦ), for He became man and not an angel.[4]

The richness of Damascene's thought is evident. However, it is impossible (and indeed unnecessary) to accommodate all his thought in this book, especially since the orientation is towards the elaboration

1. Genesis 1:26.
2. Genesis 2:8-17.
3. The underestimation or even the ignorance of the multivalence of the concept of 'according to the image' in John is very risky, since it can result in misinterpretations and can limit the scope of his writings. A very representative case of such a risky approach is Meany's *The Image of God in Man According to the Doctrine of St John Damascene*, where the discussion of the image of God in man is limited to the ontological resemblance between man and God.
4. Volunt. 30, 1-11.

of arguments regarding ethical issues of a particular character. For this reason, a selective as well as combinational approach to his thought has been chosen. This approach permits not only the development of the meaning of the biblical narration but also the proper manipulation of this meaning regarding its implications for human life and death.

I. Man, a Derivative and Relative Creature

The description of the character of humanity with a view to the elaboration of arguments regarding euthanasia must begin from the fundamentals of Damascene's theological work, namely his theological method.

Various scholars have engaged in a long discussion with respect to John Damascene's sources and the handling of Aristotle's categories in *Dialectica*,[5] the first book of his trilogy *The Fountain Head of Knowledge* (the second book of the trilogy is the treatise *Concerning Heresy* and the third is *An Exact Exposition of the Orthodox Faith*). Two points should be made for the purposes of this research. The first point is that Damascene studied Aristotle from different commentaries that had been written earlier,[6] a practice that explicitly shows that our author wanted to write a theological and not a philosophical work.[7] The second point is that, while Damascene looks at Aristotle's 'most appropriate' philosophical categories with a view to presenting the Christian faith, he does not simply introduce his own definitions for the best accommodation of philosophy to the expression of Christian truth,[8] but also presents the degree of kinship as well as the degree of distance between the philosophical and theological principles of method.[9] As John points out:

5. There are two versions of *Dialectica*; the short version (*recensio brevior*; Dial. brev.), that consists of 50 chapters, and the long version (*recensio fusior*; Dial. fus.) that consists of 68 chapters. The use of the long version of *Dialectica* is, in most cases, preferred in this chapter.
6. The dominant belief is that John uses extensively Porphyry's *Isagoge*, an introduction to Aristotle's categories. See Richter, *Philosophische Kapitel*, pp. 74-83.
7. The idea that John Damascene attempted to Christianise Aristotelian logic (Schaeder, 'Die Christianisierung der Aristotelischen Logik in der byzantinischen Theologie, repräsentiert durch Johannes von Damaskus [ca. 750] und Gregor Palamas [ca. 1359]', pp. 298-306) is not justified, simply because he was not interested in such a project. This idea is very popular among those who regard John Damascene a forerunner of scholasticism (Studer, *Die Theologische Arbeitsweise des Johannes von Damaskus*, pp. 132-33).
8. Karmiris, 'Ἡ δογματικὴ διδασκαλία τοῦ Ἰωάννου Δαμασκηνοῦ', pp. 6-7, and Zografidis, *Βυζαντινὴ φιλοσοφία τῆς εἰκόνας*, p. 68.
9. Siasos, *Πατερικὴ κριτικὴ τῆς φιλοσοφικῆς μεθόδου*, pp. 17 and 31.

> First of all I shall set forth the best contributions of the philosophers of the Greeks. . . . In imitation of the method of the bee, I shall make my composition from those things which are conformable with the truth and from our enemies themselves gather the fruit of salvation. But all that is worthless and falsely labeled as knowledge I shall reject.[10]

In other words, he is but a theologian that is interested in philosophy from a theological point of view.[11]

1. The Need for a Definition

The presentation of a Christian anthropology should start from a concise definition of what man is. As Damascene notes, the definition is used to distinguish the nature of one thing from that of another just like the land boundaries separate the property of someone from the property of someone else.[12] In the same vein the definition of man separates human nature from any other nature. This definition is given in *Dialectica* and creates in a way the relational character of the human being.

Dialectica is, at first sight, a book that deals with the five philosophical sounds (φωναί) – genus (γένος), species (εἶδος), difference (διαφορά), accident (συμβεβηκός) and property (ἴδιον)[13] and the ten most general genera (γενικώτατα γένη)[14] – substance (οὐσία), quantity (ποσόν),

10. Dial., Prooemium, 43-51.
11. Tatakis, *La philosophie byzantine*, pp. 106-16.
12. Dial. fus. 8, 38-40.
13. Ibid., 5, 94-98. In particular, '*Genus* is that which is predicated – that is, affirmed and expressed (for to be predicated is to be affirmed in respect to something) – of several things that are specifically different in respect to what pertains to their essence. *Species*, on the other hand, is that in which something is, but which is predicated of several things that are numerically different. And *difference* is that which is predicated of several things specifically different in respect to their particular sort, and it is included in the definition as essential. This is that which cannot *be* and *not be* in the same species and cannot *not be* in the species to which it belongs. . . . A *property* is that which exists in one species and in the entire species, and which is always in it and is conversely predicable with it. . . . An *accident* is that in which something is of a certain sort and which is predicated of several things differing in species but which does not enter into the definition. It can either *be* or *not be*, for, when present, it does not assure the existence of the species, and when it is absent, the species is not destroyed' (ibid., 5, 99-125).
14. A most general genus 'is that which, while it is a genus, is not a species, because it has no genus higher than itself' (ibid., 10, 136-39).

relation (πρός τι), quality (ποιόν), place (ποῦ), time (ποτέ), position (κεῖσθαι), state (ἔχειν), action (ποιεῖν) and passion (πάσχειν).[15] It must be noted that John views all these Aristotelian categories as interdependent.

In *Dialectica*, a sufficient definition must fulfil two presuppositions. First, it has to be 'a concise statement' that sets forth 'the nature of the thing in question' (*δηλωτικὸς τῆς φύσεως τοῦ ὑποκειμένου*)[16] and, second, it has to be made up by 'genus and constituent differences, that is to say essential differences' (*συστατικῶν διαφορῶν ἤγουν οὐσιωδῶν*).[17]

Two kinds of definitions for man are presented in *Dialectica*. The first definition is very precise and considers man as a separate being. According to this definition, the perfect description of man coincides with the statement that 'man is an animal, rational and mortal'. Such a statement fulfils the relevant presuppositions, since it includes terms that are considered as essentials once 'they complete man's nature, so that without them it is impossible for the man to be a man'.[18]

The second definition traverses the major issues in *Dialectica* and considers man as a being who is related to God. This definition is based on the anthropological principles of the creation of man according to the image of God.

God has created man according to His own image. This brief statement may also be expressed with a different wording: Man has been created according to the 'image of God'. The meaning of such a statement can be derived from the analysis of this statement and consists of three parts: man, the 'image of God' and the likeness between man and God. Starting from the third part, the likeness between man and God, namely the likeness of the image to its original, 'is like the relation of things which are *derivative* and *relative*'.[19]

15. '. . . a) one signifies *substance*, as, for example, man or horse; b) another, *quantity*, as, for example, two or three, two cubits long or three cubits long; c) another, *relation*, such as father or son; d) another, *quality*, such as white or black; e) another, *place*, such as in a temple or in a marketplace; f) another, *time*, such as last year, yesterday, or today; g) another, *position*, such as standing or sitting; h) another, *state*, such as being dressed or being shod; i) another, *action*, such as burning or cutting; j) another, *passion*, such as being burnt or being cut. . . . One should know, moreover, that each of the ten categories is a most general genus' (ibid., 37, 5-14).
16. Ibid., 8, 1-2.
17. Ibid., 8, 16-17.
18. Ibid., 5, 31-40.
19. This statement comes from a paragraph on the fourfold division of quality (likeness in quality) in the chapter 'On Equivocals' ('Περί ὁμωνύμων') of *Dialectica* in PG, 94, 596A-600A. The fourth division is connected with the likeness between the image and its original and with special reference to

But what do derivative and relative mean in terms of the relationship between God and man?

2. The 'Derivative' and 'Relative' in Man

Damascene, following Aristotle, presents eight different kinds of divisions between things.[20] According to the eighth and last mode of division, things are divided between those that are derivative (ἀφ' ἑνός) and those that are relative (πρὸς ἕν).[21]

The 'image of man' derives from a true cause, which is man, and therefore is considered derivative.[22] Similarly, the 'image of God' belongs to derivative once it comes from a true cause that is God. Therefore, a being that is formed according to the 'image of God' is *par excellence* a derivative being, a being that comes from God who is his true cause.

The eighth mode of the division of things also has an additional characteristic. It constitutes the only category within which, 'that which is by nature prior and posterior may be considered' (τὸ φύσει πρότερον καὶ ὕστερον θεωρεῖται).[23] John focusses on 'that is by nature prior' and, just after the discussion of the eight divisions of beings, devotes a specific section to it[24] where he explains 'what by nature prior' is:

> That is by nature prior which is implied in something else [*συνεισφερόμενον*], while in itself it does not imply this [*μὴ συνεισφέρον*]; and which takes something else away when it itself is taken away [*συναναιροῦν*], but is not necessarily taken away when the other is [*μὴ συναναιρούμενον*].[25]

John makes this abstract statement concrete by saying that the animal is by nature prior to man. When the animal is taken away, then man does not necessarily exist either, whereas when man is taken away there can still be an animal like the horse and the dog, which are certain kinds of animals.[26]

---

the likeness of man to God. Such a paragraph is the result of one of John's revisions (St John of Damascus, *Writings: The Fount of Knowledge*, trans. Chase, p. 57n). Though Kotter's critical text is the text that is used throughout this work, here an exception is made.

20. Dial. fus. 6, 45-115.
21. Ibid., 6, 103-05
22. Ibid., 6, 105-13.
23. Ibid., 6, 139-43.
24. Ibid., 7.
25. Ibid., 7, 2-3.
26. Ibid., 7, 4-12.

Applying the 'what is by nature prior' to the derivative in man, one may argue that since man is a derivative being in relation to God, such a relationship may also be represented by saying that God is 'by nature prior' to man. Consequently, if God is 'by nature prior' to man then, when God is taken away, man will consequently not exist. Whereas when man is taken away, God is not necessarily taken away. Interestingly, 'what is by nature prior' does not belong to equivocal terms (ὁμώνυμα) – those things that have a common name but which differ in their definition or description[27] – but to those that are derivative.[28] This means that what has been said about those things 'that are by nature prior' as regards the derivative in man does not imply other meanings. Thus, if God is by nature prior to man, the relationship between God and man takes on an absolute character – God only derives man. In other words, God is 'by nature prior' to man at least in the sense that God, and not another being, derives man. Obviously, such a relationship is more than an accident. Does, then, the derivative in man imply a natural relationship between God and man? The answer is given through the elaboration of the category of relative.

As regards the relative (πρὸς ἕν), it belongs, along with the derivative, to the eighth mode of division of things, and denotes those things that 'relate to one thing' (πρὸς ἕν γὰρ βλέπουσιν), such as a health-promoting drug and healthy food relate to health, and those things that are derived from someone or something *par excellence* (ὡς ἀπό τινος ἐξῃρημένου) such as the medical knife.[29] Obviously, through the category of relative, a relationship that designates a unique character to those who come under such a category (the medical knife entails a perfect relationship given that it relates to one particular thing, which is medicine) is implied. Therefore, it is not an overstatement to identify the category relative (πρός ἕν) with one of the most general genus (γενικότατα γένη), namely relation (πρός τι). As John notes, things that are in relation (πρός τι) are those things that are said to belong to other things (as a father to a son, since the father is necessarily the father of a son), or to be related to another thing (as great is to little or much to little since it is said to be 'much' in relation to 'little').[30]

27. Ibid., 32, 2-3.

28. Ibid., 60, 25-27.

29. Ibid., 6, 105-115. It seems that there is a divergence regarding the meaning of the word 'ἐξῃρημένου' between Liddell and Scott's *Greek-English Lexicon* and Lampe's *Patristic Greek Lexicon*. The former translates the word 'ἐξῃρημένως' (as an adverb, not as an adjective) as *par excellence*, whereas the latter gives transcendendly. However, both meanings want to designate the unique character of the relationship that is proclaimed by the category of relative.

30. Dial. fus. 51, 2-6.

According to Aristotle's categories, within the ten general genera, nine are accidents and only one is substance. Within such a categorisation the relative is considered an accident.[31] However, although things that are in relation (πρός τι) or relative (πρὸς ἕν) are assumed to be an accident, they have their relation either in self-subsistents (αὐθεδράστοις) or in those that are not self-subsistents. If the things that are relative are part of the self-subsistents, the relation is considered either natural, like the relationship between father and son or not natural, like the fortuitous relationship between slave and master, the artificial relation between student and teacher and the voluntary (προαιρετική) relationship between friends. If they are not part of the self-subsistents, the relation is considered either natural, like that of double and half, or not natural.[32]

Since God created man according to his own image and since the likeness of the image to its original is considered not only as derivative but also as relative, then the relative in man is by no means a fortuitous, artificial or voluntary relationship. Could, however, someone argue that the relative in man is natural as it happens in the relationship between father and son?

Coming back to the text edited by Lequien and adopted by Migne, John specifies the contents of the likeness of man to God and says that man and God have common goodness, common wisdom or even common power. However, he makes it clear that 'man is not absolutely like God, because God has these things by nature (κατά φύσιν) and we have them by position (κατά θέσιν)'.[33] In such a context the relative in man cannot be regarded as natural but rather as relative by position, namely by imitation. This implies that man's relation to God does not have a definite character. On the contrary, it is subject to change. Thus, Damascene introduces a fourth possibility in terms of the character of relative, a possibility that is not fortuitous, artificial or voluntary. While the relative by position (κατά θέσιν) is not considered a natural relationship, it is a relationship that is always present in man, since it was given at the time of creation and aims towards the imitation of God.[34] In the same vein, the derivative in man implies neither a natural nor an accidental relationship between God and man but rather a relationship towards the imitation of God.

31. Ibid., 37, 14-16.
32. Ibid., 51, 43-51.
33. PG 94, 600A. Michael Lequien published the John Damascene's works in 1717 and 1749 and Migne reprinted these editions, though he added more works attributed to the Church Father.
34. St Maximus the Confessor adopts a similar position when commenting on the 'divinised' (θεωθέν) human will of Christ that he associates with the relative (πρός τι) (PG 91, D233-236B).

In short, though there is always a difference between the natural relationship between father/son and God/man, the relationship between God and man designates a unique character that is beyond any accidental or artificial determination. In fact, this relationship is beyond any known characterisation within the empirical world. It is for this reason that John enriches the context of the Aristotelian categories by introducing a unique relationship, which is the relationship between man and God. This introduction clearly implies that all the issues relevant to human life, such as the coming of death and euthanasia, are dependent not only on the particular human being in whom they take place but also on the Being from which the human being at stake is created and to which he is related.

II. The Priority of Hypostasis over Nature in Man: Man as Composite Hypostasis

In challenging the Aristotelian categories, John is not speaking only of the relationship between man and God. He touches also on the division of beings that is very important for understanding human life as well as its end. Since death is considered the dissociation of soul and body that constitute two different natures or substances, the distinction between hypostases and natures in patristic theology becomes crucial once another element, that of hypostasis, is introduced as decisive for the knowledge of what the human being is. How does the coming of death affect our understanding of man? The answer to this question presupposes the answer to the underlying question of whether the founding of man is detected on the level of hypostasis and not on the level of natures.

We saw that, according to John Damascene, the relationship between God and man is unique and is based on the assumption that man can imitate God as an immutable possibility in human life. To avoid any misunderstanding, such a possibility does imply not only an external relation with God but also an internal one, upon which the external exposition of the relationship between God and man is based.

It is a common tenet in Christian theology that Christian anthropology has to be based on Christology, given that Christ is the incarnated Son of God who was perfect God and perfect man. What makes the case of John Damascene very interesting is the easy betrayal of the radical relationship between Christology and anthropology in his writings. This relationship, for the time being, is elaborated with regards to the ontological difference between hypostasis and nature.[35]

35. The distinction between hypostasis and nature also traces back to the

Whether hypostasis has an ontological priority over nature is a question that traces back to Christology. John, following the Greek patristic tradition, clearly points out that there is an ontological priority of hypostasis over nature just like in Christ, where human nature came into being because of the hypostasis of the Son of God. However, how does it happen in man where there is no pre-existence of hypostasis?

1. Arguments towards the Priority of Hypostasis

The ontological difference between hypostasis and nature was one of the central issues during the Christological controversies. The issue was based on the theological position that Christ is a composite hypostasis and not a composite nature and that the union of divinity and humanity in Christ was a hypostatic union.[36] It is worth noting that Damascene, though he is aware of the different character of Christology compared to anthropology, does not hesitate to draw parallels between Christ and man. Such a practice by no means eradicates the differences that exist between man and Christ. It rather expresses John's intention, on the one hand, to emphasise the priority of hypostasis over nature not only in Christ but also in man[37] and, on the other hand, to accommodate the transition from what happens to Christ to what happens to man.

Damascene explicitly considers man as a composite hypostasis. John, in *Dialectica*, designates that the outcome of the union of soul and body is not a composite nature (φύσιν σύνθετον) made from two substances (ἐκ δύο οὐσιῶν) but rather a composite hypostasis:

> It is possible, however, for one composite hypostasis [Ὑπόστασιν μίαν σύνθετον] to be made from diverse natures, which is how man is made up of body and soul. Now, even though men are said to have one nature, the individual man is not said to be of one nature. This is because, on the one hand, the one nature of

Aristotelian tradition. For the Aristotelian influence on John, as well as for John's personal treatment of borrowings from Aristotle, see Niarchos, 'Aristotelian Influences on John of Damascus' Theory of Essence (Substance) and Hypostasis', pp. 193-206.

36. Expos. 47, 54-66.
37. From St Gregory of Nazianzus, who distinguished between nature, which subsists in itself, and accident (συμβεβηκός), which subsists in another, to the Leontioi and St Maximus the Confessor, who distinguished between hypostasis that subsists by itself and nature that subsists in a hypostasis, the ontological priority of the hypostasis of Christ over human nature is proclaimed (Bathrellos, *The Byzantine Christ*, pp. 110).

> man is said to be composite, since all the composite hypostases of men come under one species; whereas, on the other hand, the individual man is not said to be of one nature [οὐ μιᾶς φύσεως ὁ ἄνθρωπος λέγεται ὁ καθ/έκαστα], since each human hypostasis is made up of two natures - soul and body, I mean - which it preserves unconfused in itself, to which fact the separation caused by death bears witness.[38]

Therefore, the union of soul and body is regarded as a hypostatic union[39] and hypostasis plays an important role regarding the status of the two natures. *Dialectica* once more offers the necessary ground for the comprehension of such a role.

First, John makes a distinction between hypostasis and *enypostaton* (ἐνυπόστατον), where the soul and body are considered as *enypostata*:

> In its proper sense, however, *enypostaton* is either that which does not subsist in itself but is considered in hypostases, just as the human species, or human nature, that is, is not considered in its own hypostasis but in Peter and Paul and the other human hypostases. Or it is that which is compound with another thing differing in substance to make up one particular whole and constitute one composite hypostasis. Thus, man is made up of

38. Dial. fus. 42, 16-25. It is quite surprising that Matsoukas chooses to characterise the hypostasis of man as a mixed (μικτή) condition following a particular passage from *An Exact Exposition of the Orthodox Faith* (Expos. 26, 26-27), where the adjective 'mixed' is attributed to man as a being that is related to both the sensible and the intellectual creature but where the character of human hypostasis is not the issue in discussion (Matsoukas, 'Φιλοσοφία καὶ δογματικὴ διδασκαλία τοῦ ἁγίου Ἰωάννου Δαμασκηνοῦ', p. 285). Such a choice presents quite an ambiguous relationship between soul and body. Matsoukas' choice is not justified for an additional reason. *An Exact Exposition of the Orthodox Faith* as the third book of the trilogy, *The Fountain Head of Knowledge*, cannot be interpreted without reference to the first book, *Dialectica* or *Philosophical Chapters*, which works in a way as an introductory terminology for a better understanding of the theological exposition of the third book. For more detail on the contents of the trilogy, *The Fountain Head of Knowledge*, and a presentation of the different assumptions regarding its original release, see Louth, *St John Damascene*, pp. 31-37.
39. Dial. brev. 50; Dial. fus. 67. It is not accidental that John completes *Dialectica* with a chapter devoted to the meaning of hypostatic union - it is the last chapter of the *recensio brevior* and the one before the last of the *recensio fusior*. If *Dialectica* is only a manual for how to correctly follow the Christian faith as represented in *An Exact Exposition of the Orthodox Faith*, placing a chapter relevant to the hypostatic union at the end of such a manual demonstrates the fundamental importance of the issue.

> soul and body, while neither the soul alone nor the body alone is called a hypostasis, but both are called *enhypostata* . . . hypostasis is that which subsists of itself by its own subsistence [καθ' ἑαυτὸ ἰδιοσυστάτως ὑφιστάμενόν ἐστί τε καὶ λέγεται].[40]

Thus, since neither the soul nor the body alone is called hypostasis, as they never subsisted either before or without one another but only in the hypostasis that is constituted by them, they are called *enypostata*.[41] Interestingly, only the hypostases subsist of themselves and it is upon the hypostases that the substances, the essential differences, the species and the accidents are found.[42] Not only in *Dialectica*, but also in *An Exact Exposition of the Orthodox Faith* towards the elaboration of Christology, John is clear that there is no nature without hypostasis once nature is only found in hypostases:

> The nature may either be taken purely theoretically, since it is not self-subsistent; or it may be taken of what is common to hypostases of the same species and connects them, in which case it is said as nature viewed in species; or it may be considered wholly with accidents in a hypostasis, in which case it is said to be viewed in an individual (ἐν ἀτόμῳ).[43]

An ontological priority of hypostasis over nature is clearly implied as the beginning of soul and body as *enypostata* is found in hypostasis.[44] This does not imply by any means any pre-existence of hypostasis in the constitution of man like the pre-existence of the hypostasis of the Son of God regarding His union with human nature; it rather implies the founding of man on the level of hypostasis.

Second, the ontological priority of hypostasis is connected with the attribution of the characteristics of the soul and body to their common hypostasis.

---

40. Dial. fus. 45, 7-16.
41. Dial. brev. o., 123-26.
42. Dial. fus. 43, 8-11.
43. Expos. 55, 4-7.
44. Rozemond, based on the same passages of John, falsely concludes that all natures are complete and what they find in hypostases is just their delimitation: 'Toute nature est complète. Aucune nature, si complète soit-elle, n'est pour autant une hypostase. Mais toute nature trouve sa concrétisation, sa délimitation dans les hypostases' (Rozemond, *La Christologie de St Jean Damascène*, p. 22). It is for this reason that he does not identify in John any ontological priority of hypostasis over nature but rather 'la signification première de la divinité du Christ', namely a priority of divinity over humanity (ibid., pp. 25-26).

According to Damascene, the hypostatic union represents a composite hypostasis of the united things. At the same time, it preserves unconfused and unchanged both the united natures and their differences, as well as their natural attributes (*φυσικά ἰδιώματα*), that are called components (συστατικὰ), and they distinguish nature from nature and species from species.[45] While the hypostatic union preserves the perfect as well as the different character of the two natures involved – that of the soul and body in man – it also ascribes to the composite hypostasis the characteristic attributes (*χαρακτηριστικά ἰδιώματα*), those that distinguish a soul from all other souls and a body from all other bodies. It is the characteristic attributes of soul and body that not only identify each hypostasis but also unite and bind (ἑνοῦντα καὶ συνάπτοντα) the two natures once these attributes characterise the hypostasis that is common to both natures.[46] Given that the soul and body as *enypostata* do not subsist of themselves but only in hypostases and that the characteristic attributes are not only those that distinguish a hypostasis from other hypostases but also those attributes that unite and bind soul and body, the hypostasis legitimately claims priority over nature.

John highlights even further the ontological priority of hypostasis over nature by arguing that the hypostatic union goes beyond death. The nature that experiences hypostatic union remains indivisible forever. Even death, though it separates soul from body, cannot disrupt their hypostasis. Thus, even after their separation, the soul and body keep the principle of their existence, which is their hypostasis:

> once the natures become hypostatically united, they remain indivisible forever [ἀδιαίρετοι μένουσιν εἰς τὸ παντελές]. And this is so because, even though the soul is separated from the body in death, the hypostasis of both remains one and the same. For the constitution in itself of each thing at its beginning of being is a hypostasis. Therefore, the body remains, as does the soul; both always having the one principle of their being and subsistence, even though they are separated.[47]

Therefore, the hypostasis is considered not only the beginning of the soul and body but also what secures their transition through death to the life 'after death'. Indeed, the hypostasis, due to the hypostatic union, is presented as being more than the union of two natures, the soul and

45. Dial. brev. o. 52-55; Dial. fus. 12, 16-20.
46. Dial. fus. 67, 2-17.
47. Ibid., 67, 17-24.

body, and it is not affected by its potential dissolution. This is what happened *mutatis mutandis* at the time of Christ's death because of the hypostatic union of divinity and humanity.

Death comes in human life as the natural dissolution of the union of soul and body. This also happened in Christ but in a unique way. While the dissolution of Christ's human nature into the soul and body took place, the union of divinity and humanity was not interrupted by death since both the soul and body remained united in the one hypostasis of Christ:

> even though as man He did die and His sacred soul was separated from His immaculate body, the divinity remained inseparable from both – the soul, I mean, and the body. This, the one hypostasis was not divided into two hypostases. For from the beginning both had existence in the same way in the hypostasis of the Word, and when they were separated from each other in death, each one of them remained in the possession of the one hypostasis of the Word. Hence the one hypostasis of the Word existed as hypostasis both of the Word and of the soul and of the body, for neither the soul nor the body ever had any hypostasis of its own other than that of the Word, and the hypostasis of the Word was always one and never two. Hence, the hypostasis of Christ was always one, since, even though the soul was separated from the body in place, it still was hypostatically united to it through the Word.[48]

Therefore, though Christ experienced the separation of His soul from the body, He did not experience any destruction thanks to the hypostatic union of the Son of God with both the soul and body.

Thus, although John Damascene acknowledges that the hypostasis of Christ is a divine hypostasis and that the hypostatic union of divinity and humanity signifies a union without change (ἀτρέπτως), confusion (ἀσυγχύτως), alteration (ἀναλλοιώτως), division (ἀδιαιρέτως) or disruption (ἀδιασπάστως),[49] he implies that whatever happens in this hypostatic union, also happens in the hypostatic union of soul and body in man.

It is remarkable that the instances of the hypostatic union of divinity and humanity in Christ, and of soul and body in man, have a parallel character and both justify the ontological priority of hypostasis over nature. This has important implications for the issues surrounding the coming of death.

---

48. Expos. 71, 18-29.
49. Ibid., 47, 60-61. See also Karmiris, *Τὰ δογματικὰ καὶ συμβολικὰ μνημεῖα τῆς Ὀρθοδόξου Καθολικῆς Ἐκκλησίας I*, p. 175.

There are two kinds of union of soul and body that can be identified. The first union refers to the union of soul and body between each other, and the second union refers to the union of each one with their common hypostasis, namely the hypostatic union. The former union secures the biological life of a human being whereas the latter union designates the consideration of human life on a level different to that of biological life. In other words, the hypostatic union proclaims that human life is something more than the biological existence of a human being.[50] The coming of death threatens the first kind of union only, a union that marks the organic life of a human being. The second kind of union, that is the hypostatic union, entirely escapes death. Such a reality is further justified by looking at the different placement of soul and body in the divisions of being.[51]

2. The Asymmetry and the Disproportional within Man

It is *Dialectica* that once more offers the necessary ground for understanding the differences between soul and body regarding the divisions of being.

It must be remembered that genus is something predicated on several things that are specifically different in respect to what pertains to their essence, whereas species is something that is predicated on several things that are numerically different.[52] As a rule, a genus may result in a species and vice versa. However, the genus that does not have any species above

50. This is in the same line of thought as Lossky, who considers the independence of hypostasis from its own nature as 'the irreducibility of man to his nature', that is, the irreducibility 'of someone who is distinct from his own nature, of someone who goes beyond his nature while still containing it, who makes it exist as human nature by this overstepping and yet does not exist in himself beyond the nature which he "*enypostasize*" and which he constantly exceeds' (Lossky, *In the Image and Likeness of God*, pp. 115-20).

51. The distinction within human existence regarding the relationship between soul and body and the relationship between the two and hypostasis frees man from the threat of the coming of death. The distinction also stresses the importance of an aspect of the human being that implies at least the possibility of a vision of man that is not dominated by his biological aspect. On the contrary, the identification of a 'biological hypostasis' along with another hypostasis such as an 'ecclesial', 'sacramental' or 'eucharistic' hypostasis made on an ontological basis (Zizioulas, *Being as Communion*, pp. 50-65) results, in a way, in a kind of metaphysics, though in an Orthodox Christian context. The focus on different 'kinds' of hypostases, though it stresses the importance of a relational character of humanity by looking at interpersonal relationships, underestimates the internal relational character of man's own existence that is also crucial for moral decisions.

52. Dial. fus. 5, 99-103.

it is the first genus (i.e. the substance), that is called most general genus (γενικώτατον γένος), whereas the species that does not have a genus below (i.e. the human being) is called a most specific species (εἰδικώτατον εἶδος):

> Substance is a most general genus. The body is a species of substance, and genus of the living. The living is a species of body, and genus of the sentient. The sentient animal is a species of the living, and genus of the rational. The rational is a species of the animal, and genus of the mortal. The mortal is a species of the rational, and genus of man. Man is a most specific species, for he is a species of the mortal and at the same time the species of Peter and of Paul, and this is just what the holy Fathers means by nature and form and substance.[53]

Obviously, the distinction between hypostasis and nature is introduced through the presentation of what exists between the first and most general genus and the most specific species. Hypostasis specifies a certain person or a thing, whereas nature signifies what this person or this thing is.[54] Therefore, man is the species of hypostases such as the hypostasis of Peter and Paul and is considered, according to the Church Fathers, as nature, form and substance.

Let us now look at how the constituent parts of man, the body and the soul, are placed within these categories and what the implications of such positions are.

While the above passage specifies that the body is a species of substance and genus of the living, it does not say anything about the soul. Though the substance as the most general genus is divided into the body and the incorporeal (ἀσώματον), John Damascene presents only the species that follow the body. This does not imply that John was unable to do the same thing for the incorporeal. The reason for doing so is that the species of the incorporeal to which the soul, the angels and the demons belong is regarded as the most specific species. Thus, soul is considered as a most specific species (εἰδικώτατον εἶδος).[55] This means that it does not contain species, but only hypostases.[56] On the contrary, the body does not belong to the most specific species since it can be either a genus or species.

53. Ibid., 47, 4-21.

54. Ibid., 18, 65-66.

55. Instit. 7, 19-21.

56. '. . . the species which are the last and the lowest and which do not have any lower species, that is, do not contain any species but only individuals, namely hypostases, are not called genera but only species. . . . For it is impossible to call that a genus since it does not contain any species. Therefore, the species which has no species but only hypostases is called a most specific species' (Dial. fus. 10, 68-80).

The first point that can be made with respect to the implication of the differences between the soul and body is that soul and body enjoy a different status in the division of being and therefore one may argue that the union of soul and body is characterised by asymmetry. Florovsky first used the term 'asymmetry' in order to describe the character of the unity of divinity and humanity in Christ. He argues that according to the Chalcedonian formula, there was no human hypostasis in the humanity of Christ and therefore human nature was in a way *anypostatos*. It is for this reason that there is an asymmetry in the unity of God and man in Christ.[57] Likewise, since soul as a most specific species contains only hypostases, and since body can simply be either genus or species, there is a profound asymmetry within their union regarding the presence or not of an immediate relationship to the hypostases.

Taking into account the fact that the union of divinity and humanity in Christ and the union of soul and body in man is not an exact analogy, the notion of 'asymmetry' is not an entirely successful description of such union. For example, in man, both soul and body are *enypostata* and, therefore, the consideration of the asymmetry within human existence is not fully justified. This is further attempted with the introduction of the notion of disproportion, which is used to designate the differentiation that exists within human existence.[58]

The assertion that there is disproportion in the relationship of soul and body to the hypostasis of man sheds more light on the discussion in progress. Both soul and body are *enypostata* and, therefore, are considered in a particular hypostasis. However, the sharing of a mode of existence (i.e. the fact that they are *enypostata*) cannot invalidate the fact that the soul as a most specific species enjoys the same status as man regarding the immediacy to hypostases in the division of being – a most specific

57. Florovsky, *The Byzantine Fathers of the Fifth Century*, p. 297. Florovsky further used the notion of 'asymmetry' that led him to the key term of 'asymmetry Christology'. For more on this see in Williams, 'The Neo-Patristic Synthesis of Georges Florovsky', pp. 287-340.

58. The notion of 'disproportion' is borrowed from Ricoeur's *Fallible Man*, where it is used to explain why it is possible for man to go wrong. Ricoeur argues that there is a basic disproportion between the finite and the infinite dimensions of a human being. This disproportion is justified by the gap that exists between *bios*, or one's spatiotemporally located life, and *logos*, or one's reason, that is able to grasp universal realities. This disproportion is revealed in every aspect of human existence. Due to this disproportion, man is never wholly at one with himself and hence he can go wrong. In this book, the notion of 'disproportion' is used for the designation of the differentiation that exists within human existence regarding the anticipation of moral issues in the medical context.

species does not contain species, but only hypostases.[59] Soul and body become hypostatically united, though such a union is disproportional. The disproportional character of such a union is very important for the understanding of the coming of death in man.

We said that, while death affects the union between soul and body and becomes apparent in the corruption of the body, it does not affect the union of the soul and body with the hypostasis. One may argue that the hypostatic union in a way preserves both soul and body from death. However, there is disproportion within this hypostatic union. Thus, though such a union may give the impression that both soul and body have always to be considered in terms of the same rationale, the disproportional nature of the character of this union must not be ignored. This means that the discussion of the issues surrounding human life and death has to take into account the differentiation that exists within human existence. In other words, arguments regarding the deliberate administration of death that results in the biological end of human existence have to consider not only the oneness of the human being due to the hypostatic union of soul and body but also the differences within the human being. Such a position directly challenges the 'undifferentiation' of sovereign bioethics regarding the inner existence of man.

III. The 'Intimacy' between Hypostasis and Nature

The belief that there is an ontological priority of the hypostasis over nature, and that man is something beyond the fate of the body, may be misleading and result not only in a belief in a bodiless human being, or a human being 'without nature', but also in an excessive emphasis on hypostasis and its subsequent sovereignty over nature. The former consequence would tend to underestimate human nature when considering the destiny of human existence, whereas the latter becomes a good argument in favour of the autonomy of the moral agent that ignores the character of human nature itself. In John's thought, even though an ontological priority of hypostasis over nature is acknowledged, there is

59. We have noticed that the soul is considered as a most specific species. It is remarkable that John, similarly, places man on the same level with the soul in terms of their immediacy to hypostasis: '. . . the *most specific species*, which is that which is immediately above the individual and contains the hypostases, as we speak of the human species [Dial. fus. 10, 13-16]. . . . Whence it is clear that Peter and Paul and John are not species but individuals, that is to say, hypostases. Nor is man the genus of Peter and all of the other individual men, but their species. Thus, man, too, is a most specific species' (ibid., 10, 169-72).

an undisputable 'intimacy' between hypostasis and nature. This idea is elaborated around the term 'will', a term that was at the centre of the monothelite controversy. The monothelites believed that Christ had a single will, whereas the dyothelites maintained that he had two. But why and in what way is the will also of central importance in understanding human existence?

God created man according to His own image and gave him a rational (λογικός) and intellectual (νοερός) soul that coincides with the intellect and the self-determining[60] aspect of man (τὸ νοερὸν δηλοῖ καὶ αὐτεξούσιον).[61] Though the terms rational, intellectual and self-determining seem to imply separate realities, the truth is that there is interdependence among them. In particular, Damascene distinguishes three kinds of life beyond divine life. These three kinds are the vegetative (φυτική), the sensitive (αἰσθητική) and the intellectual (νοερά). The intellect, and the rational and self-determining aspects of the soul, are connected with the third kind of life, where the self-determining element is considered as proper to the reason and the intellect.[62]

The two pairs of terms reason/intellect and intellect/self-determining are considered synonymous. This is not accidental, since reason and free will are directly connected with each other.[63] This connection is based on the assumption that transformation and changes are inherited in created beings and that rational beings are changed by their deliberate choice (κατὰ προαίρεσιν).[64] Since the self-determining aspect is the will[65] and since rational beings have the power to choose, freedom of will is necessarily connected by nature with the rational.[66] In other words, the self-determining element as free will is directly linked to the rational and the intellectual elements, and emerges as the critical parameter in human life.

1. Natural, Hypostatic and Gnomic Wills

In *Dialectica*, John places the will in the category of homonyms (ὁμώνυμα), which means that the will is used by different things that do

60. Here 'self-determining' signifies the freedom, the free will of the human beings, the free (autexousion), intellectual (noeron, nous) nature of ther soul, the rational, intellectual and free human being.
61. Expos. 26, 18-20.
62. Ibid., 58, 56-6.
63. Ibid., 21, 131-132; Instit. 10, 14-16.
64. Expos. 41, 2-7.
65. Ibid., 58, 61-62.
66. Ibid., 41, 11-14.

not have the same definition.[67] Consequently, it is not surprising that in *An Exact Exposition of the Orthodox Faith* John provides, on different occasions, two entirely different categorisations of the homonyms of will.[68] According to the first categorisation that is placed within the section that is devoted to Christology, the will can be either natural, hypostatic or 'contrary to nature' – the first is indicative of and is part of human nature, the second is a characteristic of a particular hypostasis, whereas the third represents the relations with those things that are destructive of the 'according-to-nature' condition of human existence.[69]

In the second categorisation things are more complex. John connects the will with the explanation of the character of man. Damascene makes a distinction only between the natural will and the gnomic will and implies that the categories of 'hypostatic' and 'contrary to nature' coincide with the category of gnomic will.[70] Is it, then, right to say that, while man has a natural will, that is 'the power to will', he does not have a particularised will, a will indicative of the 'mode of being' (*ὁ τρόπος τῆς ὑπάρξεως*) that qualifies the distinction among hypostases,[71] in order not to be self-destructive? Are humans not self-determined beings but rather driven by their nature? In other words, does man have two choices, either the denial of any particularised will, a denial that leads to a life 'according to nature', or the adoption of a particularised will that is self-destructive by definition once it is considered as 'contrary to nature'?

John, in his treatise *On the Two Wills in Christ*, gives answers to these questions, which have direct anthropological implications.[72] From such

67. 'Homonyms are those that share the same name, while each of them has a different meaning and is of different substance, that is to say, takes a different definition' (Dial. fus. 9, 5-7).
68. A lengthier version of this section is published in Bekos, 'The Image of God in Man according to John Damascene: Implications on Issues Surrounding Euthanasia', pp. 285-90.
69. Expos. 58, 77-88.
70. Ibid., 36, 132-34.
71. Volunt. 7, 18-20.
72. The fact that to focus only on *An Exact Exposition of the Orthodox Faith* negatively affects one's understanding of John's thought (though it is very common among those who study the theological work of John Damascene) is particularly evident in Frede's 'John of Damascus on Human Action, the Will, and Human Freedom'. Concentrating only on chapters 36, 41 and 58 of *An Exact Exposition of the Orthodox Faith*, Frede argues that, according to John, it is a mistake 'to identify the feature of being self-determining (αὐτεξούσιον) with the freedom of will, or the freedom of choice' (Frede, 'John of Damascus on Human Action, the Will, and Human Freedom', p. 79). He rightly says that the will is not identified with the ability to make choices (ibid., p. 73),

a treatise one may expect polemical writing with mostly Christological inferences in the defence of the presence of the two wills in Christ and in line with the treatises that were written during the Christological controversies of the sixth and seventh centuries. On the contrary, John, while he aims at the defence of the complete divinity and humanity in Christ, attempts to present a closer connection between Christology and anthropology.[73]

To start with, in the treatise *On the Two Wills in Christ* John Damascene proceeds to another distinction between the homonyms of will. According to this distinction, the will can be natural, such as the power to will and act (θέλησις-ἐνέργεια), or willing (θέλειν), acting (ἐνεργεῖν) or hypostatic, such as the different 'objects of willing and acting' (ἡ διάφορος θέλησις καὶ ἐνέργεια) and the different ways of willing and acting (τὸ διαφόρως θέλειν καὶ ἐνεργεῖν). Further, the hypostatic wills can be characterised as either good when they are 'according to nature' and obedient to the Creator, or evil when they are 'contrary to nature', driven by pleasures and intimate *gnome* (οἰκείαν γνώμην) and, therefore, against the law of God.[74] Obviously, while John views the homonyms of will in relation to the scheme natural/hypostatic, he acknowledges that among the hypostatic wills there are also those that are thrown up by intimate *gnome*. The intimate *gnome* spontaneously recalls the category of gnomic wills. Thus, one may have a particularised will, that is a will indicative of a particular hypostasis, without expressing a will 'contrary to nature' and against the law of God.

Surprisingly enough, later in the same treatise Damascene argues that those wills that follow the intimate *gnome* and are against the law of God are hypostatic and gnomic wills. He, therefore, identifies the hypostatic with the gnomic wills.[75] Does this diversity in John's statements betray a profound inconsistency in his thought?[76] Or does John follow a way of

but he fails to take into account the homonyms of the will in order to get into an in-depth analysis of what John wants to say. However, he agrees with his presupposition regarding the character of John Damascene's development of a doctrine of will, according to which 'John of Damascus tries to integrate a notion of a will into Aristotle's moral psychology and theory of action' (ibid., p. 65). Indeed, this presupposition is also in accord with the western Christian view that he was a forerunner of scholasticism.

73. The elaboration of anthropological arguments on the basis of Christological arguments is also commented on by Kallis, though briefly and without any particular reference to John's writings (Kallis, 'Johannes von Damaskus', p. 299).

74. Volunt. 6, 67-77.

75. Ibid., 25, 9-12.

76. Dyobouniotes, who is aware of this 'inconsistency', accuses John of an insufficient theological grounding that leads to the destruction of human nature (Dyobouniotes, *Ἰωάννης Δαμασκηνός*, pp. 106-10). Obviously,

thinking that presupposes a unique connection between hypostasis and nature or an understanding of this connection that may identify a unique transition from what is natural to what is hypostatic and vice versa? Or, to put it differently, is it possible that a 'gnomic' way of life may also enjoy a natural character without obliterating the integrity of hypostasis?

2. Natural 'Objects of Willing' in Man

John answers these questions by introducing the presence of natural 'objects of willing' in man. Since all human beings do not want the same things, the 'object of willing' (θελητόν) is gnomic (i.e. pertains to the *gnome* or opinion) and hypostatic.[77] While the 'object of willing' is, generally speaking, hypostatic and gnomic, Damascene believes that there are also natural 'objects of willing' (θελήματα) in man. In particular, there are two kinds of natural 'objects of willing' in man. The first is the submission to the law of God and the second is the constituents of human nature such as hunger, thirst, sleep and the like.[78] John focusses on the former, the submission to the law of God, since it comes out as a deliberate expression of the human will.

Regarding the character of 'objects of willing', John says that, although the 'objects of willing' can be either natural or hypostatic and gnomic, the gnomic and hypostatic 'objects of willing' are ascribed to man, whereas the presence of natural 'objects of willing' refers only to the Holy Trinity.[79] However, John emphasises the presence of natural 'objects of willing' in man as crucial towards the 'reconciliation' between those in the Holy Trinity and those in man. Undoubtedly, such a kind of 'reconciliation' has to pass through the gap between what is natural and comes from God, and what is hypostatic and gnomic and stands against God. It is in this context that the 'inconsistency' in the designation of the homonyms of wills must be interpreted.

This 'inconsistency' is resolved with reference to anthropology, and particularly in the way Damascene sees the 'common' and the 'different' among hypostases – the many human hypostases share the common human nature. Since man is made in the image of God and all human

---

Dyobouniotes fails to identify in John's writings the necessary foundation for a meaningful interpretation.

77. Volunt. 22, 6-8 and 23, 16-17. The 'object of willing' implies not only what someone wants by using his 'power to will' but also how one wants (ibid., 23, 20-27).
78. Ibid., 25, 6-9.
79. Ibid., 24, 10-36.

beings share the same nature, then the individuality of a human being that is revealed by hypostasis does not necessarily divide man from God and humans from one another. On the one hand, God created man in such a way that the 'common' among hypostases corresponds to the participation in that nature that is given for the joy that derives from the natural relationship. On the other, the 'different' among hypostases keeps the distinction between those that belong to the same species in order to facilitate their self-knowledge and to avoid the consideration of the 'foreign' as intimate (ὡς οἰκείῳ τῷ ἀλλοτρίῳ).[80] Consequently, the 'different' of the hypostases implies neither an attitude 'contrary to nature' and against the law of God nor the presence of only hypostatic and gnomic 'objects of willing' in man. That is to say, the preservation of the individuality of the hypostases does not exclude the possibility of having 'common' 'objects of willing' in man that deserve to be characterised as 'natural', such as submission to the law of God. This possibility is a prerequisite for the presence of the natural relationship between different hypostases. In other words, John states that the crucial thing that safeguards the 'common' of the 'objects of willing' among the different hypostases, and consequently their natural character, is the sharing of their common nature. If so, there is no obligatory connection between the reality of different hypostases with hypostatic 'objects of willing' in both the Holy Trinity and in man – in the Holy Trinity by nature, whereas in man by position (*κατά θέσιν*).[81]

The presence of natural 'objects of willing' in man is important for a number of reasons. It highlights the significance of the sharing of the same nature by all humans – the inherent natural character of not only the 'power to will' but also of 'objects of willing'. At the same time, the particularised will as indicative of a particular hypostasis is not

80. Ibid., 3, 7-24.

81. John describes this distinction by considering the difference between actuality and reason/thought regarding the perception of particular properties in man and in the Holy Trinity. He says: 'Thus, in all creatures there is an actual distinction to be seen between hypostases. Peter is seen to be actually distinct from Paul. But, that which is held in common, the connection, and the unity is seen by reason and thought. Thus, in our mind we see that Peter and Paul are of the same nature and have one common nature, for each is a rational mortal animal and each is a body animated by a rational and understanding soul. . . . The aforesaid is true of all creation, but it is quite the contrary in the case of the holy, supersubstantial, all-transcendent, and incomprehensible Trinity. For, here, that which is common and one is considered in actuality by reason of the co-eternity and identity of substance, operation and will. . . . It is by thought that the distinction is perceived' (Expos. 8, 224-50).

absent, since the presence of a natural 'object of willing' presupposes the deliberate expression of human free will. Such coexistence preserves the 'mode of being' and, consequently, the integrity of hypostasis. Thus, it may be agued that the natural 'objects of willing' have a hypostatic dimension by definition. Indeed, the natural 'objects of willing' can be considered as hypostatic natural 'objects of willing'. Although the priority of hypostasis over nature is justified once more, the 'intimacy' of hypostasis and nature is demonstrated.

In such a context, submission to the law of God as a hypostatic natural 'object of willing' bears out the intimacy between God and man in the most radical way, as it signifies that the same nature that is shared by all humans, like God the Holy Trinity, has also natural 'objects of willing'. Though man as a free hypostasis can deliberately choose whatever he wants, he was created by God to be submitted to the law of God as a servant to God and obedient to Him by nature (φύσει γὰρ δοῦλος θεοῦ καὶ ὑποχείριος ὁ ἄνθρωπος).[82] This means that the hypostatic natural 'objects of willing' coincide with what belongs to the constitution of man, whereas the hypostatic or gnomic 'objects of willing' turn against man's constitution and become suicidal. In other words, the survival of man can only be achieved through the free choice of man's submission to the law of God, namely the choice of hypostatic natural 'objects of willing'.

John exemplifies the presence of natural 'objects of willing' in man with reference to Christ. The phrase in the case of the prayer at Gethsemane, 'Father, if it is possible, let this cup pass from Me; but not as I will, but as You will',[83] and the phrase, 'For I have come down from heaven, not to do My own will, but the will of Him who sent Me',[84] leads John to state that in Christ, through His obedience to the divine will, the divine 'objects of willing' become 'objects of willing' of humanity.[85] Once the divine 'objects of willing' are natural, the presence of natural 'objects of willing' in man become possible. Furthermore, one may argue that the presence of natural 'objects of willing' in the humanity of Christ, though being safeguarded through the hypostatic union of divinity and humanity in the hypostasis of the Son of God, may also be connected with human nature. This connection is based on Damascene's consideration that every man, like the Holy Trinity, may also enjoy natural 'objects of willing'.

82. Volunt. 25, 6-8.
83. Matthew 26:39; Luke 22:42.
84. John 6:38.
85. Volunt. 41, 7-22.

In short, John, through an interplay between Christology and anthropology,[86] and without invalidating the ontological priority of hypostasis over nature, establishes the 'intimacy' between hypostasis and nature. Given that the hypostasis is connected with the particularised will that directs one's own moral choices, the fact that there is a kind of 'intimacy' between hypostasis and nature necessitates man's knowledge of his own nature for the sake of the moral character of one's own will. In such a context the absence of the knowledge of one's own nature has a negative impact on the exercising of one's own free will, given the hypostatic natural character of the 'objects of willing' in man. In a broader sense, the focus on man's knowledge of his own nature challenges the excessive interest in simply the individuality and autonomy of man characteristic of the modern age. This questioning of the accepted view is important, since it stresses the impact that anthropology should have on ethical issues, especially in modern society where the trend leads to moral accounts lacking in a content-rich anthropology, a tendency that was thoroughly discussed in the first part of this book. Moreover, the 'intimacy' between hypostasis and nature brings God and man closer together, and has important implications for the question regarding the relationship between the immanent and the transcendent. Man was created by God, and he was created by Him according to His own image, with a view to freely fulfilling his nature, as that nature was designated by his divine origin. Therefore, man's knowledge of his own nature is seen as an even more essential precondition for living a genuine human life.

The designation of man's own nature and the importance of self-knowledge place the whole discussion regarding the emphasis and the priority of hypostasis on a different level. This re-orientation is essential for the proper understanding of man's autonomy in the modern age and, in particular, in the medical context. The exercising of autonomy by a human being is no longer unconditional, but rather depends on the proper knowledge of human existence. Man has two choices, either to respect and fulfil this knowledge, or to turn to suicide.

IV. The Knowledge of Man's Own Nature

The interpersonal character of human life was established at the beginning of this chapter through the elaboration of the idea that man is a derivative and relative creature, an idea that is based on the unique

86. In the same vein, Nellas argues that the creation of man from God according to His own image proclaims the Christological basis of the anthropology of the Church Fathers (Nellas, 'Ἡ θεολογία τοῦ "κατ᾽ εἰκόνα"', pp. 295-308).

relationship between God and man established at the time of the creation of man. In the two sections that followed, the different relationships that are developed within human existence were discussed and the importance of the knowledge of man's own nature was highlighted. What follows is a more detailed discussion of the pivotal role of the knowledge of one's own nature for taking moral decisions. This is accomplished through establishing the fact that self-knowledge is of central importance for human existence (as opposed to the orientation towards self-preservation that is identified in all theories of human existence) and through discussing what the creation of man according to the image of God signifies with respect to the knowledge of man's own nature and the conditional exercising of man's autonomy.

1. The Centrality of the Knowledge of Being and Not of the Principle of Self-preservation

The centrality of this knowledge is evident in the first chapter of *Dialectica*, which is a hymn to the knowledge of being. In this chapter, John talks about true knowledge or the knowledge of the beings (ὄντων) as opposed to false knowledge or the knowledge of the non-beings (μὴ ὄντος). True knowledge is the light of the rational soul that is capable of receiving it through the intellect (νοῦς). Since the soul is clothed in the veil of the flesh and does not have knowledge of itself, the soul needs a teacher (δεῖται τοῦ διδάξοντος). Christ, in whom there is no falsehood and who is the Truth, fulfils this need.[87]

In this chapter of *Dialectica* two things emerge. First, there is nothing more estimable than the true knowledge of the beings[88] once the absence of such knowledge coincides with the non-beings, namely falsehood. Therefore, true knowledge is *sine qua non* a condition for a human being to authentically exist, an existence that is taught by the Truth, namely Christ Himself. Obviously, such an existence is not limited to biological life and cannot be considered separate from it. This assertion represents a fundamental challenge to the imperative of self-preservation, an imperative that, as was explained in chapter one, characterises all theories of human existence. Second, though the rational soul is capable

87. Dial. fus. 1, 2-21.

88. The same idea is presented in *An Exact Exposition of the Orthodox Faith*: 'Of all these thoughts and considerations, the loftiest is that which concerns ourselves – which concern our constitution, I mean, as the divine David says: "Thy knowledge from myself is become wonderful," that is to say, "from my own make-up"' (Expos. 25, 67-70).

of perceiving true knowledge, this capability depends on its relationship to the flesh (the body) and its inability to generate such knowledge. These dependences can be overcome only through God. Let us discuss how true knowledge is acquired.

God created man after His own image and likeness and placed him into the divine paradise with a view to his progressive ethical perfection.[89] For this reason, God planted in paradise the tree of knowledge of good and evil that became a trial, a test and an exercise of man's obedience and disobedience. This trial revealed a deep interdependence between the knowledge of man's own nature and obedience or disobedience to God. The knowledge of man's own nature is good for the perfect (τελείοις) and bad for those who are less perfect (ἀτελεστέροις):

> He planted the tree of knowledge as a sort of trial, test, and exercise of man's obedience and disobedience. It is either for this reason that it has been called the tree of knowledge of good and evil, or because it gave to them that partook of it the power to know their own nature – which, while it is good for the perfect, is bad for them that are less perfect and more given to their desires, as strong meat is to them that are tender and still in need of milk[90] . . . The tree of knowledge of good and evil is the power of discernment by multiple vision, and this is the complete knowing of one's own nature . . . and it is good for them that are full-grown and have walked in the contemplation of God. . . . It is not good, however, for such as are still young and are more greedy in their appetites.[91]

Therefore, the knowledge of the nature of man, that has to be the 'most estimable' of all things, becomes self-destructive once it is attempted without the proper ethical perfection and the relevant obedience to God, and given man's inclination to the care of the body:

> [the less perfect] because of the uncertainty of the perseverance in the true good and because of their not yet being solidly established in their application to the only good, are naturally inclined to be drawn away and distracted by their solicitude for their own bodies.[92]

89. Karmiris, *Τὰ δογματικὰ καὶ συμβολικὰ μνημεῖα τῆς Ὀρθοδόξου Καθολικῆς Ἐκκλησίας I*, pp. 31-32.
90. Expos. 25, 15-20.
91. Ibid., 25, 54-59.
92. Ibid., 25, 59-62.

God proclaimed the process towards man's knowledge of his nature in paradise and it is explicitly mentioned in the Scriptures:

> although before they had eaten 'they were both naked, to wit, Adam and Eve, and they were not ashamed' God wanted us to be dispassionate like that, for that is passionlessness to the highest degree. And He also wanted us to be free from care and to have but one task, that of the angels, which is unceasingly and unremittingly to sing the praises of the Creator and to rejoice in contemplating Him. He also wanted us to cast our cares upon Him, which is just what He told us through the Prophet David, saying: 'Cast thy care upon the Lord, and He shall sustain thee.' In the Gospels, too, when teaching His own disciples, He says: 'Be not solicitous for your life, what you shall eat, nor for your body, what you shall put on'; and again: 'Seek ye the Kingdom of God and His justice, and all these things will be added unto you'; and to Martha: 'Martha, Martha, thou art careful and troubled about many things: but one thing is necessary. Mary hath chosen the best part, which shall not be taken away from her', namely to sit at His feet and hear His words.[93]

If the knowledge of man's own nature is a prerequisite of his life as a being created according to the image of God, then this passage makes clearer what humans have to do in order to truly live and not to die. Contrary to the dominant principle of self-preservation, God asks man to do exactly the opposite and to be preoccupied with communication with Him. This is, for John, the only way to attain the true knowledge of being and a genuine life. It is through this communication with God that man, step by step, becomes capable of learning and of understanding properly those things that are fundamental for his own life.

2. Man as a Free Being with no Absolute Control over His Own Nature

The challenge to the imperative of self-preservation is reinforced through the knowledge of human existence. Regarding the centrality of communication and the relation with God for the knowledge of one's own nature, the biblical statement that God created man according to His own image becomes indispensable once it provides the ground for further exploration of such interplay.

93. Ibid., 25, 24-38.

Among the different meanings of the statement 'according to the image' that were presented at the introduction of this chapter is the reference to the inner state of humanity and, particularly, the relationship between soul and body. The discussion of the proper relationship of soul and body is inescapably connected with the life in paradise. This life was the life that humans experienced just after their creation and the safeguarding of this life was subject to the proper relationship between the soul and body.

Since God has given free will to man, man has to use it for the subordination of the body to the soul and against the temptation of the pleasures of the flesh. This freedom can lead either to the knowledge of the Creator, the accomplishment of His commandments, the overcoming of death and finally everlasting enjoyment in paradise or to the devaluation of the value of soul and the entry of corruption and death into human life.[94] Therefore, the proper relationship between the soul and the body becomes the criterion for achieving the knowledge of God, the knowledge of man and the overcoming of death. All these depend on the proper use of free will.

At this point, a brief physiology of the soul is necessary for the understanding of the relationship between the soul and the body.

The properties (ἴδια) of the soul – property (ἴδιον) is what is always in a species and is conversely predicable with it – can be divided into two categories. The first category includes life (ζωή), understanding (νόησις) and rational appetite (λογικὴ ὄρεξις) that is mainly will (θέλησις). The second category is represented by the coexistence of soul and body, during which the soul gives life and movement to the body and the body becomes a slave to the soul. Since the sovereignty of the soul over the body is a privilege that the angels do not enjoy, this sovereignty is said to be the most characteristic property of the soul (ἰδικώτατον ψυχῆς), a property that makes man able to enjoy what is 'according to the image' more than the angels.[95] Despite the distinction between these properties, the two categories are strongly connected to each other. Their contact link is the ruling of the soul over the body that is achieved through the proper expression of the will.

Damascene provides more details about the character of the relationship between soul and body, and says that the will rules the body and the non-rational appetite (ἄλογον ὄρεξιν), desire (ἐπιθυμίαν), anger (θυμός) and the spontaneous movement (τὴν καθ' ὁρμὴν κίνησιν)

94. Ibid., 44, 39-50.
95. Volunt. 16, 3-11.

according to its own appetite that is the will.[96] For John, the non-rational appetite is desire and anger,[97] and it is upon these that the sovereignty of the rational appetite has to be exercised. Anger has been given by God to be used against the devil and sin, whereas desire has been given by God to be directed to God and His own wills (πρὸς θεὸν καὶ τὰ αὐτοῦ θελήματα).[98] Therefore, it is the proper use of the free will that determines the proper ruling of soul over body. The use of the word 'proper' implies that the choices of the will may vary once the will, through which man understands, thinks and judges, is free.[99]

John makes this clearer by attributing to the property (ἴδιον) a double character according to which the property is always in potential (δυνάμει) and not always in act (ἐνεργεία).[100] Given this double character, the soul has the power to rule over the body. However, such sovereignty depends on the free will. Thus, the human being may either rule over the body or not by free choice.

However, even the proper use of the free will does not secure its absolute sovereignty over the body, since the free exercise of will is restrained by nature. Though the rational appetite (θέλησις) of the soul rules over the non-rational appetite by nature, there are non-rational faculties that are not obedient to the rational, and therefore the ruling of the body by the soul is limited by definition:

> One should note that the rational part of the soul governs the irrational part by nature [φύσει κατάρχει τοῦ ἀλόγου]. Indeed, the faculties of the soul are divided into those belonging to its rational part and those belonging to its non-rational part. There are two groups belonging to the non-rational part, of which one is deaf to reason, that is to say, does not obey the reason [οὐ πείθεται λόγῳ], whereas the other listens to the reason and complies with it [κατήκοόν ἐστι καὶ ἐπιπειθὲς λόγῳ]. Now, deaf

96. Ibid., 16, 5-8.
97. Ibid., 15, 8-9. It is, among others, through the non-rational appetitie that man communicates with the non-rational animals (ἀλόγοις ζῴοις) and justifies his characterisation as a microcosm or little cosmos (μικρὸς κόσμος ἐστίν), a being that with his soul and body stands between the intellect and the material and it is the liaison between the sensible and the intellectual world (ibid., 15, 1-17).
98. Ibid., 18, 31-34. This is perfectly exemplified by John Damascene in his *Sermon on the Nativity of Theotokos*. He says that the life of Theotokos pleased God since her mind was governed by God and was directed only to God, her desire was intensely aimed at God and her anger was moved against sin and its source (Nativ. M. 9, 20-24).
99. Volunt. 15, 12-17.
100. Dial. fus. 27, 7-8.

> and disobedient to reason are the vital principle [ζωτικόν], which is also called pulsating [σφυγμικὸν], the seminal [σπερματικὸν] or generative principle [γεννητικόν], and the vegetable principle [φυτικόν], which is also called nutritive [θρεπτικόν] and to which also belongs the principles of growth [αὐξητικόν] that builds up the body. For these are governed not by reason but by nature.[101]

What emerges in this passage is that those characteristics that are traditionally considered as properties of the body are also, according to John, properties of the soul. Obviously, Damascene, by saying that even those that are found in the body have their origin in the soul, ascribes a kind of relativeness to the 'sovereign role' of the soul over the body. While the soul has to rule sovereign over the body by nature, this sovereignty is not all-embracing by nature. If the sovereignty of the soul over the body is not all-embracing, a condition that implies limitations on the exercising of the free will, any absolute consideration of its power and its consequences is, by definition, rejected. In such a context, man's consideration as a being who fulfils the necessary conditions for self-preservation, namely the power claims over human life and the consequent sovereignty over it, is not justified. Therefore, it is naive, at least, to consider man as a principally autonomous and free being once he is involuntary subject to some constraints from within his own nature.

Evidently, self-knowledge has to precede any consideration of human existence. The knowledge that man does not have absolute control over his body has important implications for the issues surrounding euthanasia. This realisation challenges the fundamental assumption made in the current discussion on these issues that states that man is an autonomous being and his 'autonomous' choices have to be respected as morally acceptable.

V. The Fall and the Entry of Corruption and Death

The fact that man is free and rational, but not possessed of an all-embracing sovereignty, and always subject to the constraints of human nature makes one wonder whether the soul rules sovereign over the body and the rational rules over the irrational and, if so, what the fundamental character of the soul is. The answer to this question can be found in the fall of Adam and Eve.

The fall, as such, was a turning point in human life. In paradise, according to Genesis, the snake enticed Adam and Eve to eat from the

101. Expos. 26, 94-101.

forbidden fruit against God's command. The snake used only a single argument to convince first Eve and then Adam – 'the day you will eat this fruit, your eyes will open and you will become like gods knowing what is good and evil'.[102] For John, the snake used the hope of divinity (θεότητος ἐλπίδι) as successful bait.[103] However, this hope was actually an appetite for a fallacious form of divinity (ψευδοῦς ὀρεχθέντες θεώσεως) and as a result man became like the non-rational animals.[104] This appetite was in fact a non-rational appetite that prevailed over the rational one. It is worth noting here that John identifies this outcome with evil and sin, and uses polemical terms to show the defeat of the rational by the non-rational: 'evil [κακία] and sin [ἁμαρτία] are but the betrayal of the self-determining [αὐτεξούσιον] element and its defeat by the non-rational passions and the non-rational and brutal life'.[105]

It is through sin that death has come into the world (δι' ἁμαρτίας ὁ θάνατος εἰς τὸν κόσμον εἰσῆλθεν)[106] and thus man became worthy of death and subject to corruption (θανάτῳ κατάκριτον καὶ φθορᾶ ὑποχείριον).[107] What are the implications of the entry of corruption and death into human life? The answer to this question presupposes the identification of the character of corruption and death.

1. The Temporal and Non Essential Character of Corruption and Death

John's teaching on corruption is mainly elaborated in his treatise, *Dialogue against the Manichees*. The heresy of the Manichees or Manichaeism teaches, among other things, that there are two eternally existent principles, one good and one wicked (πονηράν τε καὶ ἀγαθήν).[108] This

102. Genesis 3:5.
103. Expos. 45, 27-28.
104. Dorm. II, 2, 24-25.
105. Volunt. 19, 36-37.
106. Expos. 45, 19.
107. Ibid., 45, 10.
108. Manichees, also Aconites, 'are the disciples of Mani the Persian, who say that Christ only appeared in a form; they worship the sun and the moon, and pray to stars and powers and demons; they introduce two eternally existent principles, one good, the other wicked; they hold that Christ was only born and suffered in appearance, and blaspheme against the Old Testament and the God who speaks in it, maintaining that it is not the whole cosmos that has been created by God, but only a part of it' (Haeres. 66). John borrowed this passage from Epiphanios' *Panarion*, a collection of heresies that were present during the fourth century (PG 42, 29A-37C).

teaching introduces, on the one hand, a dualistic interpretation of the world – there are two principles, namely the good and the evil, and the whole world is based upon and originated in these – and, on the other, the evil is eternal and therefore it possesses the same power as the good. Damascene wants to challenge these beliefs by identifying the character of good and evil.[109] The character of corruption and death is developed on this basis.

What is the character of corruption and death? Are corruption and death essential or accidental characteristics?

John, following the patristic tradition,[110] bases his thought on the idea that evil is an accident and, since evil is corruption and death (Τὸ κακὸν φθορὰ καὶ θάνατος),[111] then corruption and death are accidents.

In particular, since corruption is the dissolution of what is composite (Φθορὰ μὲν γάρ ἐστιν ἡ τῶν συντεθέντων διάλυσις) and it is visible only in the dissolution of a composite being into parts that are not pre-existent or that do not remain after the dissolution, corruption is an accident.[112] John reinforces the accidental character of corruption even further by mentioning that corruption comes after the composition of a being (Ἡ δὲ φθορὰ ἐπιγίνεται μετὰ τὴν σύνθεσιν λύουσα τὰ συντεθειμένα),[113]

109. It has been argued that John's treatise, *Dialogue against the Manichees*, is an early work since, unlike his mature writings, it is not strictly based on the words of the Fathers, but rather is in his own words, and also since only a few manuscripts of the text survived (Louth, *St John Damascene*, p. 71). On the contrary, we believe that this work is not very far from John's mature works, because a proper reading and understanding of what John says in this work presupposes at least his *Dialectica*. In addition, the argument that in his later works John Damascene is much more concerned to keep strictly to the words of the Fathers is not necessarily a guide to the maturity and chronology of John's other writings, given that his texts are each oriented to a particular historical context and each have a particular aim. (John's expression 'I shall add nothing on my own' [Ερῶ δὲ ἐμὸν μέν, *ὡς ἔφην, οὐδὲν*, Dial., Prooemium, 60] does not mean that his teaching either keeps strictly to the words of the Fathers or is not creative theology.) Moreover, the existence of only a few manuscripts of the *Dialogue against the Manichees* is more easily interpreted with reference, at least, to the minimal interest of the West in distributing a text that challenged traditional western beliefs, such as the belief that death comes from God Himself as a punishment (Augustine, *City of God*, Book XIII, ch. 15) and not as a result of man's disobedience to the divine will (see, for example, Karmiris, *Τὰ δογματικὰ καὶ συμβολικὰ μνημεῖα τῆς Ὀρθοδόξου Καθολικῆς Ἐκκλησίας I*, pp. 39-40, and Romanides, *Τὸ προπατορικὸν ἁμάρτημα*, pp. 154-55.

110. St Dionysius the Areopagite, *On the Divine Names* (PG 3, 732C-D).

111. Manich. 57, 1.

112. Ibid., 62, 1-5.

113. Ibid., 63, 13-14.

which means that it does not contribute to the birth of a being. Therefore, corruption cannot be counted as a constituent characteristic of human nature.

Indeed, if corruption is an accident, then it does not come within the definition of a species since it can either be or not be. Moreover, when it is present, it does not assure the existence of the species, and when it is absent, the species is not destroyed.[114] It is for this reason that the accident is called non-essential difference and quality (ἐπουσιώδης διαφορὰ καὶ ποιότης)[115] contrary to the essential quality that remains unchanged (ἀκίνητος).[116] Thus, if corruption is an accident, it is not a necessary condition of human life.

Once corruption became visible in human nature, it also became destined to reach an end, because it could not exist by itself, namely without reference to a particular essence or hypostasis (τὸ γὰρ συμβεβηκὸς καθ' αὑτὸ οὐχ ὑφίσταται).[117] This is perfectly justified by the fact that corruption is absolutely expressed in death, which is the end of a corruptible hypostasis and at the same time the end of corruption. It seems that death comes into human life as a necessary condition to end the fundamental ontological change in human life, which is the entry of corruption into human life due to the fall.

Any idea that considers death, suffering and corruption as constituent of human nature leads to the unacceptable conclusion that God, who created man from nothing, has also created corruption and death to fight His creation.[118] Creation and birth are counteractive to corruption – birth is the creation of a being from a non-being, whereas corruption is the transition from being to dissolution.[119] John insists that, while

114. Dial. fus. 13, 2-3.

115. Ibid., 5, 121-26. The difference signifies 'that which is predicated of several things specifically different in respect to their particular sort, and it is included in the definition as essential (οὐσιώδης)' (ibid., 5, 103-106). The quality belongs to the category of the ten general genera (γενικωτάτων γενῶν) and signifies 'that by which things are termed as being of such a sort' (ibid., 52, 2). However, when the difference and the quality are considered as accidents, then they are called non-essential differences and qualities, such as the difference between a man and another man in terms of their height (ibid., 12, 20-24).

116. Manich. 30, 9-12.

117. Ibid., 31, 5.

118. The belief that the presence of death in human life is not a constituent element of human nature as created by God is a common tenet accepted by the Church Fathers, such as St Gregory of Nyssa (Vachicouras, *Ἡ ἔννοια τοῦ θανάτου κατὰ τὸν ἅγιο Γρήγοριο Νύσσης*, pp. 153-58).

119. Manich. 63, 50-52.

everything that God created is good and very good (πάντα καλὰ καὶ λίαν καλά),[120] corruption and death are not good but rather evil, and therefore could not derive from God.

Obviously, John does not attribute any metaphysical character to the presence of corruption and death in human life. He rather places them within the sphere of human activity. Such an approach leads to two conclusions.

First, he makes a clear distinction between the source of life, that is God, and the source of corruption and death, that is man. This distinction has direct ethical implications for issues surrounding the coming of death in human life such as the issue of euthanasia. For example, one of the arguments against euthanasia is that of the sanctity of life: life has been given by God and, therefore, no one – not by any means – should take it away. It is remarkable that, while this argument highlights the value of life, it, at the same time, subordinates human life to corruption, that is an after-effect of man's choices, once corruption is left free to violate the 'sacred' aspect of human life.[121]

Second, life and corruption/death are not the two sides of the same coin. On the contrary, the former is connected with God and with the prospect of eternal life, whereas the latter are destined to end, given that they are foreign to human nature and they encroach upon the sovereignty of the rational over the non-rational elements in man. In such a context, the real problem is not when and how corruption fulfils its destiny and ends along with the corruptible human being, but rather the defeat of corruption. Given that corruption is the result of man's particular choice, namely the subordination of the rational to the non-rational that is present from the very beginning of human existence, the defeat of corruption cannot simply be a matter of the medical context once corruption concerns human existence as a whole. To raise the issue of euthanasia in such a context, while this opens up a discussion on life and death, is a distorted and ill-timed endeavour. The coming of death in the medical context is anticipated simply as a bodily experience once such a context, by definition, deals only with the somatic aspect of human nature and only when the end of the corruptible human body is approaching. From a Christian point of view, such an approach to the presence of corruption and death in human life is incomprehensible.

---

120. Ibid., 14, 6.

121. A critique of the well-known argument against euthanasia in terms of the sanctity of life is clearly implied. As was mentioned in the introduction, only brief comments on the implications of the patristic theological arguments for issues surrounding euthanasia are made in this part of the book. They are presented in full in the third part.

2. Corruption and Death as Expressions of the Divine Providence that Comes 'after' the Expression of the Human Will

Man is the cause of the entry of corruption and death into human life after the fall of Adam and Eve. God's presence in the transition of man from paradise to his fallen condition provides a further insight into the character of corruption and death. This further insight is provided by the distinction that Damascene makes between those that depend on us (τὰ ἐφ' ἡμῖν) and those that do not depend on us (τὰ οὐκ ἐφ' ἡμῖν).

Those that depend on us are those things that we are free either to do or not to do and that, therefore, incur blame or praise and to which one may be urged or bound by law.[122] John connects those things that depend on us with man's free will,[123] and points out that those things that are subject to the will are but those that depend on us.[124] Thus, the existence of things that depend on us is indicative not only of the self-determining aspect in man but also of his responsibility for his own life.

Those that do not depend on us are separated into two categories. The first category is represented by those that depend upon the divine will, whereas the second category consists of those that have their origin or cause in those that depend on us, such as the recompense for our deeds that we receive either in the present world or in that to come.[125] In such a context, those that do not depend on us are connected with divine providence – the solicitude which God has for existing things[126] – as well as with the so-called natural and blameless passions, such as suffering, corruption, the unwillingness to die, as well as death itself,[127] that have come into man's life as the result of the transgression of Adam and Eve.[128]

122. Expos. 40, 2-6.
123. Ibid., 39.
124. Instit. 10, 17-22.
125. Expos. 42, 2-4.
126. Ibid., 43, 2 and 21-24.
127. Ibid., 91, 79-83.
128. John explains what the natural and blameless passions stand for in relation to the incarnation of Christ since He assumed all of them, but without sin: '. . . those passions are natural and blameless which are not under our control and have come into man's life as a result of the condemnation occasioned by his fall. Such, for example, were hunger, thirst, fatigue, pain, tears, destruction, the shrinking from death, fear, the agony from which came the sweating and drops of blood, the aid brought by the angels in deference to the weakness of His nature, and any other things as are naturally inherent in all men' (ibid., 64, 7-12).

While divine providence and those that do not depend on us derive from God, corruption and death, which also belong to those that do not depend on us, do not derive from God, but rather man causes them.[129]

Though an internal link between those that depend on us and those that do not depend on us is easily identified, the question arises as to whether John's position is problematic, for the context within which the divine will is expressed is not clear. For example, one may argue that the interdependence between those that depend on us and those that do not depend on us is indicative of an antinomy or inconsistency within John's teaching. Are the two categories characterised by a clear-cut distinction between each other or is there interference between the expression of the human and the divine will?

While the 'antinomy' is evident in *An Exact Exposition of the Orthodox Faith*, the elements that provide the necessary ground for the appropriate answer are included in the *Dialogue against Manichees*. This interrelationship between the two works provides a strong indication against the tendency to treat the study of *The Fountain Head of the Knowledge*, as well as John's other writings, as independent of each other. Although *The Fountain Head of the Knowledge* is considered as an essential theological enchiridion, John's thought goes beyond its boundaries. Thus, the concise writing of *The Fountain Head of Knowledge* and, in particular, of *An Exact Exposition of the Orthodox Faith* is better understood in the context of the whole of Damascene's opus.

Coming back to the discussion of the 'antinomy', John explains his position, on the one hand, by making a distinction within divine providence and, on the other, with reference to foreknowledge (πρόγνωσιν) and predestination (προορισμόν). Foreknowledge is the knowledge of our inner world (ἐσόμενον) – those things that result from exercising our free will[130] – whereas predestination is the judgement and the decision based on them.[131]

According to John, divine providence is expressed in two different ways. First, through God's will for the salvation of all human beings, and that all should become part of His kingdom, and second, through His desire for the just punishment of those who sin.[132] The former is called 'antecedent will' (προηγούμενον θέλημα) and happens as an expression of God's pleasure (εὐδοκία ἐξ αὐτοῦ), whereas the latter is called consequent will (ἑπόμενον θέλημα) and concession (παραχώρησις) and is caused by

129. Ibid., 42, 7-8.
130. Manich. 79, 1-15.
131. Ibid., 78, 15-18.
132. Manich. 79, 20-23, and Expos. 43, 67-70.

us (ἐξ ἡμετέρας αἰτίας). The consequent will is referred to as the proper education of human beings for their salvation.[133] It is in this sense that God's desire for the just punishment of those who sin has to be viewed.

However, the distinction between the antecedent divine will and the consequent divine will does not only imply God's respect for man's free will or the acknowledgement of its significance for the attainment of the good. It rather introduces a more profound kind of relationship. This relationship is based on the proper understanding of the interconnection between the divine will, His foreknowledge (πρόγνωσιν) and predestination (προορισμόν) and the human free will.[134]

The key expression of John is that God foreknows those that depend on us and, therefore, designates those that do not depend on us.[135] Since God has foreknowledge of those things that will happen, He predestines justly and to the profit of each man those that do not depend on us according to those that depend on us (προώρισεν . . . κατάλληλα τοῖς ἐφ' ἡμῖν τὰ οὐκ ἐφ'ἡμῖν).[136] As such, although those that do not depend on us come from divine providence, they come into human life 'after' those that depend on us, which means that they are in a way dependent on the choices of the human free will.[137] Indeed, John calls Christians to struggle to accomplish the good in order to win eternal life once the foreknowledge of God will be His foreknowledge of such a struggle and His predestination will be according to the accomplishment of the good.[138]

133. Expos. 43, 71-73.

134. It is interesting how, as a result of its misinterpretation, John's teaching on predestination and on the antecedent and consequent divine wills can be used in theology so differently. Remarkably, this teaching has been used as a source for the development of scholastic theology (Ermoni, *St Jean Damascène*, pp. 106-07) and, specifically, of Aquinas' theological arguments (Gondreau, *The Passions of Christ's Soul in the Theology of St Thomas Aquinas*, pp. 58-66, and Svoronos, 'Παρατηρήσεις γιὰ τὴ συμβολὴ του Βυζαντίου στὴν πνευματική ἐξέλιξη τῆς Δυτικῆς Εὐρώπης: *Ἡ περίπτωση του Ἰωάννου Δαμασκηνοῦ*', pp. 142-50). While Aquinas borrows the distinction between the antecedent and the consequent divine will from John Damascene, he uses it in order to answer the question of whether the will of God is always fulfilled and not to elaborate the placement of free will in man within divine providence (Aquinas, *Summa Theologica*, FP, Q19, 6). John's teaching on divine providence is placed within the second part of *An Exact Exposition of the Orthodox Faith* devoted to the Creation and, particularly, to the creation of man. In addition, this teaching comes after four chapters, which are related to free will in man and, particularly, to what this free will stands for.

135. Manich. 22, 19-20.

136. Ibid., 78, 10-13 and 79, 1-2.

137. Karmiris, 'Ἡ δογματική διδασκαλία τοῦ Ἰωάννου Δαμασκηνοῦ', pp. 38-40.

138. Manich. 80, 20-22.

This does not imply an involuntary dependence of the divine will on the human will. According to Damascene, the antecedent will is the will of one's self, whereas the consequent will is the will that is caused by an outer event. In this context, God antecedently wills the salvation and the awareness of truth of all human beings. Since man sins, God, with his consequent will, wants to instruct him to his profit.[139] This instructive intervention of God is based on God's foreknowledge of those that will happen since God sees 'those things which be not as though they were' (Romans, 4, 17),[140] those that are caused by the free will and which God sees as already accomplished.[141] Thus, the 'dependence' of divine will on human will is the kind of 'dependence' that characterises the consequent will that, while it comes from God, is caused by us.[142] Indeed, such 'dependence' by no means unconditionally shapes human life. Rather, it establishes cooperation between man and God through which God is considered closer to man.

In such a context, Louth rightly says that Damascene, despite the fact that those that depend on us come out as expressions of human free will, places them within divine providence. Nevertheless, he falsely considers that the cooperation between God and man is limited only to those human choices that are oriented towards the good.[143] The consequent will that is related to the proper preparation of human beings for their salvation, and that betrays a particular 'dependence' on human will, justifies a kind of cooperation between God and man even when man is not oriented towards the good for the sake of man and his re-orientation towards the good.[144]

Similarly, Jugie rightly argues that John accepts a kind of antecedent predestination with which God desires the salvation of all human beings

139. Ibid., 79, 20-24.

140. Ibid., 73, 7-14.

141. Ibid., 37, 5-6.

142. Karmiris, 'Ἡ δυγματική διδασκαλία τοῦ Ἰωάννου Δαμασκηνοῦ', pp. 42-43.

143. Louth, *St John Damascene*, p. 143. Some Orthodox Christian theologians have denied even the placement of free will within divine providence, a denial that has important implications once man as a free being is placed outside that providence. See, for example, Tsirpanlis, 'The Problem of Free Will and Evil in St John of Damascus', p. 69.

144. We have already noted that, according to Pseudo-Dionysius, the beings always desire peace and friendship with God even though their actions show exactly the opposite. Therefore, is it logical that their bad choices are covered by the divine provision? Another extract from Pseudo-Dionysius is characteristic: 'the licentious man, even if he has been deprived of the Good, as regards his irrational lust, in this respect he neither is, nor desires realities, but nevertheless he participates in the Good, in his very obscure echo of union and friendship' (PG, 3, 720B).

and provides the appropriate means towards this end. Nonetheless, he wrongly views free will as a condition towards the fulfilment of God's universal antecedent predestination.[145] In fact, he misinterprets John and the placement of free will within divine providence once he misses the point of distinction between the antecedent and the consequent will.

In short, John justifies once more the importance of free will for understanding the changes that have happened in human nature due to the fall. By looking at the character of death in human life, not only the responsibility of man but also the interaction between the human and divine wills is exemplified. This interaction is characterised by the fact that the divine will as a 'consequent will' comes 'after' the human will. If so, the fate of human life in this world has to be viewed with respect to both wills in order to be properly understood. While death is considered as a natural and blameless passion and belongs to those that do not depend on us, its experience by each human being signifies that it is not only a matter of the divine will or the so-called consequent will. On the contrary, the experience of corruption and death is also dependent on the human free will in the sense that whatever happens, at whatever moment, always has to have reference to free will. Taking responsibility for death should not be based on God and His will only but also on man, who has always to take the proportional responsibility with a view to his salvation. In other words, the belief according to which there are things that man is not eligible to have anything to do with, such as the time of the end of his corruptible nature, may not be absolutely sustained.

3. Death as the Dissolution of the Union of Soul and Body: When Nature Reigns over Free Will

After the fall the divine will comes 'after' the human will, so to speak. As a result, one may expect the human will to have been strengthened. However, what really happens is exactly the opposite. While God created man with free will in order for the soul to rule sovereign over the body, and the rational to rule over the non-rational, he decided not to follow the divine will and thus his free will became subject to the disease of sin.[146]

Man is a composite hypostasis due to the hypostatic union of two essences (or natures or substances), namely the soul and body. While the hypostatic union of soul and body results in a living hypostasis, the dissolution of the union of soul and body results in death. The separation

145. Jugie, '*Jean Damascène (St)*', DS VIII, pp. 729-30.
146. Volunt. 44, 9.

of soul and body is traditionally considered as the theological definition of death.[147] Interestingly enough, for Damascene the dissolution of the union of soul and body comes as the natural effect of a composite being[148] and, consequently, death is the natural effect of the composite human being. Such a consideration is very important for the ethical issues surrounding the coming of death, since it declares that death does not belong to those that are 'contrary to nature', though it causes the end of the biological aspect of human life.

The idea that death comes as a natural effect of human nature is also supported in a different context and, particularly, in John's treatise, *Dispute between a Saracen and a Christian*. John argues that what actually happened in the death of Christ[149] or the Theotokos[150] was the natural death of a human being (ὁ φυσικὸς τῶν ἀνθρώπων θάνατος). Therefore, Matsoukas falsely says that, according to John, death is a condition 'contrary to nature' (παρὰ φύσιν) since he does not connect the entry of death into human life with the loss of the 'supernatural' communication with God that suspended death, the natural effect of mortal human nature.[151] Despite the fact that John insists that death comes as the natural effect of the composite human being, the belief that death is a condition contrary to nature (παρὰ φύσιν) is widespread. Damascene's position is absolutely consistent with the inclusion of death among the natural and blameless passions, as has already been discussed.

If death is considered as a natural effect of a human being, why is the entry of corruption and death into human life regarded as the consequence of a particular behaviour, namely the transgression of the divine will?

The answer to this question can be found in the life of Adam and Eve before the fall. Adam, before his fall, experienced only life in union

147. Ibid., 17, 8.
148. Manich. 71, 11.
149. Sarac. 9, 3-4. There is a divergence between the available manuscripts of John's treatise in terms of the subject of the particular paragraph (Sarac. 9), which is either Christ (ὅν λέγετε κύριον) or the Theotokos (ἥν λέγετε θεοτόκον) (Kotter, *Die Schriften des Johannes von Damaskus IV*, p. 436). However, since the whole treatise refers to humanity in Christ, it appears that the particular paragraph discusses the death of Christ. To avoid any misunderstanding regarding Christ, though the coming of death in Him as man is considered as a natural effect, such a coming was accomplished after its free acceptance by Christ.
150. Dorm. I, 10, 17-20. See also Anagnostopoulos, 'Ἡ περὶ τῆς Θεοτόκου διδασκαλία τοῦ Ἰωάννου τοῦ Δαμασκηνοῦ', p. 576.
151. Matsoukas, 'Φιλοσοφία καὶ δογματικὴ διδασκαλία τοῦ ἁγίου Ἰωάννου Δαμασκηνοῦ', p. 287.

(ἥνωτο) with God, and God transmitted life to his mortal nature in a 'supernatural' way (ὑπὲρ φύσιν ζωοποιοῦσαν τὴν θνητὴν αὐτοῦ φύσιν). In other words, while man as a composite being was destined to die, God put him in paradise in order for him to have the opportunity to avoid death by being united with God and by receiving life without interruption. Once man disrupted his union with God, he passed from the 'supernatural' incorruption to the 'according to nature' dissolution of his composite being (ἐκ τῆς ὑπὲρ φύσιν ἀφθαρσίας εἰς τήν κατὰ φύσιν τοῦ συνθέτου διάλυσιν), that is death.[152]

John makes here a very interesting connection between corruption and death, as natural effects, and the union of man with God. While corruption and death are natural effects in human nature, man suspends the entry of such natural effects as long as he is united with God and experiences a 'supernatural' life since what is 'supernatural' reigns over nature by definition. John makes it even clearer with reference to Christ.[153]

Since Christ took upon himself human nature, he did not only freely assume the natural and blameless passions, such as corruption and death, which he did so without sin, but he also freely chose death. However, these passions were in a 'supernatural' condition in Christ, since the natural things did not control the will (οὐ γὰρ προηγεῖτο ἐν τῷ κυρίῳ τῆς θελήσεως τὰ φυσικά). Rather, these passions existed following the voluntary permission of Christ's will' and, as such, 'He hungered by willing, He thirsted by willing, He was afraid by willing, He died by willing' (θέλων γὰρ ἐπείνασε, θέλων ἐδίψησε, θέλων ἐδειλίασε, θέλων ἀπέθανεν)[154] and not by compulsion, namely involuntary, as happens in human beings.[155] Thus, the sovereignty of the 'supernatural' and the consequent suspension of the natural dissolution of soul and body are secured once the free will reigns over natural things and is not ruled by them.

152. Manich. 71, 12-15.

153. The belief that death comes as the natural effect of the dissolution of the union of soul and body does not contradict John's position that the entry of corruption and death has a non-essential and accidental character. Death as a natural effect comes after the loss of 'supernatural' communication with God, namely the condition in which God placed man at the time of his creation, in which the natural after-effect of the dissolution of the union of soul and body was suspended, though it was a condition subject to the proper exercising of human will. On the contrary, the characterisation of corruption and death as non-essential and accidental refers to the inclusion or not of suffering and death in those constituent elements of human existence as God created it once God did not infuse death but rather life in man.

154. Expos. 64, 22-27.

155. Ibid., 67, 9-17.

Unfortunately, man has fallen and, as a result, he experiences the sovereignty of nature over free will in an extremely tragic way. Man, because of the fall, is subject to the unhindered natural progress towards death, despite the fact that he, by nature, does not want to die. This tragedy is exemplified with reference to the fear before death that is included among the natural and blameless passions.

John points out that there are two kinds of fear, natural fear (δειλία φυσική or κατὰ φύσιν δειλία) and unnatural fear (παρὰ φύσιν δειλία). The former, natural fear, is a force which clings to existence by withdrawal (κατὰ συστολὴν τοῦ ὄντος ἀνθεκτική) and is based on the assumption that those things that have been brought into existence from non-existence by the Creator do not have the desire for non-existence but rather the instinctive tendency towards those things by which they are sustained. On the contrary, unnatural fear is a fear that is caused by ruinous thinking (ἐκ προδοσίας λογισμῶν συνισταμένη), lack of faith and the ignorance of the hour of death. In this context, the unwillingness of the soul to be separated from the body because of the natural feeling of affinity and kingship (φυσικὴν συμπάθειάν τε καὶ οἰκειότητα) that are given by God at the time of Creation is a natural fear. Similarly, the fact that the soul is afraid and distressed and shrinks from death is considered as natural.[156] Thus, though the dissolution of the soul from the body is considered as a natural effect of man's composite hypostasis, the unwillingness of the soul to be separated from the body is also counted as natural. Such an obvious antinomy is the source of the tragedy within human life.

Christ experienced the fear one feels before death as well. However, he escaped this tragedy once he submitted to death voluntarily, and not involuntarily as the rest of humanity does.[157] Moreover, the way in which Christ experienced the fear one feels in the face of death shows the crucial role of the sovereignty of will over nature, along with the submission of the human will to the divine will. What humankind failed to do in paradise was achieved in Christ:

> Now the body of itself had no inclination for physical suffering, nor yet did it avoid and refuse to accept what was painful.

156. Ibid., 67.

157. To justify this position, John (ibid., 67, 24-34) borrows arguments from two treatises against Appolinarius, attributed to St Athanasius, Archibishop of Alexandria, although the author of the two treatises is not clear (see Papadopoulos, *Πατρολογία II*, p. 320) and according to which Christ's fear before death, as well as the passions He suffered, were endured voluntarily (PG, 26, 1124A and PG, 26, 1153A).

> Neither was it affected by external influences; rather, it was moved in accordance with the order of its nature, with the Word wisely willing and permitting it to suffer and do what was proper to it, so that through its works the truth of its nature might be guaranteed.[158]

Additionally, a few chapters later in *An Exact Exposition of the Orthodox Faith*, John points out:

> Consequently, while he had naturally the power of willing both as God and as man, the human will followed after and was subordinated to His will, not being motivated by its own opinion, but willing what His divine will willed. Thus, it was with the permission of the divine will that He suffered what was naturally proper to Him. And when he begged to be spared death, He did so naturally, with his divine will willing and permitting, and He was in agony and afraid. Then, when His divine will willed that His human will choose death, the passion was freely accepted by it, because it was not as God alone that He freely delivered Himself over to death, but as man, also.[159]

In other words, while in paradise man enjoyed the sovereignty of his free will over nature, that is indicative of the 'supernatural' human life united to God; after the fall he and his free will were subject to the sovereignty of human nature. The ultimate result of such a fundamental ontological change in humanity was the entry of corruption and death into human life, namely the separation of the soul from the body. Despite the natural unwillingness of the soul to be separated from the body, the dissolution of their union comes as a natural effect involuntarily, due to the fact that human nature rules over the will.

The tragedy of fallen humanity reached a peak, since it resembled the condition of non-rational animals. By definition, man as a rational and free being stands at the very opposite pole to non-rational animals that are not free. Man leads his nature rather than being led by it, whereas in animals the exact opposite occurs. The contrast between the rational human being and non-rational animals is explicitly stated in the passage that follows:

> Now, in the case of the non-rational animals, when an appetite for something arises it is immediately followed by an impulse to act. This is because the appetite of non-rational animals is

158. Expos. 59, 182-87.
159. Ibid., 62, 33-41.

> non-rational and because they are led by their natural appetite. For this reason the appetite of non-rational animals is said to be neither a will nor a volition. Will is a rational and free natural appetite and with men, who are rational, the natural appetite is led rather than leading. Thus, man is moved freely with the aid of reason, since in him the cognitive and vital faculties are joined together. Hence, he freely desires and freely wills, freely lives and inquires, freely deliberates, freely judges, freely disposes himself, freely chooses, freely moves to act, and freely acts in respect to those things which are in accord with his nature.[160]

It is remarkable that, while John exaggerates the sovereignty of free will over nature, he does not hesitate to compare man after the fall with non-rational animals. In paradise, man, through his obedience to God, drew progressively closer to God and, therefore, was dressed in incorruptibility. However, he eventually chose to become disobedient to God, like non-rational animals and, therefore, subject to death.[161] If non-rational animals are not regarded as free but are rather led by nature, then the transition from the sovereignty of free will over nature to the sovereignty of nature over free will along with the entry of death is not surprising.

In conclusion, though the entry of corruption and death are considered as non-essential and accidental characteristics of man since they do not belong to the definition of man, they affect human life itself. God has created man for life, and not death. However, death comes into human life despite the unwillingness of the soul to be separated from the body. Man suffers from the weakening of the power of his will and, therefore, he cannot command his own nature. Certainly, the will of man to rule over his own life is entirely proper. However, given the weakness of man's own will, the will for power claims over human life, as happens in the case of the self-administration of death in euthanasia, is totally unjustified, for it betrays a violation of human existence once it ignores the status of the human will in relation to human life.[162]

---

160. Ibid., 36, 84-94.
161. Ficus 3, 25-37.
162. Faucon maintains that God has endowed human nature with real autonomy since He created man according to His own image. However, he mistakenly concludes that John Damascene asserts that such autonomy and free will allows man to be revealed as an image of God's transcendence (Faucon, '*Infrastructures philosophiques de la théodicée de Jean Damascène*', pp. 382-84). He ignores the implications of the fallen state of humanity for human life and, in particular, *vis-à-vis* the power of the human will.

VI. Christ, His Church and Life-bearing Death

The description of the character of death after the fall of Adam and Eve is not sufficient to gain a proper understanding of it, given that the intervention of Jesus Christ in human history has to be taken into account. It is through Christ and the life of the faithful members of His Church,[163] such as the martyrs, that death has obtained a new meaning and now has remarkable implications for human life and death.

1. Baptism and the Death of Christ

If the fall of Adam and Eve was a turning point that resulted in remarkable ontological changes for humanity, the incarnation of the Son of God marked a new era for fallen mankind. God created man according to His own image and made him free with a view to the likeness to and union with Him. The path towards the likeness to and union with God was subject to a particular condition, that is the obedience of the human will to the divine will. Unfortunately, man did exactly the opposite. He proved disobedient to God and became subject to corruption and death. The Son of God became man in order to re-establish the obedience of the human will to the divine will and to free man from death.[164] Christ assumed human nature and he also freely took upon himself the natural and blameless passions that include death.

The case of the death and burial of Christ is very important for a better understanding of the character of death. According to Damascene, Christ, through His death and burial, wanted to put aside the natural and blameless passions, like corruption, that were introduced into human nature after the fall and man's disobedience to God.[165] In fact, it was the communication

163. Though John's theological work, and particularly *An Exact Exposition of the Orthodox Faith*, is characterised by the absence of a systematic and an explicit teaching on the character of the Church, it does not mean that John underestimated the theological issues relevant to ecclesiology. He devoted a number of his homilies to Sts and martyrs, and he would deliver his homilies at liturgical occasions in order that the monastics and laymen who were present would be encouraged to imitate the life of the Sts and martyrs. This demonstrates that John was concerned that a Christian should be directed towards a particular way of life, the life of the faithful members of the Church. These homilies formed part of the yearly panegyris (or gatherings) that were occasions for liturgical celebrations, which would include the vigil service, the Eucharist and a procession (Leemans, Mayer, Allen and Dehandschutter, *Let Us Die That We May Live*, p. 15).

164. Volunt. 40, 1-12.

165. Sabbat. 27, 2-5; Expos. 74, 2-3.

and union of man with God and the submission of the human will to the divine will that were interrupted because of the fall. God has given man a second chance so that man may enjoy a more lasting communion with God (δευτέραν κοινωνίαν ὁ συμπαθὴς ἡμῖν κεκοινώνηκεν ἀσφαλεστέραν) since Christ has the power to preserve it unbroken.[166] It was due to the hypostatic union of His divinity and humanity that death did not interrupt this communication, and both soul and body, though separate, remained united in the one hypostasis of Christ.[167] In other words, it is communication with God, and not the coming of death, that is proved, in Christ, to be of central importance for human existence.

Obviously, the death of Christ reveals the necessity to re-orient the ethical discussions surrounding human death from the focus on the event of death to the links between death and communication with God. This approach by no means entails an underestimation of death as a biological phenomenon. On the contrary, Christ's death has shown that death is now a positive prospect in human existence. This is evident in baptism, which is considered as participation in the death of Christ.

John, following St Paul's words that 'as many as were baptised into Christ were baptised into his death',[168] says that baptism is a figure of the death of Jesus Christ and the immersion into the water three times signifies the three-day burial of Christ in the tomb.[169] This participation is very important, since it links the baptised believer with what actually happened to human nature through the death of Christ:

> For, since man is twofold, being of body and soul, the purification He gave us is also twofold, through water and the Spirit, with the Spirit renewing in us what is to His image and likeness and the water by the grace of the Spirit purifying the body from sin and delivering it from destruction – the water completing the figure of the death and the Spirit producing the guarantee of life.[170]

Therefore, for Damascene, baptism is actually a tangible expression of the communication of divinity and humanity that results not only in the remission of sins but also in the deliverance from those things that sin has brought about – freedom from destruction and the renewing of the image and likeness of God in man.[171] It is through baptism and

166. Transfig. 4, 17-18; Nativ. M. 8, 6-12.
167. Sabbat. 29, 36-39.
168. Romans 6:3.
169. Expos. 82, 14-19.
170. Ibid., 82, 36-42.
171. Fortino, 'Sanctification and Deification', pp. 196-97.

the re-birth by water and the Spirit that man becomes a son and heir of God[172] and turns towards his original orientation. It is for this reason that St Paul calls the believers 'Sts'[173] and that we do not grieve but rejoice over the death of the Sts.[174] Obviously, John is writing in accordance with the Scriptures and St Paul, who says: 'Having been buried with Him in baptism, you also have been raised with Him through your faith in the power of God who raised Him from the dead.'[175]

In short, it is in the death of Christ and His life after death through His resurrection that the Christian meaning of death is completed. In such a context, death becomes something positive, which means, on the one hand, that it cannot be identified with the biological end of the corruptible body and, on the other, that it cannot be properly anticipated when it is regarded as the absolute threat to human life. However, is such a positive view of death limited only to the sacramental act of baptism? The answer to this question is given through the discussion of the life of Christ's imitators such as His mother and the martyrs.

2. The Death of the Theotokos as a Life-bearing Death

John devoted three homilies to the Dormition of the Mother of God or Theotokos, that were possibly delivered during an all-night vigil,[176] with the evident purpose of praising the person, the life and the death of Mary.

Without a doubt, the Theotokos is accorded exceptional honour within the Christian tradition, even though novelties were introduced through so-called Mariology and its development within the Roman Catholic tradition.[177] The special character of the life and death of the Theotokos provides interesting inferences about human life and death. It is worth noting that John, while he recognises the difference between the Theotokos and Sts (θεοφόροις τοῦ Θεοῦ), says that God granted to them

172. Romans 8:17.
173. 1 Corinthians 1:2.
174. Imag. I, 21, p. 110.
175. Colossians 2:12.
176. Dorm. III, 1, 1-7.
177. A critique of the development of Mariology within the Roman Catholic tradition exceeds the purposes of this study. The general comment that should be made is that most of these works interpret John's texts on the Theotokos through the eyes of the relevant Catholic dogmas, such as the absence of original sin or the belief that the Theotokos did not need redemption. Thus, it is not surprising that Greek Fathers who lived before Damascene have been accused of bad developments in the faith of the Church with regard to the Theotokos (Chevalier, *La Mariologie de St Jean Damascène*, pp. 130-36).

the 'best passage' (καλλίστης ἐκδημίας) – the end of life is considered as the transition from earthly life to another life. This 'best passage' is a passage from those things of the body to the best state (Ἐκδημοῦσα γὰρ τῶν τοῦ σώματος ἐνδημεῖς πρὸς τὰ κρείττονα)[178] and to dwelling with God (πρὸς θεὸν ἐνδημίαν).[179] Thus, Damascene proclaims two things. First, the death, or rather the Dormition, of the Theotokos is not irrelevant to human life and death. Second, the Dormition of the Theotokos introduces the idea that the biological end of a human being is in a way a passage to life after death.

Since death is regarded as a kind of passage from one 'place' to another, it does not mark the end of a being. It is for this reason that the death of the Theotokos is called Dormition (the corresponding Greek work is κοίμησις, which means falling asleep) and signifies that the end of the earthly life of the Theotokos is not the end of the Theotokos as a human being. On the contrary, the use of the word 'κοίμησις' implies that those who sleep will awake to another kind of life once their earthly life has been accomplished. Therefore, if death is merely a κοίμησις, or a 'falling asleep', then it does not designate the end of a particular being. The attribution of κοίμησις is not limited to the death of the Theotokos but rather is extended to all human beings. It is not accidental that, within the Orthodox Christian tradition, cemeteries are considered places where human beings have fallen asleep and are thus called κοιμητήρια.

John goes a step further and designates the prospect of κοίμησις as the 'best passage' towards life after death. Since in the Christian tradition death is not the end of life, then the separation of the soul from the body, as indicative of the time of death, does not interrupt life. Therefore, in the Theotokos, the experience of the natural effect of the dissolution of the union of body and soul did not result in the cessation of life. Rather, the Theotokos passed over into divine life.[180] John points out that, though the Theotokos was subject to death as a human being, the end of her earthly life is a life-bearing death (θανάτῳ ζωηφόρῳ) and a vital death (ζωτικὴν ἀποβίωσιν).[181]

To avoid any misunderstanding, John clarifies that such an intertwining of life and death is not accidental and is a result of the spiritual state of the person upon death. The death of the Theotokos was life-bearing and vital because of the particular relationship between the Theotokos and God, not only because she gave birth to God, but also because of her

178. Dorm. I, 10, 40.
179. Ibid., 10, 13-14.
180. Ibid., 10, 1-24.
181. Dorm. II, 2, 44-48.

unceasing devotion to God. Thus, a distinction can be made between the death of an evildoer and the death of a holy man. In death the former is characterised as wicked, whereas the latter is considered praiseworthy, beatified and honourable.[182]

Indeed, a praiseworthy, beatified, honourable as well as life-bearing and vital death is not actually death. While death comes, it is at the same time abolished. Thus, the establishment of a life-bearing death reinstates the whole discussion regarding euthanasia. A life-bearing death implies that one's own responsibility for one's destiny goes beyond death itself. This responsibility refers not only to life after death, that is after the biological end of one's own existence but also, as will be made clear in the chapter that follows, to the human beings who surround one. Consequently, death cannot be considered simply the end of human existence, as happens with the deliberate administration of death in the medical context.

3. The Martyrs and Voluntary Death

The death of the Theotokos reveals two very important aspects of death: the positive prospect of death (life-bearing death) as a passage from this life to eternal life; and the crucial aspect that one should have spiritual presuppositions for a death of this kind. Someone might justifiably wonder, how far may such positive connotations of death be taken? The witness of the martyrs provides the answer to this question. The martyrs are those people who have been 'baptised' with the baptism of Christ's life-giving death.[183] Let us look at how this happens.

To go back to Adam and Eve, they sinned as they turned their interest from union and communication with God to their self-preservation and false deification. All human beings face the same temptation, that is the worship of the material instead of the Creator.[184] Martyrs are those human beings who suffered torments and chose to die for the sake of Christ,[185] that is to say, those who chose to rectify the disobedience of Adam and

182. Ibid., 3, 28-32; Dorm. I, 12, 1-5.
183. 'And let us honor the holy martyrs of the Lord who have been picked from every rank and whose corps commander is Christ's archdeacon, apostle, and protomartyr Stephen; let us honor them as soldiers of Christ who have drunk of His chalice and have then been baptized with the baptism of His life-giving death, and as participants in His sufferings and His glory' (Expos. 88, 70-75).
184. Anast. 18, 13-22.
185. Barb. 19, 35-36.

Eve.[186] This choice represents the transition from a preoccupation with self-preservation to an intentness on union and communication with God that even extends to the point of a voluntary death.

The martyrs proceeded to their voluntary death in the certainty that death cannot threaten what is important for one's own life, which is union with God. As John proclaims, even though death continues to separate the soul from the body, it cannot separate the martyrs from God.[187] It is union with God and not death that really matters in human life, as was true before the fall. Furthermore, it is not accidental that, in two homilies devoted to the martyrs, St Barbara and St Anastasia, respectively, Damascene talks about the life of Adam and Eve before the fall, a life free from corruption and death, and their experience of the 'supernatural'. He also compares the martyrs with their persecutors. While the martyrs overcame nature (τὴν φύσιν νικήσαντες) and passed from the 'according to nature' to the 'supernatural' (ἐν τοῖς ὑπὲρ φύσιν γεγόνασιν) through the divine Spirit, their persecutors passed from the 'according to nature' to an inferior stage and became like the demons. The martyrs became imitators of Christ, whereas their persecutors became followers of the Devil.[188] Obviously, the end of corruptible human nature no longer holds any value when it is compared to the experience of union and communication with God. In such a context, voluntary death is absolutely justified.

To avoid any misunderstanding, John's reference to the experience of the 'supernatural' even in this life by no means involves a kind of meditation or metaphysical understanding. On the contrary, he has in mind always the union of divinity and humanity and, consequently, the most radical understanding of the relationship between the immanent and the transcendent that is experienced in the life of Christ and the life of the Church. It is for this reason that the martyrs' endurance of any torment or even death is presented as being like the endurance of the Church against those that fight it. John comments on St Matthew's phrase that the gates of Hades will not overpower the Church[189] and says that 'the gates of Hades' are considered all those torments that lead to hell and to death.[190] John explicitly implies that the members of the Church,

186. Anast. 29, 5-8.
187. Barb. 12, 28-32.
188. Ibid., 15, 12-24. John uses almost the same wording in the homily on the martyr Anastasia in order to declare the transition from the 'according to nature' to the 'supernatural' (Anast. 7, 1-2).
189. Matthew 16:18.
190. Barb. 6, 31-33.

like the martyrs, are not threatened by any kind of torment, even those that come as a natural effect of corruptible human nature, once they are united to God. He concludes that the endurance of unbearable torments, along with the miraculous healing of the martyr's ulcers, as well as their willingness to die, are indicative of this reality.[191]

The voluntary death of the martyrs does not imply any underestimation or depreciation of human life, and consequently of corruptible human nature, but it rather shows a concern for preserving the integrity of human nature. John says that, among other torments, St Barbara's breasts were cut off and that her father, who was present (it was in fact he who had denounced St Barbara to the sovereign), did not react against such an insult against nature.[192] Similarly, Damascene points out that, when the torturers of St Barbara decided to pillory her naked in public, Christ dressed her with the garments of grace, and she looked like a bride, thus protecting her from the disgraceful eyes of Christ's enemies.[193] Even though there is a distinction between the end of corruptible human nature and the preservation of union with God, this corruptible human nature always retains its value. Apparently, both must be taken into account. It is in this context that one may interpret John's call to all Christians to become martyrs by choice, even though the era of persecution and fire is over.[194] A systematic presentation of this invitation is presented through examining the work of Symeon the New Theologian in the chapter that follows.

VII. Concluding Remarks

The explanation of John Damascene's theology sheds some light on the parameters of euthanasia, such as the character of human life and death, and the responsibility of man as regards death. It is for this reason that different aspects of human existence were discussed, along with the implications of decisive moments recorded in the Old and New Testament, these are the creation of man according to the image of God, the fall of Adam and Eve, and the incarnation, death and resurrection of Christ.

191. Ibid., 12,1-17.
192. Ibid., 15, 1-10.
193. Ibid., 16.
194. Ibid., 3, 13-16. John's idea traces back to St Basil of Caesarea (PG, 31, 508B) (Imag. I, 42, p. 150) and St John Chrysostom (Imag. I, 53, *varia lectio*, p. 155). It is not accidental that this idea is also found in the context of the veneration of the icons. Given that the veneration of icons is connected not only with the praise of the prototype (Christ, Sts, martyrs) but also with the imitation of the life of this prototype, further reasons to support the idea of imitating the martyrs by choice may be cited.

John Damascene lived in an epoch of cultural and spiritual crisis, which climaxed in the confusion in the relationship between the immanent and transcendent, the cosmos and the Church, man and God. His writings were the result of his endeavours to proclaim the Christian truth with a view to establishing comprehensively what the relationship between man and God is. John participated in the iconoclastic controversy, which dealt with the question of how far the divine is allowed to impinge on the human world. The tendency to emphasise the distance between the infinite God and finite man was strongly challenged by John. In the same vein, though in a different context, this chapter has shown that John proceeded to a prudent transition from Christology to Christian anthropology that in a way brings God closer to man.

This transition was made on two levels. The first level dealt with the interpersonal dimension of human life, whereas the second level worked on the inner state of the human being.

John used Greek philosophy and Aristotle's categories in order to teach theology and not philosophy. Thus, he enriched the context of the Aristotelian categories and the relationships of beings within the empirical world by introducing the unique character of the relationship between man and God. This relationship reveals the origin (the derivative) as well as the orientation (the relative) of man. Such a relationship is neither natural, like the relationship between father and son, nor accidental, like a fortuitous relationship, and, therefore, it cannot be included in the given categories of the immanent. The consideration of man as a derivative and relative creature establishes a relationship that in an unprecedented way brings together the immanent and the transcendent and, consequently, man and God towards the imitation of God. In such a context, the death of a human, along with all those issues relevant to human life, is a matter of two beings and always subject to the dependence of one on the Other.

Additionally, Damascene challenges the Aristotelian categories and refers to the inner state of the human being and, consequently, to the division of beings. He is interested in the founding origin of man and the internal relationships that exist between hypostasis and nature. On the one hand, as in Christ, so in man, there is an ontological priority of hypostasis over nature. This is accompanied by the identification of two kinds of union: that of the union of the soul and body, and that of the hypostatic union. The hypostatic union is the union of the soul and body in a particular hypostasis that rescues both soul and body at the time of death, namely the natural dissolution of the union of soul and body, given that the hypostatic union cannot be affected by death. Though the hypostatic union of soul and body rescues both the soul and body, there is a 'differentiation' within such a union. While the oneness of man is secured, the asymmetry and disproportional character that marks the difference between soul and body regarding the hypostatic union is not invalidated. Such asymmetry and disproportionality challenge the view of bioethics regarding human existence in the medical context, according to which man is considered a mere biological existence and where a kind of an internal 'undifferentiation' is adopted. Arguments that regard the deliberate administration of death, as in euthanasia, as a simply materialistic decision cannot be sustained within the Christian tradition. Other aspects of human existence, apart from the body, have to be taken into account.

On the other hand, the priority of hypostasis over nature does not result in a kind of bodiless life. John points out the difference and relationship between hypostasis and nature, and affirms the 'intimacy' between them, an 'intimacy' that has implications for the relationship between the immanent and the transcendent in another way. John accentuates the sharing of a common nature by all human beings given that God created man according to His own image. All human beings have the same nature that has been shaped according to the image of God. Though the different hypostases constitute different 'modes of being', they are able to take advantage of their common nature and, therefore, to express the hypostatic natural 'objects of willing'. Such expression, without underestimating the particularity of each human being, highlights the importance of the knowledge of human nature, a knowledge that at least reminds man of his dependence on God and on the rest of humankind.

This kind of view of human existence also challenges the 'well-justified' modern belief that what counts is the emphasis on the individuality of each human being and the principle of autonomy without the presence of any content-rich anthropological account. For John, human life must always take into account what human nature stands for in order to avoid self-destructive decisions, that is decisions that ignore the characteristics of human existence such as the 'intimacy' that should exist between the expression of one's own will and the character of human nature. Therefore, exercising autonomy cannot be unconditional, but rather depends on the proper knowledge of human existence. The ignorance or underestimation of such knowledge inescapably leads to a 'suicidal', or self-destructive, decision. It would seem that this position of John does not offer any justification for the 'promising' project of common morality, a project that searches for the 'common' not in human nature or in a particular anthropology but rather in general, ambiguous and always subjectively interpreted principles.

Damascene reinforces the importance of the knowledge of man's own nature even further by saying that the true knowledge of beings is a prerequisite for an authentic existence, where by authentic existence he is referring to the doctrine of the creation of man according to the image of God. This knowledge of human nature must be sought in terms of and through Christ, who was made man and in whom there is no falsehood but only truth. Therefore, man's only preoccupation must be his communication with God that progressively leads to the true knowledge of his being and, consequently, to proper self-knowledge. Apparently, John does not consider man's self-preservation as the first priority in human life, even though it has been the most common principle in human life throughout the centuries. The principle of self-preservation is challenged even more by the knowledge that man cannot fulfil, by definition, the necessary condition for his self-preservation, namely his power claims over human life. According to John, while the soul has to rule over the body, it, through the will, does not have absolute control over the body. Consequently, the absolute power of the human will cannot be justified. Therefore, the consideration of man as a principally autonomous and free being once he is involuntary subject to constraints from within his own existence is risky.

John completes the description of the character of corruption and death in human life with reference to the causes of their entry into the world. This is necessary, since the idea that man should assume proper responsibility for the time of his death may be misleading and may be viewed as a 'deification' of the human will. Such misunderstanding is avoided with the acknowledgment of the fallen condition of the human will. As a consequence of the fall, the human will and its power to reign over nature and non-rational desires are weak. Even though the human will by nature does not want death to come, death comes. This is an indication of the sovereignty of nature over the human will. Since the cause of this sovereignty was the disobedience of the human will to the divine will, Christ became man in order to reestablish the obedience of the human will to the divine will and, consequently, the power of the human will to rule over nature. In this context, the tendency of human beings to claim power over human life throughout the centuries lacks the appropriate ground, since the human will still suffers from profound weaknesses. In fact, such power claims are nothing else than disguised self-interest that would deliberately ignore the human condition.

Without a doubt, the meaning of death and its proper placing in human life is not possible without taking into account the incarnation of God and the life of the faithful members of His Church. Christ as man freely suffered from the so-called natural and blameless passions, including death. Due to the union of divinity and humanity in the hypostasis of the Son of God, Christ did not experience the dissolution of the body and the enslavement of His soul to death,[195] even though He died a natural death. On the contrary, He preserved united both the soul and body in His hypostasis. Thus, the preservation of the communication of human existence with God displaces death from its central position in human existence. What now is important is the preservation of the union of humanity with God. This union changes the character of death and attributes a positive connotation to it. This is obvious in baptism, where participation in the death of Christ results in the renewal of the image of God in man, an image that signifies the newly restored relationship between man and God from the beginning of human existence.

The positive consideration of death in human existence is perfectly exemplified in those who have been proved to be faithful to God. Damascene points out that the death of the Mother of God, the Theotokos, is a life-bearing death. This death is viewed as a passage from this life to the life after death, which means that death leads to endless life. However, not all deaths are life-bearing, since not all of them share the same ground, which is communication and the union with God. Once more, particular conditions justify the designation of a particular moral status regarding a fact or an action.

The positive view of death culminates in the life and the death of the martyrs. In this case, death is not considered simply as an unavoidable event in human life. Rather it is a voluntary action, since the martyrs choose death over life. Obviously, the voluntary death of the martyrs brings the whole discussion closer to the debate around euthanasia and the voluntary administration or self-administration of death. For the martyrs, death does not hold any value when compared to the experience of union and communication with God. Therefore, their willingness to die is absolutely justified, a willingness that is never accompanied by an underestimation of human life and corruptible human nature. The martyrs, through their voluntary death, want to defend their orientation towards God by not assigning an absolute character to their biological end and, at the same time, to safeguard the integrity of human nature. This book now turns to a deeper exploration of the character of voluntary death in the Christian tradition.

195. Acts 2:27.

Chapter 4
St Symeon the New Theologian and the Character of Man

Introduction

The exploration of the character of voluntary death in the Christian tradition clearly raises the possibility of a Christian form of individualism – voluntary death as such implies the deliberate willingness to die on the part of a particular individual. The theology of Symeon the New Theologian, in an epoch that is characterised by the emphasis on the subject of human actions, offers suitable ground for a thorough description of such a Christian individualism.

The place of Symeon within his era was extensively discussed in the general introduction to this work but some additional points justifying the choice of Symeon in a work that deals with a challenging ethical issue are considered necessary.

Engagement with a difficult issue presupposes the contribution of a challenging thinker. By the tenth century the Byzantine intellectual tradition, justly called 'encyclopedic',[1] had regularised and we see within Byzantine society efforts towards its systematisation.

The most classic example of this endeavour is the case of Emperor Constantine VII Porphyrogenitus, who wrote four books, which are best described as an 'imperial or political encyclopedia'.[2] It was in the

1. Lemerle, *Le premier humanisme byzantin*, pp. 267-300.
2. The first book is *The Life of the Founder of the Dynasty of Basil I* and the three other books are a three-part descriptive chronicle of the empire that deal with, respectively, the ceremonies of the imperial court, the goals of Byzantine

tenth century that the first religious encyclopedia also appeared. This encyclopedia was a religious almanac composed by Symeon Metaphrastes and called *Μηνολόγιον*, or Menologion. This collection includes the lives of the Sts, according to the order their feast occurs in the ecclesiastical year (no more than one biography per day). Common to all these efforts is an absence of originality that betrays a fear of innovation. This is not surprising, since the traditionally theocratic Byzantine culture would not permit any rearrangement of the divine order, at least openly.[3] In such a context, Symeon the New Theologian, like all the great Church Fathers, was to prove a prophetic personality. Confronting the dominant formalistic and conservative character of the Christian theology, and life, of his era, without ignoring the ideological environment of his epoch, was a great challenge for him. This was 'a conflict between a scholastic theology removed from the spiritual life, with intense formalistic and conservative elements, and a theology understood as an expression of the Holy Spirit'.[4]

Thus, Symeon, who lived during the first quarter of the eleventh century, and who was aware of the new trends in human life, witnessed the power of the incipient individualism and felt a responsibility as a spiritual father properly to express Christian teaching on the matter. The association of Symeon with individualism does not correspond to his characterisation as a representative of monastic individualism, which would claim that Symeon underlines the individual way to salvation, and considers that to be occupied with society or other monks is a distraction.[5] On the contrary, the link that is made between Symeon and individualism is connected with his presence in a society where the emphasis on the individual is a point of reference in ideological discussions and social norms. It is for this reason that, in order to properly understand his ideas, his theological arguments need to be set side by side with those of Michael Psellos, who represents the ideological principles of the eleventh century and who is considered 'a philosopher who took the trouble to give the subject a more substantial role in intellectual life'.[6]

---

diplomacy and the themes of the empire – *De cerimoniis* (Περὶ βασιλείου τάξεως), *De administrando imperio* (Περί τὸν ἴδιον υἱὸν Ρωμανόν) and *De thematicus* (Περὶ θεμάτων) (Lemerle, *Le premier humanisme byzantin*, pp. 248-54).

3. Ibid., pp. 269-76.
4. Krivocheine, *St Symeon the New Theologian*, p. 45. The conflicts between Symeon and the incumbent ecclesiastical authorities as well as with his fellows in the monastery of St Mamas have been extensively discussed. See, for example, Spidlik, 'Syméon le Nouveau Théologien', DS XIV, pp. 1395-97; Turner, 'St Symeon the New Theologian and Dualist Heresies: Comparisons and Contrasts', pp. 363-64.
5. Kazhdan and Epstein, *Change in Byzantine Culture in the Eleventh and Twelfth Centuries*, pp. 90-92.
6. Duffy, 'Hellenic Philosophy in Byzantium and the Lonely Mission of Michael

It is within such a context that Symeon's contribution to a modern moral issue such as euthanasia has to be viewed. Symeon is presented as challenging the sovereign role of individualism through the introduction of the 'Trinitarian' consideration of human existence and a Christian view of the inner state of human existence. The challenge to individualism by no means represents a devaluation of each person's own individuality. On the contrary, man's individuality reaches its highest point in the Christian consideration of the willingness to die and voluntary death.

I. The Trinitarian Character of Human Life

The importance of knowledge and, in particular, of self-knowledge, that is the knowledge of the character of one's own existence, has already been discussed with reference to the theology of John Damascene. John prioritises self-knowledge through the communication with and the union to God over self-preservation, since one's own self-knowledge is a condition *sine qua non* for a human being authentically to exist. In the works of Symeon, the role of a particular kind of knowledge, namely of self-knowledge through the proper knowledge of God, is emphasised even more so. Mainly in his *Hymnes*, but also in his *Theological Orations*, Symeon attempts to deal with human life by drawing a direct parallel between God and man. It should be mentioned here that Symeon was a representative of mystical theology, which expounded direct personal communication with and the vision of God through proper ascesis. Therefore, he is interested in establishing a way of life that would bring the divinity and humanity, the immanent and the transcendent, together and in fighting against any metaphysical orientation.

For Symeon, the knowledge of God is life itself and, therefore, anyone who wants to live must know God. This knowledge of God is the knowledge of the doctrine of the Trinity, and particularly the knowledge of the three hypostases along with their personal properties (unborn, begotten and proceeding). Moreover, the knowledge of God is the knowledge of the truth that God is the Creator and Maker of all things and beings that coincides with the awareness that God is the Principle and the Cause (ἡ ἐπίγνωσις τῆς ἀρχῆς καὶ αἰτίας) of all things and of human beings.[7] Indeed, since the beginning of human existence traces back to God, the knowledge of God is necessary for a human being to exist. This idea is extensively discussed in Symeon's theological orations.

Psellos', p. 154.

7. Hymn II, ll. 77-115.

God has created man according to His own image. Accordingly, man is endowed with divine properties that allow him to know the things about God (τὰ περὶ Θεοῦ) as well as that God is the Father and the Creator of man. This knowledge is possible because the parallelism between God and man is possible as well. This correspondence is not only based on Christology but also on the doctrine of the Trinity.[8] Before presenting Symeon's thought it is necessary to set the historical context of his era and understand the contemporary ideology and its implications for human life.

The doctrine of the Trinity featured in discussions in Symeon's era, even in the secular context. During the tenth century the presence of Islam on the Byzantine borders resulted in philosophical clashes between the two worldviews, such as worries that the doctrine of the Trinity violated the Divine Monad. This issue was also debated in the philosophical circles of the Byzantine capital, as is apparent from the writings of Michael Psellos and the equivalence that he attempts to draw between the Holy Trinity and the soul. As was pointed out in the general introduction to this book, Psellos' philosophical and theological thought is considered representative of the ideological environment of the era in which Symeon lived.

Psellos says that the character of the soul resembles the Holy Trinity since it has a threefold character – mind, word and spirit. However, while he emphasises the fact that the Holy Trinity is made up of three hypostases and is characterised by a monarchy (μοναρχία), he fails to draw the same conclusions about the soul, since he thinks that the soul before the fall is different to the soul of the fallen man and, thus, the parallelism between the soul and the Holy Trinity may refer only to the condition of the soul before the fall. The monarchy of the Holy Trinity indicates that the Holy Trinity has one nature and is characterised by a unity of opinion (σύμπνοια γνώμης) and a sameness of movement (ταυτότητα κινήσεως). On the contrary, the presence of the oneness of the nature, the unity of opinion and the sameness of movement characterises the soul only before the fall.[9] Therefore, fallen man has in fact a fragmented soul, which in its fallen state is unable to use God's prototype or archetype for his salvation. Though the Holy Trinity is the most radical anti-individualistic model, a human being who is shorn of the possibility of profiting from God's prototype is a human being with a fragmented soul and, therefore, one perfectly adaptable to an individualistic and individualised society.

Symeon is aware of the theological speculation that rules out applying the doctrine of the Trinity to the human realm. Therefore, Symeon's use

8. Theol. II, 63-190; Theol. I, 217-39.
9. Theol. Ps II, 3, 585-629, and Theol. Ps I, 62, 242-46.

of the parallelism between the Holy Trinity and the soul is not accidental. Though he does not directly enter into a detailed discussion about this parallelism, he refers to its important implications for understanding humankind.

Just as the three hypostases of the One and Trinitarian God are co-eternal and co-essential, without confusion or division, and are conceived as one sole Principle of all things, similarly, the image of God in man signifies the tripartite soul, that also includes mind and reason, and where there is no pre-existence or division or confusion between the three parts (ψυχὴν ζῶσαν καὶ ἐνυπόστατον . . . αὕτη δὲ τριμερίς ἐστι, νοῦν καὶ λόγον τὰ συνεπόμενα ἔχουσα).[10] Symeon, while he makes it clear that the soul is tripartite, is careful not to introduce any kind of trichotomy by pointing out that:

> in yourself the mind, the reason and the soul [*τὸν ἐν σοὶ νοῦν σὺν τῷ λόγῳ καὶ τῇ ψυχῇ*] are of equal honour [ἰσότιμον], of the same honour [ὁμότιμον] and consubstantial [ὁμοούσιον] since they are of the same essence and of the same nature [ὡς μιᾶς ὄντα οὐσίας καὶ φύσεως].[11]

Since the knowledge of the Triune God becomes indispensable for the understanding of human existence, those human beings who ignore their Creator lack reason and resemble non-rational beings.[12] Such a person ignores that he has fallen into a condition that is characterised by the loss of rationality, the loss of self-knowledge and the ignorance of God. It was the fall that resulted in the blindness of the soul and, therefore, the blindness of the divine properties in man and in man's unwillingness to gain the knowledge and the vision of God.[13]

Thus, regarding the parallelism to the Holy Trinity, while Psellos identifies the problem of fallen man in the inevitably fallen human nature,[14] which implies that any parallelism between the Holy Trinity

10. Theol. II, 63-190.
11. Ibid., 138-40.
12. Hymn XXIII, ll. 527-41.
13. See, for example, Hymn XLV, ll. 50-76, and Hymn LIII, ll. 133-83 and 228-33. The idea of the blindness of the soul is central to Symeon's thought given that he deals with the possibility of the vision of God even in this life. Krivocheine has systematically elaborated Symeon's ideas regarding the vision of the divine light (Krivocheine, *St Symeon the New Theologian*, pp. 215-38).
14. The emphasis on the role of nature in the writings of Michael Psellos has been widely acknowledged. Meyendorff says that Psellos, whose thought system is based on Ancient Greek philosophy, acknowledges the competence of the

and the soul refers to the condition of man before the fall and is not applicable to the fallen state of humanity, Symeon points out that what makes the difference between the paradisiacal life and the life of the fallen man is the use of the reason with which God endowed man. For Symeon, an argument from the nature cannot justify the elimination of the Trinitarian character of human life, a character that corresponds to the most radical anti-individualistic model of human existence.

The relevance of the Trinitarian life to human life is further established in Hymn XLIV, which, according to its epigraph, is devoted, among other things, to designating the meaning of the creation of man according to the image of God.[15] In this particular hymn, Symeon reinstates the likeness between the tripartite soul and the image of God, and the Holy Trinity, in man, in order to reach the knowledge of God and the proper self-knowledge that secures the rational character of man. Yet, in this hymn, the Holy Trinity is not only a prototype for the unity or the distinctive character of the constituent parts of the human soul. It rather signifies the possibility of imitating God and particularly of becoming gods by grace.[16] This idea is stressed even more in a catechetical sermon by Symeon:

> How great the marvel! Man is united with God both spiritually and physically [ἄνθρωπος Θεῷ ἑνοῦται πνευματικῶς τε καὶ σωματικῶς], since the soul is not separated from the mind or the body from the soul. Through such union man becomes, in essence [οὐσιωδῶς], a three-hypostases being [τρισυπόστατος] like the Holy Trinity by grace [κατὰ χάριν]. He becomes one with God in position [θέσει], with his body, his soul, and the divine Spirit of whom he partakes.[17]

Needless to say, Symeon does not want to violate the Christian dogma that states that it is not possible for man to participate in the essence of God. He simply attempts to show that such a union leads to the restoration

---

ancients in understanding the natures of beings and is in favour of 'a basis for a natural knowledge, a knowledge of the Creator through the creatures' (Meyendorff, *Byzantine Theology*, p. 61). In the same vein, Kazhdan and Epstein point out that Psellos' thought is characterised by an appreciation of the material life that leads to a kind of naturalism (Kazhdan and Epstein, *Change in Byzantine Culture in the Eleventh and Twelfth Centuries*, pp. 210-20).

15. The epigraphs to Symeon's hymns were added after his death by Nicetas Stethatos and his fellows and function as introductions to the text that follows. (Afentoulidou, 'Οἱ ὕμνοι τοῦ Συμεὼν τοῦ Νέου Θεολόγου: σχέσεις τῶν ἐπιγραφῶν μὲ τοὺς ὕμνους', p. 128).
16. Hymn XLIV, ll. 28-165.
17. Cat. XV, 72-77.

of the image of God as well as to the Trinitarian interpretation of human existence and he, therefore, wishes to highlight the proximity between the divinity and humanity.

Returning to Hymn XLIV, though man has been endowed with the image of God and, therefore, can become like God, this can take place only once man has been cleansed of his passions, has become full of self-sacrificial love towards others, and loves his enemies and is concerned for their salvation. Love of one's enemies is a precondition *sine qua non* for man to proceed along the path of deification. Once such a condition is fulfilled the Holy Spirit as unspeakable light teaches man the intelligible things. As a result, man becomes an imitator of God and God by grace. Interestingly, the love of one's enemies has to extend up to the point of sacrificing one's own life for the salvation of others as an imitation of God (ὑπέρ πάντων δὲ τιθέναι τὴν ψυχήν σου καθ' ἑκάστην).[18] Obviously, Symeon accepts the voluntary self-relinquishment of one's own life, though for a particular purpose.

In other words, though man has been endowed with divine properties and his soul can be considered as parallel to the Holy Trinity, such a parallelism makes sense and its potential is accomplished when, and only when, man becomes able to love his enemies. Consequently, the Trinitarian character of the soul implies a Trinitarian interpretation of human life that is designated not only by each individual and God but also by other people, such as one's enemies. Such a Trinitarian view of human life culminates in the inclusion of God Himself in the definition of man, for 'God, soul and body are the man, who is created according to the image of God and made worthy of becoming God'.[19] This inclusion of God in the definition of man lays the foundations for a genuine human existence that by definition has a double orientation, namely towards God and one's fellow human beings.

To sum up, Symeon establishes the relationship between God and man according to the most radical relational model. The resemblance of man to God, and particularly to the Holy Trinity, is not limited to the constitution of the soul, but rather it is represented in the loving relationship between all human beings including the enemies in one's own life. Man does not completely depend on his fallen state as Psellos believes. On the contrary, he is able properly to use the divine property of reason to imitate God and become God by grace. In any case, human life has to pass through the stage of exercising love towards God and one's fellow men, given that God is the common Principle and Cause of all things. It is for this reason that self-knowledge and the knowledge of God become crucial in Christian life.

18. Hymn XLIV, ll. 40-164.
19. Eth. VI, 176-78.

II. The Inner State of Man and Man's Double Character

While reason in man is of great importance for human life, it does not coincide with the definition of man, since man is more than a soul. Symeon, following Christian tradition on this issue, says that man is the only creature who consists of soul and body. He borrows the idea that the double character of man signifies a union of the visible and invisible worlds that makes man a mortal and immortal animal (ζῶον θνητὸν καὶ ἀθάνατον), who is visible and invisible (ὁρατὸν καὶ ἀόρατον), sensible and knowledgeable (αἰσθητὸν καὶ νοούμενον), and supervisor of the visible and wise of the knowledgeable (ἐποπτικόν τῆς ὁρωμένης κτίσεως, γνωστικὸν τῆς νοουμένης).[20] However, he also attributes to man a kind of relationship between the immanent and the transcendent. For example, Symeon connects the presence of soul and body in man with the experience of the shining of two suns, namely the visible sun and the invisible Sun that is God Himself. The former, the sensible sun, shines over the visible world (i.e. the body) whereas the latter, God, shines over the knowledgeable world (i.e. the soul).[21] Consequently, what is particularly important is the identification of the relationship between soul and body in man, and both of them with God. A discussion on the relationship between the soul and body follows in the next section.

1. The Union of Soul and Body: against Dualism and Rationalism

The description of the relationship between soul and body always risks the loss of balance regarding the dual character of humanity and the proper placement of reason within it. The attribution of a double character to the constitution of man and the designation of the proper relationship between the soul and body has been an issue that has occupied not only Christian theologians but also philosophers and a variety of thinkers throughout the centuries. It may be traced back to ancient Greek philosophy and the tradition of Plato. In the Church different interpretations developed. Some of these resulted in the so-called dualistic heresies. Symeon's era also saw the appearance of such heretical doctrines.[22] These heresies, along with the rise of individualism and the consequent tendency to base human life on the power of reason

20. See, for example, St Gregory Nazianzus' Oration 38 (PG, 36, 324A) and John Damascene's *An Exact Exposition of the Orthodox Faith* (Expos. 26, 24-30).
21. Cent. 2, ch. 22-23.
22. Hussey, *The Orthodox Church in the Byzantine Empire*, pp. 156-66.

reveal an interplay between dualism and rationalism. Symeon developed his theological work within this context. Once more, Psellos' writings are very indicative of the ideas regarding the relationship between soul and body that dominate this era.[23]

Psellos' writings present thoroughly the common ground that both dualism and rationalism share. Given that Psellos accepts the existence of a tripartite soul – mind (νοῦς), word (λόγος) and spirit (πνεῦμα),[24] he elaborates his main assumption that the mind has greater value even compared to the soul. The mind is considered eternal and immovable as well as a principial essence (οὐσίαν ἀρχικήν), whereas the soul is thought of as self-moved and changeable. The mind is neither a servant to the soul, a power of the soul, nor the eye of the soul.[25] Inevitably, the overemphasis on mind leads to rationalism. As a consequence, the transition from rationalism to dualism is to be expected.

We saw that Psellos, when discussing the tripartite character of the soul before the fall, notices that the soul had a character parallel to the Holy Trinity in such a way that it was not divided into three separated things, but rather it was united into one in terms of the sameness of opinion and movement. Psellos also points out that the soul was united with the body, and both of them were considered as one in relation to God.[26] Though such union and oneness is in fact an indication that both soul and body are oriented towards the union of man to God, this interpretation is quite foreign to the thought of Psellos. Rather, he favours rationalism and believes that the vision of God is possible only through the soul, and after successful efforts have been made for it to break away from the body. According to him, the proximity of man to God is proportional to the distance between soul and body.[27] Interestingly, Psellos goes a bit further and says that the union with God is only possible through the mind and by those who consider themselves as only mind.[28] He blames

23. The consequences of the absence of a synchronic consideration even of Psellos' arguments are visible in Karahalios' 'Michael Psellos on Man and His Beginnings'. Karahalios, although he presents a number of Psellos' phrases regarding his anthropology, fails to realise the implications of such phrases not only for Psellos' theological arguments but also for understanding the cultural environment of Psellos' era. For example, while he talks about 'a clear dividing line between the two' (ibid., p. 83), namely soul and body, he does not draw attention to the self-evident dualism that governs Psellos' thought.
24. Theol. Ps II, 3, 585-97.
25. Ibid., 21, 95-96.
26. Ibid., 62, 67-70.
27. Theol. Ps I, 30, 121-26.
28. Ibid., 64, 89-95 and 247-52.

the body for the tripartite character of the soul, which was a consequence of the union of the soul with the body. It is for this reason that the soul must be separated from the body. This division liberates the soul from the non-rationality of the body, and is a prerequisite for the union of the soul, the reason and the mind with the perfect mind.[29] In other words, it is the union of the soul with the non-rational body that keeps man away from God, since the proximity between man and God depends upon the free and uncommitted expression of the human mind, which is rationality.

Undoubtedly, Symeon wanted to fight against such widespread trends in Byzantine thought. He therefore denounced any dualistic approach within the Christian tradition. To start with, on the basis of the parallelism between the Holy Trinity and human life that results in the imitation of God that has already been discussed, Symeon declares that the imitation of God by man has an immediate impact on the body, which becomes incorruptible.[30] Though the image of God in man is only connected with the soul, which is the starting point towards the deification of humans, it finally entails also the second element of human nature, namely the body, given that the body is not excluded from receiving the divine grace that is given if one follows a proper way of life.[31] This idea is further stressed in another idea that has already been discussed, that the image of God in man also should be seen in terms of God the Trinity. Symeon points out that God Himself is included in man, since he has been endowed with the divine image, an image that is connected with the bodily aspect of humanity as well.[32]

Soul and body are not simply placed side by side with regard to the relationship between God and man. For Symeon, there is a special relationship and interaction between the soul and body, which is very important for man to draw towards God. What is crucial in order to understand the relationship between soul and body is the way in which they change and, consequently, influence human life. Symeon has devoted one of his *Catecheses* to this issue. He states that both soul (along with the mind) and body change but in a different way and for different reasons:

29. Ibid., 30, 105-08.
30. Hymn XLIV, ll. 141-65.
31. In the same line of thought Ware says that: 'Symeon insists with great emphasis upon the unity of man's nature: Christ and the Holy Spirit take possession of the *whole* man, body as well as soul; salvation is not for the intellect alone, but man's material nature is redeemed and glorified along with his soul' (Ware, 'The Mystery of God and Man in St Symeon the New Theologian', p. 233).
32. Eth. VI, 176-78.

> The body in particular is subject to much change that, for the most part, takes place by nature [ἐκ φύσεως . . . μεταβολή]. The soul is by nature and essence immutable [ἄτρεπτος], and so is the mind, which the Creator has formed simultaneously with it. Both of them are moved by free intention [τῇ προαιρέσει ἀγόμενα], and by their own will [τῷ ἰδίῳ θελήματι] they lay hold on virtue or vice . . . the soul and the mind adhere to the one or the other of these by their own free will and intention, as I have said, either to goodness, so that they become good, or to wickedness, and so become wicked. The body, however, is by nature subject to change [τρεπτόν] because it is composite [σύνθετον]; in essence it is changeable since it is created out of corruptible and changeable matter, being a mixture or a compound of mutually opposite elements. . . . As such the body has neither liberty nor will [ἐστέρηται καὶ προαιρέσεως καὶ θελήσεως], and, if I must say so, not even movement, unless one were to call its mutability and its tendency to move toward corruption a natural movement of its substance, which would be a non-rational [ἄλογος] one. But if it is non-rational, it is clear that it is also non-sinful and without condemnation before God.[33]

What makes the difference between the soul and body, in terms of their changeable character, is the presence of free will in the soul and its absence in the body. On the one hand, since the body changes by nature, the alterations are towards its absolute corruption. On the other hand, even though the soul does not change regarding its nature and essence, it is moved by the free will and changes in terms of its ethical status. Therefore, the soul can turn from goodness to wickedness according to its own intention and will. This conclusion is a clear indication that the total responsibility of any decision is attributed to the soul once the changes of the body are considered as non-rational (changes that are not subject to reason). As a result, the body cannot be blamed, even for those actions that are accomplished through it.[34] Obviously, any argument that derives from the bodily condition in order to justify particular actions by human beings is not legitimate. Any justification for any action has to be primarily linked with the movements of the soul and mind and not those of the body. This statement opposes dualistic beliefs, such as those of Psellos, since it reveals that the body is not connected with what is 'good' or 'bad' and, therefore, it is not responsible for the destiny of man.

33. Cat. XXV, 53-73.
34. Ibid., 72-84.

The Christian tradition posits that free will, and not nature, determines the character of human life, and that free will is responsible for whatever happens in human life, whether good or bad.

While the body should not be blamed for any human action, it is the body that affects both soul and mind:

> Sometimes the vicissitudes that take place in the mind cause the soul to become oppressed. . . . Sometimes the mind shares in the sufferings of the soul, and so is compelled to be in the night. . . . Sometimes both [soul and mind] are tyrannically oppressed by the vicissitudes of the body, at times burdened from without, yet while they are aware of their burden they keep intact their peace. At other times they are agitated and perturbed from within are totally subject to passions, to the extent that the sufferer loses hope of ever returning to his past equilibrium and calm. So then the soul and the mind are troubled by the body, the mind by the soul itself, and the soul in turn by the mind and the body.[35]

There is, at first sight, an inconsistency in Symeon's thought, since, on the one hand, he states that the body is not responsible for its movements, while, on the other, he says that it is considered responsible for any afflictions that are placed upon both the soul and mind. The latter statement may imply that the body becomes in a way the cause for taking particular decisions regarding one's own life, such as limiting the afflictions from body on soul by any means. However, what Symeon wants to do is to highlight the crucial role of the soul with respect to the ethical orientation of each human life.

God created man from soul and body in order to be the master of the soul and the sovereign of the body.[36] Regardless of the movements of the body, the soul has to rule over it and not to be governed by it. Though one may argue that the fall has disturbed the course of human life, for Symeon, the soul remains able to fulfil its purpose. Symeon reminds his reader of the case of Job, who, while he was suffering afflictions in his body, did not experience suffering in his soul due to the fact that his soul was protected by God. For anyone whose soul is not protected by God and is poisoned by sin, his suffering is ten times worse than the plague of Job.[37] Similarly, everyone, through his relation to God and the spiritual health that is given to the heart by God, can prevent the afflictions of the body from touching his soul, since the joyfulness of the soul that results

35. Ibid., 177-92.
36. Ibid., 85-92.
37. Cat. XXIII, 53-57.

from its health does not derive from this world, and as such cannot be influenced by the health of the body.[38] In other words, it is through God that man, even in his fallen state, can challenge the afflictions that are imposed on the soul by the body. Once spiritual health is secured, the corruptible body, though real and existent, may not perturb the peace of the soul. This does not imply that the body is the prison of the soul from which the soul has to be freed. It rather implies that the body is an indispensable constituent part in the human journey towards union with God and the vision of God.[39]

Such a position has immediate implications for issues relevant to the afflictions of the body, such as unbearable suffering during an illness. Since the soul should rule over the body, any decision on euthanasia should not be based on illness and suffering that derive from the body. Such decisions have to be founded on other arguments. Similarly, since the changes of the body have their cause in nature and not in free will, they should not be allowed to shape human life. The soul and its free will must do so. However, the soul is changeable, and so is its temper, which may vary from the desire to die to uncontrollable rejoicing.[40] Therefore, decision-making on the administration of death in the medical context has to take a sceptical approach, given not only that these decisions deal with the destiny of human existence but also that the desire of the soul may change.

The modern discussion on euthanasia revolves around the character of the medical context, which is based on the coexistence of dualism and rationalism. While it would tend to support the autonomy of the patient, and, consequently, the authority of his free will to decide on matters related to the destiny of his life, the medical context is at the same time occupied with the destiny of the body only. Though such an environment, by definition, can only elaborate arguments that are strictly connected

38. Ibid., 112-23.

39. Symeon notes that the heaviness of the body is an expression of the divine Providence and its educational orientation towards the virtue of lowliness (Cat. XXV, 156-59). This virtue is prerequisite regarding the relationship of man to God. The following passage is very indicative: 'The very weight of our body, which apart from any other cause, solely on account of vanity, or pride, or the mutual accusation of carelessness, or for many other reasons, delivers us to this demon for the destruction of our flesh and the affliction of the soul. But it is also for the testing and the greater training of the soul, in order that we recognize God's compassion and mercy towards us, and turn our whole love toward Him with full purpose, and attain to an exclusive desire for Him' (ibid., 159-67).

40. Ibid., 21-25.

with the bodily condition, it bases arguments on the patient's free will, a matter that is out of its context. Without a doubt, this environment is not the most suitable one for taking a decision regarding the end of life.

2. The Separation of Soul and Body on Death: Mercy or Punishment?

Despite the relationship between soul and body, their separation comes inevitably. Thus, in order to reach a better understanding of what soul, body and death stand for, it is necessary to identify the character of this division.

One may argue that, due to the fall, the entry of corruption and death that is particularly visible in the body is indicative of the natural trend towards the dissolution of the union between the soul and body. Therefore, what is natural (natural in the sense that it has been given by God) coincides with the separation between the soul and body. If so, Psellos' argument that the soul has to be freed from the body as a necessary precondition towards the vision of God is closer to the Christian tradition than Symeon's position. However, both the hypothesis and the conclusion are far from true.

Death entered into human life after Adam and Eve disobeyed God's commandment not to eat the fruit of the tree of knowledge of good and evil. Adam and Eve first suffered from the death of their souls, that is called a 'psychic' death (ψυχικόν θάνατον), and later from the death of their bodies, that is called bodily death (σωματικόν θάνατον).[41] At first sight, the entry of death into human life appears to be a form of punishment from God, because His rational creatures were disobedient to Him. However, Symeon does not consider death in human life as a punishment. Rather, bodily death, the dissolution of the union between the soul and body has a merciful character.

The idea behind this assertion, that of 'merciful death', is that death, as the dissolution of the union between the soul and body, is much preferred to the coupling of the corruptible with the incorruptible (the coupling of the corruption that entered human life after the fall with eternal life). Symeon exemplifies the merciful character of death with reference to the lepers who plead to God to free them from their body, since their suffering made their life intolerable in such a way that life was worse than death. It is for this reason that what is generally considered as a punishment, i.e. death, is in fact merely mercy and divine economy.[42]

41. Eth. II, ch. 7, 82-92; Eth. I, ch. 3, 66-69.
42. Hymn LIII, ll. 270-89.

It must be noted that in the thought of Symeon, death is synonymous with the end of the life that resulted from the fall. This life is not the kind of life that man was created for but it is rather indicative of the fallen state of humanity and man's subjection to suffering.[43] Therefore, death that puts an end to a life that is characterised by suffering is nothing but mercy. It is not accidental that Symeon says elsewhere in the same hymn that, while death is mercy, it has been considered by all as punishment (καὶ τοῖς πᾶσιν ἐλογίσθη ἄφυκτος ὡς τιμωρία),[44] implying a view that was very popular and widely accepted at that time even within the Church, a view that he wanted to challenge. Thus, he gives a detailed account of the merciful character of death:

> The death of human beings is the death of difficulties; death is the deliverance from cares; death is freedom from diseases and passions; death is the severance from sins and injustice; death is the remission from all bad things in life; it is the cause of endless joy, of eternal luxury, of the eternal light.[45]

Interestingly, considering this quote in terms of Symeon's wider thought reveals much more than simply the attribution of a merciful character to death. It was argued above that the parallelism between the Holy Trinity and human life signifies, among other things, man's voluntary choice to imitate God in order to become God by grace. Also, this orientation entails even the voluntary self-relinquishment of one's own existence. In such a context, the Christian life is a life of voluntary decisions, where man has always to pursue whatever brings him closer to God or makes him like God. If so, the fact that Symeon calls death 'freedom from diseases' or 'remission from all bad things in life' clearly implies that death falls into the spectrum of human responsibility. Consequently, decisions on euthanasia, as decisions that deal with the deliberate administration of death in the medical context, are not *a priori* to be excluded from consideration in terms of the Christian point of view, though the context in which euthanasia is discussed today is quite different from the context of Christian thought, such as that of Symeon.

In the same vein, if God brought death into human life as a form of punishment, He is the only Being responsible for fulfilling the process of corruption in human life up to death. This means that man has no legitimate right in that process and, therefore, no responsibility with

43. Genesis 3:17-18.
44. Hymn LIII, ll. 239-42.
45. Ibid., 290-302.

regard to the decisions on euthanasia. Man must only endure this punishment. According to such a line of thought, not only is God accused of being responsible for the presence of something bad in human life, that is corruption and death, but also man is deprived of his free will in the most crucial and decisive dilemmas of his life – dilemmas that have spiritual implications as they affect the human being as a whole (the endurance of bodily suffering is not irrelevant to the condition of the soul, given their internal interdependence). On the contrary, if death is not a punishment but a form of mercy, then death must be viewed positively once it is considered as a passage towards endless joy, eternal luxury and the eternal light. In such a context, man takes full responsibility to treat death and the coming of death through the progressive presence of corruption as a means towards God. Indeed, death is not only the end of a procedure but also the last means to accomplishing the purpose of Christian life in this world. Therefore, the role of free will in the coming of death is justified and the widespread belief that Christians have to let things happen as they come, especially those things that are related to the uncontrollable corruption of the body, is at least disputable.

In short, since the entry of corruption and death into human life does not have its principle and cause in God Himself, it cannot be considered as 'natural', but rather it should be seen as a merciful action of God. Given that the life of man should be a voluntary movement towards God and that the coming of death is a form of mercy, just like all gifts of God to man, then man has to adopt the proper approach even towards his own death.

III. Recommended Voluntary Death

The proper treatment of one's own death is exemplified in Symeon's recommendation to voluntary death (κατὰ προαίρεσιν, κατὰ πρόθεσιν). One could easily conclude that Symeon equates voluntary death with spiritual death or the death of the passions. Could voluntary death also include the death of the body and the acceptance of a kind of euthanasia (*εὐ-θάνατος*), namely a good kind of voluntary bodily death?

The recommendation to voluntary death has its roots in the death of Christ. Symeon devotes Ethical Oration XI to the meaning of the death of Christ and its possible implications for the life of Christians. The title of this oration, 'On the Life-giving Mortification of Jesus and God that is Experienced with Keen Perception [*εὐαισθήτως*] by the Perfect Ones',[46] includes a phrase that was extensively discussed by scholars in the field. The whole discussion regarding this phrase has been elaborated in terms

46. Eth. XI, title.

of whether Symeon, not only in this oration but also in other writings, characterises the experience of God in this life as an experience that takes place εὐαισθήτω' (with keen perception or feeling) or αἰσθητῶς (with the sense, sensibly). Krivocheine argues that those who publicised Symeon's writings deliberately replaced the latter with the former in order to prevent the accusation that he was a follower of the Messalian resonance[47] – a teaching that maintained that the Holy Spirit manifests his presence perceptibly and visibly (αἰσθητῶς καὶ ὁρατῶς).[48]

As far as it is known, there are no manuscripts of Ethical Oration XI that use the term αἰσθητῶς, as happens in Catechesis II[49] and Catechesis XXIV.[50] However, regardless of whether Symeon used either the term αἰσθητῶς or the term εὐαισθήτως, or both of them interchangeably, it can be argued that he attached the same meaning to both in his mind, namely the emphasis on the real experience of God by man even in this world. Indeed, what is problematic is not the use of a particular term that could possibly be used by the representatives of a heresy (heresies have always been elaborated on the misunderstanding or misinterpretation of a crucial theological term) but an interpretation that ignores the theological presuppositions behind such use. Since Symeon has been shown to be profoundly anti-dualist, the accusations of a supposed link with the Messalian heresy reveals that his accusers were, though unconsciously, dualists, if they interpreted terms like αἰσθητῶς on dualistic grounds.

In such a context, the 'sensible' experience or the experience 'with keen perception' of the life-giving mortification of Christ by the 'perfect ones', as is proclaimed by the oration's title, is easily identified with Symeon's recommendation to the imitation of the death of Christ and the death of the martyrs through so-called voluntary death, a death that includes not only the soul but also the body.[51] In other words, Symeon, through the use of either the terms αἰσθητῶς or εὐαισθήτως, wants to avoid limiting the experience of God to a 'spiritualised' Christian life, a kind of life that ignores the simple truth that man is not a mere soul but also has a body, and that the two are united without division and confusion.

In short, any aspect of the Christian life, including voluntary death, that limits the involvement of a human being to one of his two constituent natures (either soul or body) is, by definition, dualistic.

47. Krivocheine, *SC*, 96, pp. 151-54.
48. See, for example, John Damascene's treatise on the heresies (*Haeres.*, 80, 140-42).
49. Cat. II, 423.
50. Cat. XXIV, 64.
51. Cat. XII, 252-62.

Similarly, the belief that the presence of God in human life, such as the imitation of the death of Christ, is not something that is experienced αἰσθητῶς and the belief that such an experience is merely a spiritual experience without any participation on the part of the body are also indisputably dualistic.

Let us discuss thoroughly Symeon's thought on the subject of voluntary death. This discussion starts with the spiritual aspect of humanity and proceeds to its bodily aspect.

1. Voluntary Death and the Involvement of the Spiritual and Bodily Aspects of Humanity

The voluntary death that is identified with the imitation of the life-giving mortification of Christ is not an easy endeavour. It is accomplished by the perfect ones (τέλειοι) or those who have achieved significant spiritual progress. Thus, voluntary death could be considered as irrelevant to the great majority of Christians, since it is the end of a procedure that is marked by the successive attainment of a series of virtues that follows spiritual stages. However, at least some of these stages are within the capabilities of all Christians. Symeon notes that to deny that voluntary death is applicable to all Christians derives from a contemporary heretical belief, according to which the period of the great Sts and Fathers had passed, the Holy Spirit does not give the same grace in all historical eras and the communication and union with God in the present life is not possible. Symeon's argument is based on the fundamental assumption that anyone who wants to (θέλων), or has the intention to (προαιρούμενος), is able to become holy and to imitate Christ by adopting the mind of Christ (νοῦν Χριστοῦ) and Christ's way of thinking and life.[52] For Symeon whatever applies to the 'perfect ones' applies also, *mutatis mutandis*, to all Christians.[53]

The first and most crucial stage in this procedure is the attainment of blessed humility (ἡ μακαρία ταπείνωσις) that is achieved through voluntary death.[54] For Symeon, 'blessed humility' does not simply represent a particular disposition at a particular time that ends with so-called voluntary death. It rather entails a whole process whereby, through

52. Cat. XXXIV, 202-27.

53. Symeon devotes Catechesis XXIX to the heresy that states that is not possible for those who wish to reach the summit of virtues and to emulate the Sts of old. Krivocheine in the French translation of the text in *Sources Chrétiennes* identifies this heresy with pusillanimity (SC, 113, p. 165).

54. Eth. XI, 49-53; Eth. IV, 369-72.

the bearing of suffering and shame that usually accompanies the coming of death, man is oriented towards a godlike mind and against a devilish mind. As Christ endured suffering and shame, similarly, man must also go through the same torment.[55]

Symeon identifies humility with the renunciation of man's own will and of the entire world for the sake of God's commandments.[56] It is then not accidental that voluntary death is identified with the mortification of man's own will. Symeon points out that the attainment of holy humility is the end of a task that is accomplished by God Himself, implying the difficulty of this task.[57] Given that the humility that is granted by God is a fundamental presupposition for voluntary death, the latter could be considered as a voluntary project on the part of man and at the same time of God. Thus, voluntary death becomes the outcome of the cooperation between man and God.

This cooperation entails a particular use of free will that is the cornerstone of Christian life. Symeon, based on the Scriptures, clarifies from the beginning of his oration that only those who comprehend with clarity St Paul's words on the proper anticipation of this world understand the experience of the life-giving mortification of Christ by the perfect ones[58] and, consequently, the voluntary death of men:

> And I say this, brothers and sisters: the time is short. So then those who have wives should be as those who have none, those with tears like those not weeping, those who rejoice like those not rejoicing, those who buy like those without possessions, those who use the world as though they were not using it to the full. For the present shape of this world is passing away[59] . . . as dying and yet – see! – we continue to live . . . as having nothing, and yet possessing everything.[60]

---

55. Cat. XXVII, 276-85. Symeon, like St Paul – 'Redeeming the time of our present lives' (Ephesians 5:16), argues that the most proper buying off of the present life is man's courageous and patient bearing of the pains, the sorrows and the tribulations that come upon him (Eth. XII, 87-135). As he states: 'He [God] is aware that he honors his servants with dishonor, enriches them with abject poverty, glorifies them through insults and abuse, and restores them to their heritage and participation in eternal life by means of death [διὰ θανάτου τῆς αἰωνίου ζωῆς μετόχους αὐτοὺς καὶ κληρονόμους ἀποκαθιστᾶ]' (Cent. 3, ch. 70).
56. Eth. I, ch. 12, 172-78.
57. Cent. 1, ch. 91, and Eth. VI, 85-96.
58. Eth. XI, 1-19.
59. 1 Corinthians 7:29-31.
60. 2 Corinthians 6:9.

Symeon combines these two passages from the New Testament in order to show that voluntary death is a death that allows man to reach a proper understanding of life and, consequently, to learn what is the proper way to live one's life in this world. Before man there are two realities, life and death, two worlds, the visible, dissoluble and present world as well as the eternal, invisible and indissoluble one, and two principles. These two principles express two entirely opposite ways of life. There is God, who cares about man's salvation and eternal life, and there is the devil, who, through temporary pleasures, attempts to bring about the death and perdition of all human beings.[61] Therefore, man is called to choose the world upon which he will base his life, given that a mortified will towards one of these worlds leads to a will that is alive towards the other. In this context, the mortification of man's own will is the disposition of being 'dead' to this world and its pleasures. But how is such mortification achieved?

Symeon works out his response to this question based on the Old Testament. He considers the mortification of man's own will as a kind of offering to God and compares it with the offerings made by the Jews at their feasts. Therefore, the mortification of man's own will resembles the sacrifice of the goat, which was one of the offerings on the Day of Atonement. Just as the blood of the goat was brought to make atonement in the holy place and was then taken outside the camp,[62] so each person must die voluntarily outside the Kingdom of Heaven and kill his will before he enters into it and therefore imitates Christ,[63] who suffered outside the camp to sanctify people with his own blood.[64] The 'killing' of the will is the voluntary attachment of man to God and His will contrary to man's attachment to this world.

The attachment of man to God's will along with the vanquishing of his own will is perfectly presented in the distinction that Symeon makes between the 'mortal' (θνητόν), 'fleshly' (σαρκικόν) or 'earthy' (χοϊκόν) way of thinking (φρόνημα) and the spiritual way of thinking. The former represents the attachment of man to evil thoughts, the passions and sin, whereas the latter represents the freedom of man from all these.[65] It is remarkable that, though the spiritual mode of thought represents the particular use of one's own will, it does not signify an individualistic action but rather an action that encompasses all human beings. Symeon

61. Eth. XI, 560-75.
62. Leviticus 16:27.
63. Hebrews 13:12.
64. Eth. XI, 51-61.
65. Cent. 3, ch. 38; Cat. V, 1068-85; and Cat. XII, 6-13.

explains the communal understanding of voluntary death in *Ethical Oration IV*, which is dedicated to the perfection of the Christian life or, as its title indicates, to 'the perfection of the spiritual stature according to Christ' (ἡ τελείωσις τῆς κατὰ Χριστόν πνευματικῆς ἡλικίας).[66]

Once more, humility is the starting point in the way towards voluntary death, a parallel procedure to the construction of the human body. Symeon demonstrates step by step the construction of the spiritual body, which is completed with the head.[67] The head coincides with the exercising of love as Christ exercised it. Thus, the demonstration of this love is the perfection of the spiritual stature according to Christ. This perfection is fulfilled in voluntary death for the sake of Christ, His commandments and the whole world.[68] In other words, voluntary death is oriented towards God and all other people, and therefore, it is profoundly anti-individualistic. Then, could it be argued that in such a context the participation of the body is also identified?

We saw that the voluntary attachment to God's will is a prerequisite for voluntary death. However, this voluntary attachment to God requires man to entrust himself to God. Symeon, like St Paul, says, 'we ourselves had the curse of death within ourselves so that we would not trust in ourselves but in God who raises the dead'.[69] When man stops putting his trust in himself and starts putting his trust in God, he is ready to die the voluntary death. As a result of entrusting oneself to God, when man is disposed towards a voluntary death this penetrates even the bodily aspect of humanity as well. This is evident in the case of St Anthony the Great. Symeon refers to the case of this St to justify the necessity and feasibility of voluntary death, which must happen with eagerness (προθυμία) and will (προαίρεσις).[70] Here is the passage:

> Has he not shut himself up in the tomb as though he were a corpse [ὡς νεκρόν ἑαυτόν ἐν τῷ μνήματι ἔκλεισε], bringing with him nothing of the world, without any anxiety whatever in himself? Was he not dead as a whole [ὅλος ἦν νεκρός] to the world? As he lay in the tomb [κείμενος ἐν τῷ μνημείῳ] was he not seeking God, who was able to give him life and raise him up? Was he not satisfied with dry bread and water? Did he not suffer much harm from the demons and lie half-dead from their unbearable beating [ἡμιθανής ἔκειτο ἐκ τοῦ ἀφορήτου δαρμοῦ]?

66. Eth. IV, title.
67. Ibid., 369-544.
68. Ibid., 548-642.
69. 2 Corinthians 1:9, in Eth. IV, 625-29.
70. Cat. VI, 52-53.

> He was taken into the church as though he were dead [ἐν τῇ ἐκκλησίᾳ ὡς νεκροῦ ἀπενεχθέντος αὐτοῦ], but once he regained consciousness did he not of his own accord go back to face his adversaries? Had he not returned to them and persevered to the end, but stayed in the world though he had delivered himself to death in intention and will [εἰς θάνατον ἐκδεδωκώς ἑαυτόν τῇ προθυμία καὶ προαιρέσει], he would not have been found worthy of the vision of the Master, which he so greatly desired, nor would he have heard His sweet voice. But he sought with all his heart, he knocked without growing weary. He persevered to the end and received the reward of which he was worthy. Since, as we have said, he died in will for Christ [ἀποθανών γάρ, ὡς εἴρηται, τῇ προαιρέσει ὑπὲρ Χριστοῦ], he lay as though he were dead [ἔκειτο ὡσεί νεκρός] until He came who gives life to the dead. He raised him up from hell – by which I mean the darkness of the soul [τοῦ σκότους φημί τοῦ ψυχικοῦ] – and brought him out into the wondrous light of His countenance.[71]

Obviously, at least in the case of St Anthony, even the body participates in the experience of voluntary death. Even though St Anthony did not have to experience the end of his bodily life, something that the martyrs did, he participated in voluntary death as a whole.

Generally speaking, voluntary death expresses the deliberate choice of man to follow God and His will, or the selection of the so-called spiritual way of thinking over the fleshly. This choice is a very difficult and crucial one for human life, just like the choice between life and death, given that it is through voluntary death that eternal life may be obtained as God designated it: 'Die and you will live. You do not will it? Then, you are dead.'[72] For Symeon, the journey towards voluntary death is something that may be traced back to the Scriptures and the sacrifices to God, and it entails both aspects of humanity, that is the soul and body. Though voluntary death is a voluntary task, its accomplishment is a result of cooperation between man and God by virtue of trusting oneself to God. Moreover, this accomplishment encompasses all people since it requires the virtue of love. In short, Symeon systematically liberates man from the individualised and dualistic society of his era and places him in a life that is, by definition, communal, and in which he preserves a unique individuality, where all aspects of a human being and all free beings are involved.

71. Ibid., 42-60.
72. Eth. XI, 46-48.

2. Presuppositions for Voluntary Death

Symeon's belief in the inclusion of bodily death in the context of voluntary death is based on two assumptions. First, bodily death is not a 'definite' death[73] and the willingness to die has as an absolute criterion the belief that the end of life in this world does not signify the end of life. While he supports the willingness to die, he does not consider this as an 'absolute' death since bodily death is not identified with the end of life. Second, the experience of the union of man with God is possible in this life, though it is not permanent and is followed by the breaking away of the soul from God. This separation is so painful that one may wish to seek death in order to be united once more with God.[74] Indeed, both assumptions de-dramatise bodily death and consider it of relative value or as a necessary passage towards everlasting union with God. In this context, the willingness to undergo bodily death seems to be absolutely justified. However, what is of great importance is the designation of particular presuppositions regarding this willingness to die.

The first presupposition is that the 'willingness to die' must always be in constant reference to God. Since God seems to be the only factor that may give meaning to death, Symeon notes that this death has to happen face to face with God (ἀποθανεῖν ἐνώπιον Θεοῦ).[75] This presupposition shows that the 'willingness to die' does not imply a death that is unrelated to the presence of God. It is this presence that Symeon calls the 'vision of the divine light', a vision that must accompany the 'willingness to die'. Despite the fact that all human beings want to live and not to die, Symeon points out that the experience of the 'vision of the divine light' is identified with the acquisition of a seed worthy of dying even if it is required to die several times.[76] Obtaining this 'grain' reminds Symeon of the parable of the mustard seed (κόκκω σινάπεως), according to which the Kingdom of Heaven resembles a mustard seed that a man took and sowed in his field. Despite the fact that this seed is the smallest, when it is fully grown it becomes like a tree so that the wild birds come and nest in its branches.[77] Similarly, Symeon implies that, while the vision of God may be considered as a short-lived experience, such an experience coincides with the experience of the Kingdom of Heaven in this life. Given that death has already been overcome due to this experience, that

73. Hymn XXVIII, ll. 42-47.
74. Ibid., ll. 90-105.
75. Ibid., ll. 1-10.
76. Ibid., ll. 78-99.
77. Matthew 13:31-32.

transgresses death by definition, and that such an experience is worthy of dying, then, the 'willingness to die' is absolutely acceptable. This is principally evident in the death of the martyrs, who died 'in front of God' in a way that would be considered as an offering to God, who is the ultimate judge of all human actions. This disposition is explicitly pictured in the icons of martyrs, such as that of St John the Baptist, in which he is presented as offering his head to God on a platter (ἐπὶ πίνακι τὴν κεφαλὴν).[78]

The second presupposition does not declare something entirely new. It rather stresses even more the importance of the quality of the relationship between man and God regarding the meaning of death. In particular, man has to pass through this death unshamefully (ἀνεπαισχύντως), something that can only be achieved through God. Otherwise, death is not of profit to man.[79] Interestingly enough, Symeon connects the coming of death with a kind of expedience. What is important is not when and how death comes but whether man, through God, has secured the necessary gain for himself. Passing through the doors of death (παρελθεῖν τοῦ θανάτου τὰς πύλας) profits man only when he is in a position not to feel shame for his own life and not to be afraid as Adam was after his disobedience to God.[80]

The absolute character of these presuppositions for achieving a legitimised 'willingness to die' within the Christian context is self-evident if one takes into account what the absence of such presuppositions signifies. This is the case of a Christian who exercises *metanoia* (repentance) with great suffering, and whose relationship to God is characterised by hesitation and double-mindedness (ἐν δισταγμῷ καὶ διψυχίᾳ) and not by absolute trust in the power of God and in God's providence *vis-à-vis* all human beings. As Symeon notes: 'Double-mindedness consists in not giving oneself over completely, even to the point of death, for the Kingdom of Heaven, but being anxious, however little, for the life of one's flesh.' Following the definition of double-mindedness, Symeon suggests that the only thing that man has to care about is that 'he does not kill himself by any means and become a suicide, such as by casting himself down from a precipice or by hanging himself, or by committing some other crime'.[81] One may easily argue that what Symeon says is that God cares even for the body and therefore everyone must avoid suicide. However, it could also be argued that Christians with

78. Mark 6:24-28; Matthew 14:8-11.
79. Hymn XXVIII, 195-203.
80. Genesis 3:10 II.
81. Cat. XXX, 226-239.

double-mindedness are at risk of suicide, whereas those who are willing to give themselves 'over completely, even to the point of death' do not face such a risk. Symeon, with direct reference to the New Testament, justifies both arguments and emphasises not only the interest of God for the needs of the body ('seek first the Kingdom of God and His righteousness and all these things will be added to you'),[82] but also the obligation of every Christian to carry the curse of the death of Christ that implies the imitation of Christ's death in both the soul and body ('we felt that we had received the curse of death; but this happened that we might not rely on ourselves but on God, who raises from the dead').[83]

Importantly, the 'willingness to die' with respect to bodily death is justified for an additional reason. This states that, before death, man can experience the future blessedness only with his soul, whereas after death the body changes to a spiritual body and man experiences God with both his soul and body. The following passage is very representative of Symeon's thought:

> For while they do not receive all the promises here below [οὔτε γὰρ τὰς ἐπαγγελίας ἁπάσας ἐνταῦθα ἀπολαμβάνουσιν], yet neither do they remain without any portion or taste of the things to come by hoping for everything there and merely existing here. . . . It is indeed through death [διά θανάτου] that God arranged to give us the kingdom of the Resurrection, and incorruptibility and all of life everlasting. . . . It is right here already that we receive it all [the future blessedness] by the perception and knowledge of our soul, unless we are in some respect untried with respect to our faith or lacking in our keeping of the divine commandments. In the body, however, we do not yet receive it [σωματικῶς δὲ οὐκέτι]. Just as Christ before His resurrection, we carry around our body as corruptible, and, encompassed and bound by it with respect to our soul, we cannot now accommodate receiving the entire glory, which has been revealed to us. In reflecting that ineffable ocean of glory, we believe we see a single drop of it [ρανίδα βλέπειν ἐκείνου μίαν ἡγούμεθα], and for that reason say that for the moment we see as in a mirror and obscurely. . . . After the resurrection, though, just as He Himself raised His own body from the tomb transformed by His divine power, so shall we, too, all receive our body as itself spiritual, and, having first been likened to Him in our soul, we shall then become like Him in both soul and body

82. Matthew 6:33.
83. 2 Corinthians 1:9; *Cat. XXX*, 241-52.

> [ὁμοιωθησόμεθα αὐτῷ καὶ τότε σωματικῶς τε ἅμα καὶ ψυχικῶς]. This is to say that we shall be like him, human being by nature and gods by grace, just as He Himself is indeed God by nature Who in His goodness has taken on the nature of man. How must those who have accurately understood this mystery long for and desire death [πῶς μὴ ποθοῦσι καὶ ἐπιθυμοῦσι τὸν θάνατον]! As the Apostle says: 'For while we are still in this tent, we sigh with anxiety, awaiting the revelation of the sons of God'.[84]

Thus, after death, man has a complete experience of God and becomes God by adoption while remaining man by nature. Consequently, the 'willingness to die' becomes meaningful once man's participation in the future blessedness by both his body and soul is a prerequisite to become like God. This prerequisite justifies, in the best way, first, the belief that man is not only soul and, second, the certainty that the experience of God by man also passes through the human body. Therefore, given that God created man according to His own image in order to lay the foundations of the deification of man, and that the participation of the body in the future blessedness is necessary for this, the 'willingness to die' becomes not only a legitimate desire but also a task that has to be fulfilled.

In short, both the death of the soul and the death of the body can be placed within so-called voluntary death, a death that does not coincide with any kind of suicide or self-administration of death for three main reasons.

The first reason is that suicide or the self-administration of death are not subject to any pre-condition – apart from one's own existence – such as the spiritual presupposition of the experience of the presence of God in one's own life and the entrustment to God. The Christian 'willingness to die' makes sense only when it is a result of proper spiritual progress and a desire for complete union with God. This assertion means that such a 'willingness to die' is developed within a meaningful context, in which modern individualism is abandoned for a kind of Christian individualism. Though voluntary death is nothing other than the 'individual's' deliberate choice to die, it is a choice made for the sake of God, His commandments and one's fellow human beings. Thus, neither one's individuality nor the societal character of human life is violated. In contrast, suicide or the self-administration of death, at least in the context within which the current discussion on these issues is developed, is basically supported on the grounds of universal principles such as autonomy and self-determination that do not entail any meaningful or societal orientation.

84. Eth. X, 703-37.

The second reason is that the Christian 'willingness to die' is not tied either to a 'spiritualised' consideration of human life or to man as merely a body or physical entity and, therefore, it escapes both Scylla and Charybdis. Indeed, although in this aspiration the 'differentiation' within human existence regarding the status of the soul and body is retained, one also finds a holistic view of human life, either before or after death. On the contrary, the fact that the modern discussion on suicide or the self-administration of death is shaped by remarkable developments in medicine and not, for example, in philosophy, demonstrates its attachment to a particular aspect of humanity, namely the 'creation' of a 'new' human being by bioethics.

The third reason is even more fundamental. Recommended voluntary death clearly implies the proper exercising of the human free will that has to be oriented towards cooperation with God. This cooperation is a condition *sine qua non* for a meaningful and justified 'willingness to die'. What is not necessary is the cooperation with nature and its laws, such as respect for the process of the unavoidable corruption of the human body that results in the dissolution of the union of the body and soul and death. This is a very important point, since it exemplifies that, even though the sovereignty of nature over the human free will is evident (nobody wants to die, yet all men die without exception), nature can be bypassed so that man, through his free will, directly refers to God and His will. This choice implies that the fulfilment of a natural procedure must always be subject to the cooperation of the human free will and the will of God – it need only be repeated in passing that such cooperation is based on the mortification of one's own will for the sake of the divine will and the love of others. The tension that exists between the authority of free will compared to the inescapable authority of human nature as regards the destiny of human existence is easily betrayed, drawing parallels with the thought of Michael Psellos and Symeon the New Theologian.

On the one hand, Psellos, in his philosophical writings, identifies three principles or causes that lead to the dissolution of the union of soul and body. These are the creative word (δημιουργικός λόγος) of God, natural ties (φυσικοί δεσμοί) and man's own choices (κατά προαίρεσιν), such as the choice to die through hanging.[85] These principles or causes represent the three factors that designate the destiny of human life. These factors are providence (ὑπό προνοίας), (human) nature (ὑπό φύσεως) and the disposition towards a particular choice (ἐκ προαιρέσεως).[86] What man

85. Phil. Ps II, 22, 96-98.
86. Ibid., 47, 162.

has to do is to consider all three of them together as much as possible,[87] since it is impossible to distinguish one from the other.[88] In other words, human nature as a decisive factor in human destiny cannot be ignored, or better, cannot be isolated from divine providence and the human will.

On the other hand, taking into account Symeon's theological arguments as presented above, he focusses on the decisive role of the divine and human will. Yet he by no means underestimates human nature, and, in particularly, the human body, for he includes the bodily aspect of humanity in the path towards, and final state of, deification. Even though he acknowledges that the entry of corruption and death is inescapably part of the fallen state of humanity, in his opinion corruptible human nature is not a decisive parameter of human destiny. Obviously, properly exercising one's human will transgresses the natural process through the free disposition of human existence, in both the spiritual and bodily aspects, towards voluntary death.

IV. Recommended Voluntary Death and Life within the Church

The centrality of free will in human life and death is also evident in daily life within the Church. Two examples may be cited. The first is that of the martyrs and the second is participation in the sacraments. The former example is the voluntary death of Christians during periods of persecution, whereas the latter is the sacramental participation of Christians in the voluntary death (ἑκούσιον θάνατον) of Christ. In what follows, the discussion of practical aspects of the Christian life will lead to a further understanding of the 'individualistic' disposition towards voluntary death.

1. The Fearless Approach to Death and the Death of Martyrs

The discussion around euthanasia draws attention to our understanding of death, since euthanasia deals with the coming of our end, which usually provokes unpleasant and undesirable feelings of threat and of being in danger, namely the fear of death.

Given that Symeon is in favour of voluntary death (always in the context of man's orientation towards union with God and the experience of future blessedness in both his soul and body), Symeon's approach towards the fear of death sheds more light on his thought.

87. Ibid., 22, 98.
88. Ibid., 22, 97.

It has already been pointed out that Symeon does not hesitate to say that all Christians may arrive at the summit of virtue and emulate the Sts of old at all periods in the life of the Church. Similarly, he does not see any inconsistency in comparing, on the one hand, the crucifixion and voluntary death of Christ, or the voluntary death of the martyrs, and, on the other, the life of Christians in a peaceful society. However, if the common ground in all these instances is the mortification of one's will, could someone argue that Symeon's focus is limited to the spiritual aspect of human existence?

> I have learned from Scripture and from experience itself that the cross comes at the end for no other reason than that we must endure trials and tribulation and, finally, voluntary death itself [τὸν θάνατον αὐτόν τόν ἑκούσιον]. In times past, when heresies prevailed, many chose such a death through martyrdom and various tortures. Now, when we through the grace of Christ live in a time of profound and perfect peace, we learn for sure that the cross and death consist in nothing else than the complete mortification of one's own will [τὴν παντελῆ τοῦ ἰδίου θελήματος νέκρωσιν]. He who pursues his own will, however slightly, will never be able to observe the precept of Christ the Saviour.[89]

Obviously, the parallel made between the bodily death of Christ and of the martyrs, and the mortification of one's own will by no means excludes the body from the discussion in hand. In addition, this parallelism does not designate that the mortification of one's own will does not entail a bodily death since, according to Symeon, there is no clear-cut distinction between the constituent parts of a human being. For him, there is always an interpenetration between the parts. This is made more explicit in one of Symeon's orations where the parallel between the death of the martyrs and the life of a Christian in an epoch without persecution is drawn. This time Symeon goes a step further and leaves the door open with respect to bodily death accompanying spiritual death:

> they [the martyrs] from the shedding of their own blood, we from the cutting-off of our own will, and by remaining steadfast and keeping before us the curse of death, and by expecting death hourly, readily stretching our necks out to die for every commandment of the Master rather than expecting its

89. Cat. XX, 36-43.

> transgression by even the merest word. We ought, brothers, to despise the present life equally with them [ἐξ ἴσης ἐκείνοις τῶν παρόντων καταφρονῆσαι ὀφείλομεν].[90]

Thus, though the cutting-off, namely the mortification, of one's own will, is a prerequisite for the imitation of the martyrs, it is not sufficient, for one must also 'die' to all things in this life as the martyrs did. The martyrs depised this present life, including even their own bodily death, and so all Christians should do the same, and to the same extent.

In such a context, the fear of death could be considered a permanent state in the life of a Christian, although the disposition towards voluntary death has to always be present.[91] However, the mortification of one's own will, which is the starting point towards voluntary death, abolishes the fear of death:

> Why then, brethren, do we not run toward the merciful God who has so loved us? Why do we not give up our souls to death for Christ our God who has died for us? Why are we fearful and why do we dread our departure from the body? Surely hell is not about to receive or take possession of the souls of those who have hoped in Christ? Can death have any power over the souls that have been sealed by the grace of the all-Holy Spirit and the Blood of Christ? . . . Therefore, as many as lack the seal [ἀσφράγιστοι], run to Him, all who have not been signed [ἀσημείωτοι], hasten to be marked with the sign of the Spirit. But who is he who lacks the seal? He who is frightened of death. . . . Accordingly, let us recall ourselves by salutary repentance [σωτήριος μετάνοια], and do and perform all the things that are well pleasing to Christ, so that we may be marked with His seal and from henceforth live without fear.[92]

For Symeon, the fear of death is abolished when the mortification of one's own will is accompanied by trust in Christ and *metanoia*

90. Eth. X, 598-606.
91. The fear of death coincides with the fear experienced in this life as a conscious or an unconscious feeling, as discussed in the first part of this book. Man is always oriented towards his self-preservation and, consequently, the defeat of his enemies (whoever or whatever they may be) that threaten human existence as a whole, just as bodily death threatens its biological aspect. The belief that facing up to death becomes a problem only when the biological life of a human being is threatened is an illusion.
92. Cat. II, 123-48.

(repentance) as a permanent state of mind.[93] Such interplay derives from a funeral catechesis that Symeon devotes to a monk who deserves to be imitated:

> But not that we have all once again looked over the life of our brother, let us, I entreat, imitate his faith, his struggles, his confession, his penitence, so that we too, when we arrive at our departure from the body, may like him, without fear and perturbation, depart from the body and go off to God. Let us thus dwell in Him with good hope and find our rest in eternal tabernacles, the dwelling place of all those who rejoice where the choir of our blessed and holy fathers abides.[94]

In other words, the abolition of the fear of death depends on the proper use of the human will, faith in God and *metanoia*. The freeing of man from the fear of death depends on the freeing of man from his own will. Once more, Symeon de-dramatises the presence of death in human life and places it within the context of the relationship of man with God. Thus, it is the quality of such a relationship that reveals the meaning of death within human life.

2. Voluntary Death and Participation in the Sacraments

The tripartite norm of will-faith-*metanoia* is also considered as *sine qua non* a condition for proper participation in the sacraments,[95] such as baptism, which is another way to imitate the voluntary death of Christ.

Whoever is baptised is actually baptised into the death of Christ and buried as Christ was buried before his resurrection.[96] However, to be baptised is not an end in itself. Participation in baptism is just the beginning of a process that is completed later. Symeon compares baptism to engagement in order to show that it does not assure either the marriage portion or intercourse. These are ensured after marriage when the faithfulness of the bride to the bridegroom is tested.[97] This comparison shows that participation in the voluntary death of Christ is not completed through baptism. On the contrary, voluntary death

93. Sotiropoulos, *Συμεὼν ὁ Νέος Θεολόγος*, p. 114, and Sotiropoulos, *Οἱ νηπτικοὶ Πατέρες περὶ τῆς κατὰ Χριστὸν τελειώσεως τοῦ ἀνθρώπου*, pp. 80-93.

94. Cat. XXI, 98-106.

95. Konstantinidis, *The Recognition of the Sacraments of Heterodoxies in the Diachronic Relations between Orthodoxy and Roman Catholicism*, p. 58.

96. Romans 6:3-4.

97. Cent. 3, chs 47-52.

concerns the whole, spiritual and bodily, life of a human being, and it goes beyond the event of the sacrament of baptism itself. Baptism is an event in time, but its meaning and implications extend outside time into the whole life of a person.

In the same vein, while Symeon follows St Paul ('For all of you who were baptized into Christ have clothed yourselves with Christ'),[98] and talks of the sensible character of participation in baptism,[99] at the same time he considers the implications of participation in baptism conditional. Once more, the role of the human will becomes crucial. The fact being clothed in the 'image of the Heavenly' is conditional is based on the assumption that, even though man is purified through baptism and can preserve himself undefiled in accordance with the image of God who made him,[100] God does not want to take man's free will away, and for this reason baptism does not involve the provision of perfect grace from God.[101] On the contrary, the grace that comes through the Holy Spirit in baptism is contingent upon accomplishing God's commandments and, as such, it is contingent the particular use of free will.[102] Therefore, despite the fact that Christ became man and that baptism has been given for man's deliverance from the dead, man faces the same dilemma with which Adam and Eve were confronted, that is the choice either to accomplish the commandments of God or to turn away from God.[103] Thus, the redemptive character of baptism does not change human nature itself. Rather, man changes according to his free will:

98. Galatians 3:27; see, for example, Eth. III, 354-61.
99. Symeon argues that those who think that in baptism one is clothed with Christ in a non-sensible way are truly dead and naked regarding their spirituality: 'If the baptized have put on Christ, what is it that they have put on God. He then who has put on God, will he not recognize with his intellect and see what he has clothed himself with? The man who has clothed his naked body feels the garment that he sees, but the man who is naked in soul will not know that he has put on God. If he who is clothed with God does not perceive Him, what has he put on in fact? According to you, God would be nothing at all. For, if He were something, those putting Him on would know it. When we put nothing on, we feel nothing, but whenever we are clothed by ourselves or by others, so long as our senses are intact, we are quite aware of it. Only the dead feel nothing when they are clothed, and I am very much afraid that those who say such things are the ones who are really and truly dead and naked' (Eth. V, 60-73).
100. Cat. XXX, 129-32.
101. Cent. 3, ch. 45.
102. Ibid., ch. 89.
103. Eth. XIII, 184-213.

> If men give way to the promptings of the evil one [τοῦ πονηροῦ θελήμασιν εἴκοντες] after their baptism and put these decisions into effect, they cut themselves off from the holy womb of baptism in accordance with the saying of David.[104] But no one can become something else or change his nature. It has been fixed from creation itself. Each man is created good by God because God has never made evil. Each is created unchangeable in nature and essence. Each wishes and wills according to his own voluntary opinion [ἐξ' ἑκουσίου γνώμης προαιρεῖται καὶ θέλει], either for good or for evil. Whether a sword be used for good or for evil does not change its proper nature: it remains steel. And it is the same when a man stirs into action, as I have said; he does what he wills [ἅπερ βούλεται], but he does not change his own nature.[105]

As in the death of the martyrs, similarly in baptism, exercising one's free will plays the most crucial role. Even though baptism represents the death of Christ and participation in it coincides with the imitation of the death of Christ, such an act involves both the body and soul and it is subject to one's willingness to fulfil its implications to the necessary extent.[106]

To sum up, practical life within the Church is a good indication of the character of voluntary death in the Christian tradition. Both the imitation of the death of martyrs and participation in the sacraments reveals that the Christian life is not limited to any particular aspect of the human being. On the contrary, such a way involves every part of man and covers human life as a whole, without excluding even the extremes of life, namely the coming of death and death itself. Such a holistic approach is characterised by the freedom of man to decide to live either an individualistic life or a life in which the aim is the experience of God and eventually union with Him. The union with God coincides with

104. 'The wicked turned aside from the womb, speakers of lies go astray from the womb' (Psalms 58:3).

105. Cent. 3, ch. 90.

106. The same idea is identified in the Eucharist, which is another way of bringing together human life and the voluntary death of Christ ('For every time you eat this bread and drink the cup, you proclaim the Lord's death until he comes', 1 Corinthians 11:26). Symeon says: 'Through Holy Baptism and the Communion of His undefiled Mysteries, His body and His precious Blood, He cleanses us and gives us life, and restores us to holiness and sinlessness. More than that, He sends us forth to enjoy the honour of liberty, so that we may not appear to serve our Master by compulsion, but out of free choice' (Cat. V, 436-41).

the Christian form of individualism, which is discussed in detail in the third and last part of this book, along with its implications for the issues surrounding euthanasia. Before making the transition to the next part of this book, where we will study the impact of all those things that have been discussed regarding the issue of euthanasia more systematically, we will focus the discussion on the environment of the 'clinic'.

V. The 'Physician' and the Treatment of the Will of the 'Patient'

Without a doubt, Symeon's cardinal interest is the spiritual health of Christians that would lead to salvation and union with God. However, given that Symeon does not share any ground with dualistic perspectives, one may legitimately draw lessons from his arguments relevant to the soul in terms of those related to the body. Thus, it is not an overstatement to say that his thought is connected with the health and disease of the body. In Ethical Oration VI, Symeon refers to the relationship and the communication between the 'physician' (the spiritual father) and the 'patient' in a spiritual context. [107] Following this, a parallel is drawn between the character of the relationship and the communication between the 'physician' and the 'patient' in a spiritual context with that of the physician and the patient in the medical context. [108]

The relationship between the 'physician' and the 'patient' benefits all those involved on the basis of a fundamental condition, namely that of 'natural sight'. It has previously been noted that, since God created man according to His own image and bestowed him with divine properties, the task of every man is to acknowledge the character of his own creation, a process that leads to self-knowledge and the knowledge of God. This is possible only through the proper use of free will and the acknowledgement of God as the Principle and the Cause of all things. Any autonomous consideration of human life is, by definition, self-destructive. In other words, the duty of every human being is to view and, consequently, know himself as God created him. Such a 'natural' vision of reality is very important, especially in the medical context, since it protects man from viewing pivotal things wrongly and, therefore, from

107. The quotation marks are used to indicate that, while the terms 'physician' and 'patient' are used mainly in the medical context, they can easily be applied to the spiritual context as well.

108. The quotation marks are used to indicate that, while the terms 'physician' and 'patient' are used mainly in the medical context, they can easily be applied to the spiritual context as well.

taking incorrect decisions on issues such as euthanasia. Unfortunately, this 'natural sight' is what man has lost because of the fall of Adam and Eve. Fortunately, the recovery of this 'natural sight' (τὸ βλέπειν κατὰ φύσιν) is connected with the preservation or the recovery of the image of God in man.[109] Whoever fulfils such a condition is not subject to the superficial elements of this life, since he is able to see and focus on those things that are essential and stable:

> Such a man therefore goes about his life in becoming fashion as in broad daylight. He sees everything for what it is by nature. He does not wonder at the surface glitter of things, but beholds their essence and quality and so remains unmoved, paying attention only to what is stable and enduring. He sees gold and pays no mind to its gleaming, but understands that it is stuff which comes from the earth and is mere stone and dust, incapable of ever being changed into anything else.[110]

Such clear sight or, according to Symeon, 'natural sight' is very important for spiritual guidance as well as for the medical treatment of a 'disease' for both the 'physician' and the 'patient'.

'Natural sight' is the necessary ground upon which the experienced spiritual father, as well as the experienced physician, may clearly and naturally see and, consequently, not be deceived by the 'patient' and his or her desires as well as the 'disease'. A physician with 'natural sight' may know exactly what happens in a particular 'disease'. The 'patient' experiences confusion regarding his illness, its causes and its cure and may desire things that are bad for his health. Since the 'patient' does not know the cause of his suffering and the appropriate treatment for his illness, the presence of a 'physician' with 'natural sight' is necessary:

> Someone ill comes to the spiritual physician. He is overcome by suffering, troubled in all his intellect, and, rather than what heals, he is looking for what is injurious, that is, what gives rise to

109. Eth. VI, 217-219.

110. Ibid., 219-226. The forgetfulness of the temporal and changeable character of all created things is a characteristic of pseudo-knowledge (fleshly knowledge). All things in this life are changeable. Therefore, founding human life upon changeable things for pleasure is not prudent (Hymn X, ll. 6-14). Therefore, the aim of man to enjoy the pleasures of the present life eternally is, in fact, a deception (ἑαυτούς πλανῶσιν) (Hymn I, ll. 128-31). Moreover, ignorance of the temporal character of this life is a common deception among human beings. Symeon exaggerates this trend and argues that man quite often does not want to be reminded that he is mortal, although he is aware that people die (Cent. 3, ch. 42).

> suffering and brings on death in short order. The physician, who is loving and compassionate, examines the man, understands the brother's weakness, the passion's inflammation, its burden, and sees that the one who is sick is quite at the point of death.[111]

While the identification of the character of a 'disease' is a step towards its cure, it should be accompanied by the proper treatment. The 'physician' must not only examine and also clearly see the nature of the 'disease' of the 'patient' but also how such a 'disease' should be treated. Once 'natural sight' is secured, the 'physician' is informed that the healing of the 'patient' is not only subject to the treatment of the 'disease' but also subject to the other aspects of human nature such as the need for love and compassion:

> When the spiritual and knowledgeable physician sees the brother in the condition we have described, he does not immediately argue or shout, or say: 'You are asking for something bad and lethal, and I will not give it to you,' lest, on hearing this, he take to flight and go off to someone else who has no experience of such afflictions and be dead within the hour. He welcomes him instead, holds on to him, comforts him, shows him at once all affection and simplicity, in order to reassure him that he will undertake his treatment with the same medicines that he has asked for and so fulfil his desires . . . but he does promise to fulfil all his desires.[112]

This is the second indispensable step in curing the 'patient'. The 'patient' does not only suffer from what is identified at first sight, since the 'patient' comprises more than one constituent element. Therefore, a human being is more than the changeable and corruptible nature that results in a variety of 'diseases'. A 'physician' with 'natural sight' can see that, behind a patient's particular behaviour or demand, such as his self-destructive demands, there are other needs that should be fulfilled.

Even then, the cure of the 'patient' is not ensured. What is also needed is the 'natural sight' of the 'patient'. Otherwise, the 'physician' and the 'patient' would define health and medicine differently. It is not accidental that the 'patients', due to their lack of 'natural sight', associate their desires with what they think is best for them. Since these desires originate in a vision of life which lacks natural sight or of the knowledge of what is beneficial, they are not in a position to take a right decision. It is then imperative that the 'patient' be convinced that to recover 'natural sight' is not an impossible feat:

111. Eth. VI, 279-85.
112. Ibid., 298-310.

> They [the 'patients'] imagine rather that it is healthy to accomplish the wishes of the flesh, and to practise all its lusts and desires. . . . For they are blind, and neither do they believe that anyone else can see. Thus, they live deprived of sight and unconvinced they can lift up their eyes. If they were so convinced, then they would look up and, looking up, would clearly see and recognize those who are crucified to the world.[113]

The 'patient' is convinced only when he identifies and imitates those whose lives are oriented towards voluntary death. Given the different interpretation that voluntary death has in the Christian tradition, the relationship between the 'physician' and the 'patient' does not have a procedural character. On the contrary, it covers the whole of human existence and not only the corruptible 'body' of the 'patient' or purely 'medical' treatment because of this understanding of 'natural sight'. Man, either as a 'physician' or as a 'patient', must always acknowledge that 'natural sight' is not possible without the presence of God, given that God created human nature and bestowed it with divine properties, and that the Holy Trinity and the character of His own existence is embedded in human existence itself.

In short, from a Christian point of view, because of the fall of the ancestors, human beings suffer from the absence (partly or fully) of 'natural sight' (one need not mention that, due to Symeon's consideration of human existence as a whole, 'natural sight' affects all aspects of humanity). In the medical context this coincides with the absence of the clear vision, by both patients and physicians alike, of the reality of the character of the disease and of suffering, the features of the condition of the patient and the needs that such a condition entails, as well as with the competence of the physician to have a holistic perspective of the disease and of the patient. Obviously, such a vision is not easily acquired and, therefore, the moral agents involved in the medical context must always have some reservations regarding their possession of 'natural sight' and, consequently, how they treat the coming of death in human life.

VI. Concluding Remarks

The theology of Symeon has been criticised by some and praised by others. His critics have interpreted the mystical theology and the efforts towards a personal experience of God as an extreme form of individualism, whereas those who have praised him viewed his conflicts

113. Ibid., 334-46.

with the ecclesiastical representatives of his era as a reaction against the dominance of a formalistic and conservative tendency in Christian life.[114]

The idea that Symeon laid the foundations for an individualistic approach to Christian life is right to the extent that it takes into account the fact that Christian individualism constitutes, for modern thought, an anti-individualistic account of human existence. Symeon attributes to humanity a Trinitarian aspect that is connected, on the one hand, with the character of the soul and the deification of the whole man and, on the other, with the most radical rapprochement of divinity and humanity, namely the fact that God becomes part of human existence itself once man is considered as God, body and soul. This last statement in a way challenges the traditional belief that man simply consists of a soul and a body. Thus, Christian life cannot be individualistic in any of its aspects, since the Triune God is not indicative of any kind of individualistic life. In such a context, the life of a Christian that is a life lived by voluntary choice, has voluntarily to be made subject not only to God and His divine will but also to the development of a loving relationship with one's fellow men. Even though the efforts at achieving a personal experience of God, as Symeon promotes them, give the impression that they are an individualistic endeavour, a distinction should be made between modern individualism and a Christian approach to individualism. Such an approach reveals the appropriate implications for the modern way of life that is individualistic *par excellence.*

The interpretation that Symeon's conflicts with the ecclesiastical 'establishment' were merely an effort against 'the legalistic and minimalistic view of Christianity' signifies that Symeon did not hesitate to challenge the well-established Christian mentality of his time through, in a way, a prophetic form of warning.[115] This mentality had been founded on a stereotypical perception of the Christian tradition that favoured a kind of formalism within the Church, in which even the personal encounter with God had to be controlled with the fear of a

114. Krivocheine points out that Symeon's era was marked by 'a conflict between a scholastic theology removed from the spiritual life with intense formalistic and conservative elements and a theology understood as the expression of the Holy Spirit' (Krivocheine, *St Symeon the New Theologian*, p. 45).

115. Symeon was accused of not accepting the objectivity of ecclesiastical ordination because he questioned the performance of the sacraments by an 'unworthy' priest. Though such questioning implies 'anti-hierarchical' tendencies, Symeon wanted to caution 'against a too easy conception of the high office of priesthood' (Rossum, 'Priesthood and Confession in St Symeon the New Theologian', p. 224). See also Meyendorff, *Byzantine Theology*, p. 75.

heresy.[116] In such a context, the relationship between God and man and, consequently, the relationship between the Kingdom of God and this world were subject to objective rules and controllable practices. In other words, both the free will of man and the divine will were unconsciously underestimated and limited. Thus, the efforts to avoid Scylla, that in this context is the risk of heresy, resulted in Charybdis, or the devaluation of divine and human cooperation in human history.[117]

Symeon, without rejecting the tradition of the Fathers, went a step further. This was necessary in order to go beyond those elements that, while they were part of the Christian tradition and had come down from the past, were not sufficiently robust in order to confront the ideologies and culture of a particular time. It is through these lenses that the theological contribution of Symeon should be assessed, which is what has been attempted in this chapter. Symeon maintained a balance regarding the unconditional exaggeration of the rational character of humanity and fought against any dualistic element in human nature. On this basis, he emphasised the role of free will and its relation to the divine will, and showed how the cooperation between both touches upon the most controversial and serious issues in human life, such as the anticipation of the coming of death. Finally, Symeon explained the real possibility of a close relationship between man and God even in this life by fighting against those beliefs that were oriented towards compromises with the 'world', while taking into account the limitation of the power of the human will. In any case, Symeon highlighted the priority of the free will over nature and rejected any voluntary subjection of human freedom to fallen human nature. If formalism is the scholastic and lifeless approach towards human life, then Symeon went beyond formalism, given that some of his theological points are regarded as unusual and suspicious even today.

Without a doubt, the most profound challenge to Christian formalism, however, is found in Symeon's view of the character of so-called voluntary death. For him, voluntary death is not simply an isolated fight against one's own passions and sins, that occurs at a remove from the rest of human existence. Rather, it signifies a practice that involves the whole of humanity and, consequently, the human body as well as the rest of

116. Spidlik, 'Syméon le Nouveau Théologien', DS XIV, p. 1398.

117. Ware notes that the ending of the great Christological and Iconoclastic controversies that resulted in the 'Triumph of Orthodoxy' was followed by formalism. Christians tended towards a passive and mechanical acceptance of tradition, instead of making creative efforts towards a better understanding of it (Ware, 'The Mystery of God and Man in St Symeon the New Theologian', p. 230).

one's fellow men. Though in Symeon's era the persecution of Christians was over and the disposition towards a bodily death was not necessary, everyone's spiritual integrity was in danger, as happens in every era and despite the possibility of participation in the sacraments being there. Interestingly, one's spiritual integrity cannot be separated from the whole of human existence, once safeguarding it becomes a lifelong procedure that involves all aspects of humanity.

Symeon's refusal clearly to separate the soul from the body signifies that, whatever happens in the spiritual sphere of a human being applies, *mutatis mutandis*, to his bodily life as well. Since voluntary death deals with both the soul and body, and since voluntary death is considered as crucial for the proper treatment of spiritual diseases, it is not, therefore, out of context to speak of voluntary bodily death, although of course always given that certain particular conditions are fulfilled.

Conclusions to Part Two

At the end of part one we wondered whether there was any way out of the vicious circle that keeps man, by definition, subject to the tendency for self-preservation through power claims over human existence. Let us see whether the second part of this book has anything to contribute to this question.

Even though John Damascene and Symeon the New Theologian have different historical starting points and theological orientations, they both bring together the immanent and the transcendent, man and God. On the one hand, John lived in an era of spiritual crisis in which apocalyptic literature proliferated and which was characterised by the dominance of the Church, and, in particular, of monasteries, over Byzantine society. In this context, John accommodated the beginning of Byzantine 'humanism' and the re-orientation of Christian theology towards the worldly aspect of human life without violating the proper relationship between the Church and the *cosmos*. This is easily visible in his attempted transition from Christology to anthropology and in the fact that he centres on the meaning of an image or an icon for understanding the Christian life, such as focussing on the implications of the image of God in man. On the other hand, Symeon experienced the peak of Byzantine 'humanism' within a secular and individualistic society. Accused of extreme individualism, Symeon's endeavours were oriented towards a Christian form of individualism that is marked by a transition from the security of imprisonment in one's own self to the ecstasy of love for God and all other people. This transition is manifested in his efforts against the ecclesiastic formalism that was applauded in his era and that safeguarded the deception that the Christian life could be practised without the risk of the heresy. Within such an individualised society an agreed conduct in the Christian life was necessary. However, for the Church, such an approach towards human existence gives rise only to a lifeless life.

It is the rapprochement of the immanent and the transcendent, of divinity and humanity that leads to the need to properly understand the character of the nature of man and, consequently, the relationship between God and man. It is for this reason that self-knowledge, as opposed to self-preservation, emerges as the cornerstone of human life. Both John and Symeon place emphasis on the knowledge of human nature, or, in other words, on the character of humanity. John connects the true knowledge of being with human existence, since the absence of such knowledge coincides with falsehood. For John, what matters is self-knowledge and not self-preservation. Though John starts out from the Aristotelian division of beings, he goes beyond such a system of division, especially regarding the relationship between hypostasis and nature. Without departing from the patristic belief that there is an ontological priority of hypostasis over nature, he highlights the 'intimacy' between them. Thus, he succeeds not only in preserving the hypostasis as indicative of the particularity of each human being, but also in stressing the cardinal role of the sharing of common human nature by all human beings. Such an anthropology is explicity visible in Symeon's Trianitarian consideration of the human being. The creation of man according to the image of God corresponds not just to the rational and the intelligible in man but also to man's resemblance to the Holy Trinity, a likeness that Symeon identifies in the constitution of man as soul, body and God. It is for this reason that self-knowledge is a prerequisite for the true knowledge of God. The fact that the presuppositions for the true knowledge of God exist within man, given that he is gifted with divine properties, has two implications. On the one hand, self-knowledge and, consequently, the safeguarding of one's own existence is an aim within this world and, on the other hand, God becomes part of human existence itself and, therefore, the most radical rapprochements between the immanent and the transcendent are provided. This by no means implies a kind of pantheism.[118]

One may argue that, in such a context a kind of 'divinisation' of man by nature is promoted, that implies a misappropriation of the divine power and divine sovereignty from man. In such a case, the orientation towards

118. Farantos, *Δογματικὴ καὶ ἠθική: εἰσαγωγικά*, pp. 169-71.

power claims over human life would be an inevitable outcome. However, the whole argument is false, since it ignores a fundamental condition regarding the Trinitarian aspect of humanity, namely its fallen state.

In particular, in such a context, any power claims of man suffer from subjectivity, given that all human beings are free and, therefore, are capable of thinking, deciding and acting according to their will, though within the constraints of human nature. However, for the Christian tradition, it is not only natural necessity (nobody wants to die, but nevertheless all die) but also the capability of the free will due to its fallen state that limits the spectrum of the human will. The fallen state of humanity reveals a profound weakness in the human will in man in his lack of ability to rule even over his own life. It is then self-evident that there are grounds neither for objective assertions nor for power claims. Obviously, it is the continuous process of self-knowledge that secures such a reality and lays the foundations for self-relinquishment up to the point of voluntary death.

Even voluntary death cannot be considered as power claims over one's own body or over one's own fellow men. On the contrary, voluntary death is conditional upon the human will, and, in order for it to be properly exercised, certain conditions must be present. Man may completely give himself over even up to the point of death, but this must be always for the sake of God and others. This practice is associated with man's own individuality, as happens in the case of martyrs. The martyrs imitated Christ, the incarnate Son of God, and all Christians are called to imitate Christ.

Obviously, it is interesting to apply these theological findings to bioethics and, particularly, to the issues surrounding euthanasia. This is the aim of the third part.

Part Three

Christian Tradition and the Issues Surrounding Euthanasia

The third part of this book sets out the fundamentals of Christian individualism and contrasts them with those of modern individualism. The Christian form of individualism is applied to the current debate on euthanasia, and a critique is made of the most popular arguments used either in favour of or against euthanasia. In this way the common ground that all these arguments share, as well as their inadequacy from an ethical point of view, is revealed. This will lead to a series of concluding remarks that will summarise the main arguments of the discussion in this third part. The main question of this book – whether euthanasia is considered to be self-sacrifice or murder both in non-religious modern society as well as within the Christian Tradition – will then be addressed in the conclusion of this book.

Chapter 5
Christian Individualism and Decisions on Euthanasia

Introduction

The first part of this book raised the issue of the polemical character of all theories, and, particularly, of the power claims of bioethics over human existence, through the application of Kondylis's descriptive theory of decision. These claims are evident in the 're-creation' of the human being, a 're-creation' that entails particular ideological principles and, therefore, a particular anthropology. Eventually, the power claims of bioethics are shown to be unjustified, given that they are deeply subjective and that they are motivated by the desire for self-preservation and, as a consequence, for sovereignty in the public arena.

The second part of the book effects the transition from a descriptive approach to bioethics, and particularly euthanasia, to a normative account of moral life through the development of the anthropology of the patristic tradition. This anthropology is based on the biblical narration that God created man according to His own image, the interdependent meanings of which constitute what the Christian tradition considers fundamental to understanding the character of human existence. It is on this basis that human existence is considered an existence oriented towards union with Christ and the imitation of the martyrs. This orientation is fulfilled by voluntary self-offering in its various meanings for the sake of God and others. Despite the fact that the Christian tradition, as a normative approach to moral life that entails an orientation towards self-preservation, is subject to the critical analysis of the descriptive theory of decision, it does not regard self-preservation as the cornerstone of human life.

If so, what could be the contribution of an approach to human existence that in a way goes beyond the character of bioethics? It has been argued that the Christian tradition may be able to shed more light on the modern understanding of humanity and provide the ground for a critique of the fundamentals of bioethics, and, particularly, of those surrounding the decisions around euthanasia. The third part of this book is devoted to this potential contribution that the Christian tradition may offer.

By prioritising self-knowledge over self-preservation, the Christian tradition abandons the 're-created' human being of bioethics and puts forward a human being who wants to know himself and not to be affected by externally imposed principles, which is an aim and practice that was thoroughly discussed in the first chapter. The priority of self-knowledge that is justified by the patristic tradition is of great importance because of the centrality of internally (i.e. the image of God), rather than externally, imposed elements. Indeed, this is a challenge to the traditional rationale of all theories relevant to human existence that presuppose the sovereignty or the self-preservation of a subjective 'worldview' in the name of objectivity and universality. Since for the Christian tradition the starting point of any consideration of human life is the individual or the hypostasis, as is suggested by the ontological priority of hypostasis over nature,[1] what matters is the appropriate knowledge of man's own existence.[2] Otherwise, man is controlled from other sources and not from the knowledge of his own existence. In such a case, a particular hypostasis bases himself on externally imposed principles when taking his own decisions.[3]

In a society that is increasingly marked by individualism while, at the same time, consciously underestimating the significance of anthropology for the sake of so-called common morality, the Christian tradition proposes Christian individualism.[4] Such a kind of individualism not only substantially values each human being and his freedom but it

1. 'The nature . . . may be considered wholly with accidents in a hypostasis, in which it is said to be viewed in an individual [ἐν ἀτόμῳ]' (Expos., 55, 6-7).
2. 'Nothing is more estimable than knowledge, for knowledge is the light of the rational soul. . . . By knowledge I mean the true knowledge of things which are, because things which have being are the object of knowledge' (Dial. fus., 1, 2-11).
3. This idea of the relationship of the 'intimacy' between hypostasis and nature and, consequently, the dependence of one's own autonomy on the knowledge of human existence was elaborated in the previous part of this book.
4. Christian individualism is what derives in the patristic tradition from the consideration of human existence as a hypostasis and not as an autonomous individuality. For a very interesting account of this distinction that has profoundly affected the foundations of Christian ethics, see Reed, *The Genesis of Ethics*, particularly pp. 1-57 and 183-252.

also introduces an interdependent relationship with all other human beings. The characteristics of Christian individualism are highlighted with reference to the issues surrounding the decisions on euthanasia. Moreover, the application of such an approach to the issues regarding the administration of death redesignates the whole discussion of these issues. The redesignation of the discussion is charted in the following section.

I. The Fundamentals of Christian Individualism

The second chapter of this book referred to the fact that the whole discussion on the decisions around euthanasia is based on the assumption that human beings are moral agents who accomplish procedures.[5] Along with this assumption comes the focus of bioethics on the definition of principles and the provision of consent between the moral agents involved in a particular case. All these have to be secured for the sake of man's individuality and in order to respect his autonomy.

Another assumption of bioethics is related to one's own power over one's own existence due to the technological power in the medical context. This assumption has resulted in an ideology of control, since the physician is considered as capable of controlling death, and the patient is also able to assume such control.[6] This book has already discussed the fallacious character of such an assumption, which entails the transition from the human being to the autonomic being and, consequently, the self-determination of man on the grounds of autonomy.

The third assumption of bioethics that designates discussions around various bioethical issues and, in particular, euthanasia centres on the cardinal role of suffering and death in one's own existence. The whole argumentation in this context is elaborated with reference to the best possible 'treatment' of suffering and death by means of the voluntary decisions of every individual (physician, patient and relatives) involved.

It is a generally accepted belief that these three assumptions are the sole means of reaching moral decisions in modern societies. However, what is often ignored is the fact that these assumptions reflect the sovereignty of an individualistic ideology founded on a subjective worldview. It is, consequently, entirely justified to challenge such an ideology. This is attempted through the presentation of a kind of individualism that is inspired by the fundamentals of the Christian tradition as elaborated in the second part of this book.

5. The main ideas that are developed in this section are also discussed, though in a different context, in Bekos, 'Tò κακὸ σήμερα'.
6. McKenny, *To Relieve the Human Condition*, pp. 25-32.

1. A Universalistic Account of Man's Individuality: beyond Procedures and Communities

Those who defend the rationale of bioethics declare that man is not so autonomous at the point when reaching consensus among, and effecting cooperation between, the moral agents becomes unavoidable. In order for procedures to be accomplished, other people must necessarily be involved, which means acknowledging the limited autonomy of all moral agents. To make it clearer, if the procedure is considered to be the only legitimate precondition of moral actions within a world of moral diversity and that is without moral consensus, and if the involvement in such a procedure is viewed as the minimal necessary contribution of all moral agents, then the relational character of human life and the relational interdependence among human beings emerges as an inescapable reality. However, due to sovereign bioethics, the relational disposition of a human being is in a way divorced from all those elements that make a decision meaningful, for fear of establishing moralities of a divisive character, a fear that is totally unjustified, since a particular morality does not necessarily constitute a danger to society. Quite apart from the fact that a particular morality may claim the same authority in the public discussion of moral issues as any common morality. Let us see how the Christian tradition, in particular, may respond to such a reality.

John Damascene proposes that man is a derivative and relative being, which means that man comes from somewhere or someone and refers, by being related, to something or someone.[7] For example, each human being comes into this life, biologically, through his parents and grows up within a particular cultural context. Moreover, man, as a relational being, builds societies and his life develops as relationships with his fellow men develop. Obviously, it is clear that human existence is something more than the accomplishment of procedures and, therefore, the proper understanding of human existence is required. As a consequence, a quest towards self-knowledge and self-understanding is initiated.

Both John and Symeon the New Theologian break all conventional boundaries regarding the sources and points of reference in man's quest for self-knowledge.

John's belief in the derivative and relational character of the human being implies that man is a being characterised by a kind of interdependence with either rational or non-rational living beings.[8]

7. Dial. fus., 6, 45-115.
8. The idea that man is a microcosm or little cosmos (μικρός κόσμος), for he recapitulates in himself the whole universe, both rational and non-rational

Therefore, an external means for gauging the proper self-knowledge and self-understanding of the human person is necessary.[9] This is further elaborated by Symeon, who views man as a Trinitarian being, a being that is something more than the union of two parts, namely soul and body. Symeon says that there is also a third part in the substance of humankind that is not simply another element such as the emotions or a spiritual faculty. This third part is nothing else than God Himself, on the basis that God created man according to His own image.[10]

This vision of humanity obviously looks beyond what traditionally is regarded as the limits of a human being and his individuality. This expansion of the horizon results in the inclusion of other being(s) in one's own existence. As a result, man's individuality transgresses any relational account of humanity, which is oriented only to a sort of exteriority. Consequently, the source of man's relational life is not only external but also internal and, therefore, man's relations, either external or internal, become constituent parts of his own existence.

The view of man as a derivative and relational, as well as a Trinitarian, being lays the foundations for a universalistic account of individuality. An immediate consequence of this consideration must be the redefinition of the context in which decisions on euthanasia in this era are taken. From a Christian point of view, the medical context violates the character of human existence because it is seen as the most appropriate framework for the taking of such decisions, despite the fact that its character does not correspond to the fundamentals of human existence. This assertion is not to question the crucial role of medicine in the service of human life. It is rather to question its 'inhumane' character. However, in a context where procedures and individual rights rule sovereign, a universalistic account of man's individuality sounds strange.

---

beings (Expos., 26, 82-85), and that he is a being whose death coincides with the partial end of this world (ibid., 15, 16) is very indicative of such interdependence. As the death of each human being results in the partial end of this world, likewise the life of each human being constitutes a part of the whole life of this world. This assertion clearly implies that there are deep relationships between each human being and the rest of the living beings, either rational or non-rational, in this world. Damascene, in fact, follows a long-standing patristic tradition that considers human existence as an image of the universe (see, for example, St Gregory of Nazianzus, PG, 36, 57A).

9. Ricoeur, 'Intellectual Autobiography', p. 16.

10. 'Father, Son, and Holy Spirit are the one God we worship. God, soul and body are the man who is created according to the image of God and made worthy of becoming God' (Eth. VI, 176-78).

It is the universalistic account of individuality that could reshape the nature of the medical context, such as the character of the relationship between physician and patient. Such a rationale transgresses the traditional scheme of sameness/otherness that constitutes the basis for metaphysical accounts, as happens in Levinas's moral account. It also breaches the scheme of friend/enemy that represents an inescapable reality in human life in which sovereignty over the other is sought, and that goes beyond the practices of the attainment of consent in the medical context. A medical context that treats a human being as derivative, relational and inclusive of other being(s) in his own existence takes into account the interdependence between human beings in the most radical way and, consequently, recognises a shared responsibility. Such responsibility does not only refer to the moral agents who are usually present at the clinic, i.e. the physician, the patient and the relatives. On the contrary, the universalistic account of individuality as found in the Christian tradition implies going beyond the conventional limits of the context that is usually legitimate for taking decisions on euthanasia. This Christian universalistic account also recognises a common responsibility that goes beyond the medical context and even beyond the particular community to which the patient belongs. Therefore, it penetrates the life of all communities in a particular society and steps beyond a communitarian consideration of human life. This is the first fundamental element regarding man's self-knowledge, a step towards a Christian form of individualism and a transition from bio-politics to a kind of bioethics that truly deserves its name.

In short, in the first chapter of this book it was argued that bioethics, instead of being the ethics of human life, turns into a kind of bio-politics. It does so in that it restricts its horizons by focussing only on the medical context, which results in the concern for providing the appropriate justification for accomplishing procedures that represent the health policy of modern society. On the contrary, the proposal of a universalistic account of individuality places the relevant discussion in a wider context, in which the emergence of bioethical issues in modern society is seen as a matter of responsibility for the whole of society. Such a consideration, at least, widens the discussion regarding the fundamentals of modern civilisation.

2. Individuality and the Chimera of Control: the Inner State of Humanity

The second constituent element for the understanding of self is linked with the inner state of human existence. As a reminder, chapter two above considered the division and the 'undifferentiation' within the inner reality of mankind that characterises the 're-creation' of the human being by bioethics. There it was argued that such a reality is connected with dualistic (the division of man into two fundamentally different parts such as body/soul and mind/matter) and materialistic (the absence of the separation between, for example, mind and matter) views that are evident from a philosophical point of view. In a non-religious and a morally fragmented world, the bodily aspect of humanity becomes the generally accepted ground for taking such decisions. At the same time, the presence of reason in man and his consequent ability to exercise his will and choose whatever he wants, gives the feeling not only of power claims over others but also over one's own life.

The theological part of this book has explicitly shown that man's rationality or free will is of central importance to understanding human existence. What makes the difference between the Christian tradition and the sovereignty of rationality in bioethics is placing the human ability to exercise one's will, choose and decide in a context that cultivates an ethos of self-limitation. The absence of such an ethos in modern societies is of cardinal importance, for it shapes human life as a whole and founds it on imaginary elements. The ethos of self-limitation is laid aside on the basis of an imaginary sovereignty of rationality.[11] As a result, man is not willing to recognise his self-evident mortality, for he assumes that what has value and coincides with his own existence necessitates the exclusion of whatever he thinks is not part of himself.[12] In other words, it is the absence of such an ethos that results in the alienation of man from his inner reality.

In the Christian tradition, while primacy is attributed to the so-called hypostasis, that is free and capable of choice due to the faculty of reason, this primacy is not absolute and unconditional as in God. On the contrary, it is a primacy in transition, which means that, even though it must rule sovereign over human nature and the fate of human existence, it can accomplish its mission only partially, due to its fallen state. The word 'partially' signifies man's unwillingness to die and his failure to escape from it. An immediate implication of the idea of partiality is the necessary acceptance of the fact that man is not capable, by definition, of

11. It is worth noting that in ancient Greek the word 'mortal' (θνητός) and the word 'man' (ἄνθρωπος) are synonyms. For Castoriadis, the absence of the ethos of self-limitation is nothing but an insult (ὕβρις). In the ancient Greek context, the insult signifies supercilious behaviour that does not respect the limits of human nature and the norms of ethical and divine law. Castoriadis believes that the ethos of self-limitation has to be the main anthropological component of both real philosophy and democratic society (Castoriadis, *Ὁ θρυμματισμένος κόσμος*, pp. 79-96).

12. Castoriadis, *Le monde morcelé*, pp. 27-41.

exercising absolute control over his own life.[13] Indeed, once man accepts such an indisputable reality, he loses the ground for power claims over his own life. One may, therefore, argue that these claims are conditional and limited. Nevertheless, the recognition of limits that result from the presence of death undermines one's own power claims over death, once death is also credited with having power claims over one. Moreover, it follows that death, therefore, may designate limits on one's own power claims. Though it is on the basis of empirical reality that the ethos of self-limitation is founded, a further clarification of the implications of this ethos for human existence is necessary.

The necessary clarification is provided by the careful consideration of the different constituents of the human being, along with the designation of the relations between them. On the one hand, John has stated that, while there is an ontological priority of hypostasis over nature, there is also a unique 'intimacy' between them. On the other hand, Symeon does not subscribe either to any account of dualism or to any form of sovereignty of the rational. Both Church Fathers make it clear that it is beneficial for man neither to overestimate his rational faculty by being impressed by his power to reason nor to underestimate the body upon which the power of the free will is exercised. This suggestion is not based on a normative account of human life but rather on the inner state of human existence itself.

Nevertheless, the union of soul and body does not eliminate the different status of soul and body. According to John Damascene, there is a kind of asymmetry within both since the soul and body enjoy a different status in the Aristotelian division of beings, while their union with hypostasis is characterised by a kind of disproportionality regarding their proximity to hypostasis. The difference between the status of soul and body should not be considered as indicative of an absolute distinctiveness among them and an excuse for unlimited, legitimised and justified power claims of one over another. Yes, the temptation is always there, but the task of a rational being is not to give in to it. On the contrary, his task is to override such a temptation for the sake of his union as a being. Otherwise, man becomes the cause of his inner alienation and of the inescapable superceding of his

13. Man suffers from a profound antinomy that, according to John, is evident, on the one hand, in the dissolution of soul from body that is considered as a natural effect of man's composite hypostasis and, on the other hand, in the unwillingness of the soul to be separated from the body that is also counted as natural. Such unwillingness is not sufficient for the avoidance of death, namely the separation of the body from the soul. This did not happen in Christ, who escaped this tragedy once He voluntarily, and not involuntarily, experienced death as the rest of human beings do (Expos., 67).

own limits. Such an outcome, however, is not simply unethical but also self-destructive for man, as is evident in the fall of the ancestors where the hope of divinity (θεότητος ἐλπίδι), the successful bait on the part of the snake,[14] signifies not only the forgetfulness of the real status of human nature but also a willingness to make an unconditional transition from humanity to divinity.

The inner alienation in human nature, as well as the confusion with regard to the limits of one's own existence in terms of decision-making, is also exemplified in the application of rights regarding the best possible 'treatment' of end-of-life decisions such as euthanasia. The use of the rationale of rights for arguments in favour of euthanasia is incomprehensible, for the institution of rights is oriented towards the protection of the person from whatever or whoever threatens what is generally accepted as fundamental for human life. Such an orientation, when applied to the inner state of humanity, constitutes the foundation of man's inner alienation, as is evident in the 'right-to-die' argument, which implies the absolute authority of one's own freedom over one's own existence. The Christian tradition does not encourage deepening the alienation in man with the adoption of whatever is considered as a threat to human life, such as the belief that the corruption of the body does not allow man to be seen as an autonomous being. On the contrary, this tradition aims at overcoming any alienation for the sake of the wholeness of humanity. Along the same lines, the imperative of self-determination in the autonomous being that characterises modern ideology is merely an unwise imperative. Self-determination makes sense only when it secures one's own life against those foreign to it and who have power claims over it. Consequently, the self-determination regarding the destiny of one's own body through the exercising of power claims over it as an enemy (one's own body becomes an enemy of one's own existence!) can hardly be considered as prudent and justified.

3. Suffering, Death and the Christian Individual: the Focus on Life

Within the Christian tradition a universalistic account of individualism and the orientation towards overcoming the alienation of man from his own existence have been identified. Now the ability of Christian individualism to confront morally important issues in human life comes under the spotlight. Two interrelated issues, suffering and death, are central to this investigation.

14. Expos., 45, 27-28.

Right after 1960, death was 'rediscovered' as an issue deserving of attention and discussion. Because of developments in medicine and technology, and the fragmented state of man's moral world, medicine claimed the authority to designate the significance of death in human life and the power to separate man from suffering and the fear of death.[15] It is not accidental that at the same time the ideology of the autonomous being that rules sovereign in modern society resulted in the emergence of human rights, up to the point of claiming rights over death. The easy transition from the right to live to the right to die betrays a moral confusion regarding life and death in human existence, once both are considered as equally dependent on the imperative of rights. Despite the fact that life and death are mutually exclusive - death comes when life ends, death is presented as being a maidservant of and not an enemy to life - the foundation of rights are oriented to the service of human existence. Therefore, the right-to-die is, by definition, the maidservant of human life integrity. However, nobody would fight against - and, particularly, with the most modern weapons, as happens in the medical context regarding the threat of coming death - an enemy that is not considered serious, important and real. It is then a paradox that death, which in a way is viewed as something that serves life, is fought against as the worst enemy of human life.

Within the Christian tradition, things are clearer. The biological end of a human being is seen relatively. From a Christian point of view, corruption and death have a temporal and not an essential character in the sense that they are not constituent of human existence and, therefore, they cannot threaten human existence.[16] This concept is very important, since it does not justify the focus on the elimination of suffering and death. On the contrary, other things in human life are more important. Thus, the temporal and accidental character of suffering and death offer the grounds for fundamentally redirecting the orientation of human interest. In such a context, the endless efforts towards establishing control over suffering and death do not make sense. Such an approach challenges not only the sovereignty of modern medicine and its role in human life, namely bioethics, but also the cardinal role of technology

15. Hauerwas supports the idea that it is not the technological revolution but rather the fragmented moral world that has resulted in the power claims of medicine over human existence and the rise of bioethics (Hauerwas, *Suffering Presence*, pp. 1-2).

16. For John Damascene, corruption and, consequently, death are accidents and non essential characteristics of the human being (Manich., 62, 1-5). This belief implies that these characteristics are not constituent of human existence (the character of the entry of corruption and death was discussed at length in chapter three).

and its power claims over human existence. Can it then be argued that such a position demonstrates the indifference of the Christian tradition towards threats to mankind such as corruption and death?

Modern society considers death and suffering of central importance and as real and serious enemies, while it fails to see that such a notion is an after-effect of the particular worldview that this society has adopted and not an uncontested objective truth – the application of the descriptive theory of decision to bioethics in the first part of this book revealed the fallacy of objectified ideologies. This failure is crucial, since it results in the belief that death and suffering cannot have any meaningful place in human life and, therefore, that their 'elimination' is imperative. It has been argued repeatedly throughout this book that the orientation towards content-less and general principles and not towards a content-rich anthropology produces an ethical discussion that is fundamentally subjective, but which, nevertheless, is accompanied by objectification claims. In such a context, the recognition of any meaningful relationship between the presence of suffering and death in human life and the ideological choices of human beings is almost impossible. However, establishing such a link is necessary in order to challenge the current imprisonment in the rationale for the elimination of death in the service of human life!

Christian theology provides an interesting way out of this 'sentence', for the presence of corruption and death is connected with the particular use of the human will. In this tradition, there is a meaningful relationship between the choices of Adam and the experience of suffering and death by all human beings. This relationship is by no means indicative of any blame or guilt that man has to bear as it passes down through the generations to all humans. On the contrary, once this order of things is acknowledged, the focus of human interest is redirected from death to life and to the particular choices of man that are always based on a particular account of morality. Thus, the ultimate outcome of accepting a connection between the human will and the experience of suffering and death is the stressing of, on the one hand, the importance of a content-rich anthropological account that stands behind all human actions and corresponds to a particular morality and, on the other, the taking of responsibility for a meaningful confrontation of suffering and death. Thus, suffering and death are placed in a meaningful context and one acknowledges one's own indebtedness regarding the proper designation of decision-making on issues surrounding suffering and death. This double aim is perfectly fulfilled within the Christian tradition.

The confrontation of suffering and death in the Christian tradition is designated by the imitation of the paradigms of Christ and the martyrs,[17]

17. To avoid any misunderstanding, for the Christian tradition presented in this book,

paradigms that are representative of the way of life that is put forward in the Church, and the cultivation of loving relationships with all human beings, not only with the members of the particular community to which someone belongs – a Christian is conscious that he is not only a member of the Christian community but that he is also part of the universe that is not necessarily Christian. Indeed, the Christian narrative does not imply any conscious or unconscious indifference to the narrative(s) of the wider society. On the contrary, each human person has a personal responsibility towards the rest of humanity, including one's enemies, taking into account all one's possible dependences. This is what is really threatened in the medical context by sovereign bioethics. In such a context, the real enemy of man is not suffering and death but rather the narrow orientation of the principles that shape the current debate on euthanasia.

To sum up, the Christian foundation of a universalistic account of individuality stands at the very opposite pole to the individualism that characterises modern societies and which, according to de Tocqueville, is a process of cutting oneself off from the wider society and of withdrawing into the circle of family and friends with a view to taking care of this little society. Christian individualism proposes a process that works the other way around. Even though Christians start from their own Christian environment, their morality embodies the whole of society through the widening of their worldview in order to incorporate those human beings who are outside their own particular world. This procedure challenges in the most radical way the orientation of modern life. It is within this universalistic worldview that Christian morality makes sense.

II. Christian Individualism and the Current Debate on Euthanasia

The application of Christian individualism to the current debate on euthanasia follows the presentation of its fundamentals that was completed in the previous section. This application by no means underestimates the approach that other theological trends take towards bioethical issues. On the contrary, the focus on Christian individualism, by taking into account simultaneously all these theological trends, attempts to engage in a more precise discussion of a bioethical issue, namely euthanasia, an issue that is identified with the individualistic and autonomous human being like the other side of the same coin.

---

the life of the martyrs does not constitute the only paradigm of a Christian life. Continuous referral to the life of martyrs is made in this book because of the special relevance this way of life and death holds for the issues surrounding euthanasia.

What became evident in the theological part of this book is that the character of an Orthodox Christian approach to bioethics has at the same time a Christological orientation[18] (the imitation of the life and death of Christ), a Church-centred rationale[19] (the imitation of the life of the martyrs and participation in the sacraments), along with a liturgical understanding of Christian life,[20] an anthropological foundation (the identification of the character of humanity)[21] and an eschatological point of reference (the orientation towards the fulfilment of the relationship between God and Christians in His Kingdom to come).[22] Nevertheless, Orthodox Christian bioethics must also be properly oriented within the secular rationale in order to gain a proper voice in the public debate on these issues.

Without doubt, such an endeavour must not be shaped by the rationale that has already shaped bioethics. For example, Orthodox Christian bioethics has been thought of as an ethical approach that is marked by orientations and principles and not by limits and barriers, a consideration that obviously resembles popular principlism.[23] Contrary

18. Phidas, 'Bioethical Issues with Respect to Scientific Interventions to Avert Death', pp. 3-6.
19. Guroian, 'Euthanasia and Care for the Dying in the Orthodox Tradition', pp. 44-47.
20. Eber, 'Orthodox Christian Bioethics', pp. 139-41.
21. Breck, 'Bioethical Dilemmas and Orthodoxy', pp. 6-8. Breck, in his systematic work on bioethics, along with the need for an anthropological foundation, attributes a teleological as well as an eschatological character to Orthodox Christian bioethics and attempts to make a distinction between an Orthodox teleology and utilitarianism (Breck, *The Sacred Gift of Life*, pp. 16 and 246). In my view, it is not clear how a teleological character may contribute to a Christian consideration of the bioethical issues. On the contrary, it entails the risk of underestimating man's individuality and responsibility regarding human life in this world as well as in the world to come. It is remarkable that Breck's first idea regarding the character of Christian ethics and, consequently, of bioethics also included a deontological orientation in order to focus on the present obligations of moral agents – 'Christian ethics is eschatological and teleological as well as deontological' (Breck, 'Bio-Medical Technology: of the Kingdom or of the Cosmos', p. 23). Even in such a case, the inclusion of the major branches of moral theories becomes slightly confusing, for his ethical considerations are based on different presuppositions and are oriented towards different ends. Since there is a clear-cut distinction between deontology and teleology from an epistemological point of view, their use in Christian ethics implies a distance between the ultimate ends and the present obligation. There is no need to say that such an implication is far from the very meaning of Orthodox Christian ethics.
22. Scouteris, 'The Sacredness of the Human Person in Itself, with Reference to the Bioethical Dilemmas', pp. 9-13.
23. Hatzinikolaou, 'Ἀρχές ὀρθόδοξου βιοηθικοῦ προβληματιμοῦ', pp. 2-3. However, the dilemma is not an ethics of limits or an ethics of principles (the

to this, this book argues that the richness of the Christian tradition can provide a context that takes into account the ideological priorities of modern society while also remaining faithful to the fundamentals of the Christian faith. In other words, Orthodox Christian bioethics must deal with every aspect of Christian theology and Christian life as well as the essential issues in contemporary secular society. It is for this reason that an approach towards a Christian form of individualism was chosen, an approach that has to be well balanced and far from any unilateral (not taking into account the different aspects of Christian ethics) or confused (the inability to keep each aspect, secular or Christian, in its own domain) ethical consideration. One example will serve to justify the above.

Two of the most eminent Orthodox Christian bioethicists, Fr John Breck and Stanley Harakas, when dealing with the issue of euthanasia, consider euthanasia, or 'good death',[24] in the Christian tradition, and, particularly, in the medical context, as something 'that preserves a maximum of consciousness with a minimum of suffering, together with the peaceful surrender of one's life into the merciful hands of God'.[25] This definition brings in both elements of the current debate on euthanasia (maximum of consciousness, minimum of suffering) and elements of the Christian tradition. However, such a definition of 'good death' moves away from the Christian tradition at least as it is presented in the teaching of John Damascene and Symeon the New Theologian in the second part of this book. These Church Fathers refer to other indicatives of 'good death', such as the proper spiritual condition of the patient, his loving relationships with all his fellow men as well as his responsibility as a free being towards the proper passage from this life to the eternal life. These characteristics are evident in the life and death of Christ and martyrs, whose life and death should be voluntarily imitated by all Christians.

---

insufficient foundation of principlism has been extensively discussed in the first part of this book) but rather a substantial dialogue with and a critique of the worldview of bioethics.

24. The expressions 'good death' and 'euthanasia' are used interchangeably for two reasons. First, they have already been used in such a way by a number of Christian bioethicists who consider euthanasia as an expression of the 'good death' of a human being. Secondly, if the deliberate administration of death in the medical context, namely euthanasia, signifies the administration of a 'good death' that is counted as a positive development in one's own life, then the expression 'good death' can also be used interchangeably as indicative of the same reality. Within a secular way of thinking, euthanasia is quite often identified with the 'good death' of a suffering patient. However, this is not possible within a Christian way of thinking for the same reason that voluntary death cannot be identified with the practice of euthanasia in the medical context.

25. Breck, *The Sacred Gift of Life*, p. 224.

Since the adopted definition of the issue under discussion designates the character of the relevant ethical discussion, the theological presuppositions of the Christian tradition regarding the designation of the context in which moral issues such as the issues surrounding euthanasia are encountered should be clear and well-founded. In this book, this is accomplished through a critique of the most popular arguments in the current debate on euthanasia that are used by either the proponents or the opponents of euthanasia, as well as through the identification of their common ground. For practical purposes, these arguments are categorised into a series of groups, and they are presented immediately below.

1. Autonomy, Heteronomy and the Argument for the Sanctity of Life

The first group includes the arguments that derive from autonomy or heteronomy. The proponents of euthanasia see the human being as an autonomous being. The opponents of euthanasia consider man a heteronomous being, given that he is not the creator of his own life and, therefore, he is not entitled to govern this life independently from either the giver of this life or the significance of life itself. Both rationales betray the imprisonment of those involved in the current bioethical debate. Without doubt, this reality undermines the complexity of human existence with regard to not only the internal life of the human person but also the interrelational life of human beings. It also assumes that the choice of either extreme (autonomy or heteronomy) is imperative and sufficient as a basis for a moral decision that would be considered as justified and controllable. However, this assumption is an illusion, when one takes into account, on the one hand, the self-evident truth that man is subject at very least to the law of corruption and death (man is a mortal being) for, if so, the autonomy of a human being is in question. On the other hand, according to the descriptive theory of decision, each moral agent, in taking his decisions, is always dependent on his own worldview and, therefore, cannot be absolutely heteronomous. The Christian tradition abandons both autonomy and heteronomy for a kind of interplay between the two[26] and eventually for a form of Christian individualism.

The ineffective discussion around the bipolar scheme of autonomy/heteronomy is easily betrayed in one of the most popular arguments against euthanasia, namely the sanctity of life. All Christian Churches

26. Mantzarides, *Εἰσαγωγὴ στὴν Ἠθική*, pp. 30-33, and Mitsopoulos, *Θέματα ὀρθοδόξου ἠθικῆς θεολογίας*, pp. 17-20.

have used this argument extensively. According to this reasoning, life has a divine source that is found outside man and, therefore, man is not eligible to carry out any action that may violate the preservation of life.

At first sight, the argument for the sanctity of life seems to be well-founded on the rationale that whatever goes beyond man (man cannot create life and his life has been given to him as a gift) is by no means subject to his authority. This is expressly proclaimed in the encyclical, *Evangelium Vitae*:

> Human life is sacred because from its beginning it involves the creative action of God, and it remains forever in a special relationship with the Creator, who is its sole end. God alone is the Lord of life from its beginning until its end: no one can, in any circumstance, claim for himself the right to destroy directly an innocent human being.[27]

Obviously, such a statement emphasises the absolute authority of God over man, an authority that is justified to the extent that God rules sovereign over man by nature and by definition. At the same time, the sovereignty of God over man is considered a special kind of relationship. Without denying the absolute authority of God over man, the establishment of a special relationship between God and man implies a sort of responsibility on the part of the free human being regarding the 'treatment' of 'sacred' human life.

In the same vein the Bioethics Committee of the Church of Greece proclaims, 'Our life is a supreme gift of God, of which the beginning and the end are in His hands only ("in God's hand is the spirit of all human beings" [Job 12:10]). . . . Every effort to designate the limits of life only by the human will, thought, decision or ability strips life of its sanctity.'[28] However, a thorough examination of this statement reveals an inconsistency. As this statement says, 'life is a supreme gift of God,

---

27. John Paul II, *Evangelium Vitae*, chapter III, 53. The inadequacy of the argument that 'God alone is the Lord of life from its beginning' is evident in the discussion around the bioethical issue of cloning, a technological achievement that in a way creates life.

28. The Holy Synod of the Church of Greece, *Βασικές θέσεις ἐπὶ τῆς ἠθικῆς τῆς Εὐθανασίας*, § 4. The same idea was expressed by the Jubilee Bishops' Council of the Russian Orthodox Church, *Bases of the Social Concept of the Russian Orthodox Church*, XII, 1, and XII, 8. There is no need to say that the argument for the sanctity of life is not only used by the Orthodox Christian Synods but also by other Christian Churches, as well as secular thinkers who focus on the importance of life as such. See, for example, Doucet, *Les promesses du crépuscule*, pp. 84-99.

of which the beginning and the end are in His hands only'. At the same time, it declares that the designation of the limits of life is in the hand of humans as well ('every effort to designate the limits only by the human will. . .'). Therefore, the doctrine of the sanctity of life is violated only when man sets such limits. This clearly implies that the sanctity of life has to be subject to a kind of coordination between God and man. If so, the absolute character of the argument for the sanctity of life as an argument that establishes an absolute prohibition on man's intervention in the process of human life is exposed.[29] The weakness of such an argument is evident in human history, where the justified or unjustified interventions of the human will that cause death in cases such as so-called just wars or terrorists attacks, cases that cannot be attributed to any kind of absolutism that believes that the end of human life is in God's hands only.

The absolute character of the ideas of the sanctity of life and of heteronomy in human life is, consciously or unconsciously, violated by their most faithful supporters. The acceptance of exceptions in the obligation to preserve human life, where the administration of death is considered as a just or an unintended harm, proves such violation.[30] Additionally, the fact that the life of every creature in this world is a gift that comes from God, but that only human life is sacred, is another reason that this argument is not convincing.[31] Moreover, the Christian

29. It is not accidental that the argument for the sanctity of life in the statement of the Holy Synod of the Church of Greece is placed at the top of a list of theological statements regarding the character of life and death. What may be considered as accidental is the implication of this particular use of the argument for the sanctity of life, a use that leaves the door open for the intervention of the human will in the process of human life and death.

30. The relation between the just-war theory, the doctrine of double effect and bioethics was extensively discussed in the first part of this book. The implication of this relation for the validity of the argument for the sanctity of life is one among others and is implicitly present in documents that are oriented against euthanasia. In the document, *Βασικές θέσεις ἐπὶ τῆς ἠθικῆς τῆς Εὐθανασίας*, of the Church of Greece, it is proclaimed that the application of the doctrine of double effect and the consequent acceleration of death is justified (§ 50). Similarly, according to the *Bases of the Social Concept* of the Russian Church, 'While recognizing war as evil, the Church does not prohibit her children from participating in hostilities if what is at stake is the security of their neighbors and the restoration of troubled justice. Then war is considered as a necessary though undesirable means' (VIII, 2). In the same vein, Grisez, an eminent Catholic scholar on morality, says that 'Israel's law recognizes life as sacred and established protection for it, but its sacredness is qualified by the presumption that God authorizes killing in some cases' (Grisez, *The Way of the Lord Jesus I*, p. 218).

31. Zizioulas, 'Εὐθανασία: Ἀποφάσεις κατὰ τὸ τέλος τῆς ζωῆς', pp. 15-18.

tradition believes that 'there are values that are weightier than that of life' and these values are exemplified in the lives of the Sts and the martyrs, who 'have given up their lives for the sake of higher values embodied in their faith'.[32]

In such a context, the development of the idea of the sacredness of a person, rather than of human life, is considered as an interesting step forward in the discussion surrounding euthanasia. Zizioulas declares that the sacredness of human life must be based on the consideration of man as a person, as an image of God. In such a case, death is viewed not in an individualised context but rather in a relational environment.[33] Likewise, Skouteris argues that the sacredness of a person is associated with the uniqueness of every human being, a uniqueness that is not connected to his biological difference but rather to his ability to reveal Christ through his personhood until he reaches Sthood or *theosis*. This ability is based on the creation of man according to the image of God, an image that signifies the divine origin as well as the relatedness of man to God.[34] However, even such a concept is not a panacea, since it raises a series of questions. For example, neither the limits in the freedom of a person when faced with a bioethical dilemma such as euthanasia, nor the character of the relationships of those involved in the medical context in a variety of cases in taking decisions (i.e. the role of relatives acting for a patient in taking end-of-life decisions) are clear. Moreover, the fact that every person lives in contemporary society, which is governed through the application of laws and medical practices, does not assure the preservation of the character of the person.[35]

Can it then be argued that there is an incompatibility between secular society and the Christian tradition? And, if yes, is there any philosophical alternative towards which the Christian may choose to orient himself within modern society?

The proposal of the Christian form of individualism is a response to these questions. This proposal attempts to provide the proper orientation of Christians, along with a critique of the fundamentals of such a rationale. The belief that Christians, as well as the rest of humanity, are

32. Committee on Medical Ethics, Episcopal Diocese of Washington, DC, *Assisted Suicide and Euthanasia*, p. 29.
33. Zizioulas, 'Εὐθανασία: Ἀποφάσεις κατὰ τὸ τέλος τῆς ζωῆς', p. 16.
34. Scouteris, 'The Sacredness of the Human Person in itself, with Reference to the Bioethical Dilemmas', pp. 3-5.
35. Zizioulas, 'Εὐθανασία: Ἀποφάσεις κατὰ τὸ τέλος τῆς ζωῆς', p. 18. Having in mind the uncertainty that exists in the anthropological content of our civilisation, Manent wonders: 'How does it [the state] recognize my humanity if it does not recognize the content of my humanity?' (Manent, *A World beyond Politics?*, p. 195).

free and self-determined beings that enjoy a kind of interdependence is a good starting point for the reconsideration of the real but suppressed character of the principles of modern society. Neither the sanctity of life nor the sanctity of a person, but rather the undisguised declaration of the limits of one's power claims, in terms of the interdependence between people, is the best alternative in attempting to reconsider the character of an individualised society and of an autonomous being.

2. The Evilness of Suffering and Respect for Dignity

Another group of arguments is characterised by the pivotal role of suffering. Those who are in favour of euthanasia argue that there is no meaningful suffering, whereas those who are against euthanasia consider suffering as meaningful and profitable to human life. According to the former argument man should not be subject to the process of corruption in human life since it is an affront to human dignity. According to the latter argument, man is considered as something more than his body and its functioning. Both arguments reveal a lack of knowledge regarding human existence, for they consider suffering as powerful enough to threaten human life and human integrity either by permission, though the accomplishment of the process of corruption in human life, or by intention, in the intentional ending of human life before the self-accomplishment of the corruption process. Both considerations attribute to suffering a decisive role regarding human life, though with different orientations.

The decisive role of suffering for issues surrounding euthanasia is widely recognised. What is often ignored is the role of suffering when considering whether a life is worth living or whether a person retains his dignity in his life. Indeed, an attempt has been made to look at both suffering and respect for dignity isolated from human life as a whole. However, this isolation is artificial and results in assumptions such as: 'The suffering associated with a terminal condition assumes the status of the greatest evil arising out of the human condition in public discourse, judicial reasoning and medical morality.'[36] While such an assumption generates arguments in favour of decisions that may result in ending a human life, it does not take into account what actually constitutes a life worth living.

The choice of bioethics, either consciously or unconsciously, to be shaped by the rationale of modern medicine and the medically-defined character of the medical context has been criticised throughout this book. This choice, however, has imposed a system of anthropology on

36. Campbell, 'Suffering, Compassion, and Dignity in Dying', p. 110.

the public debate and, therefore, it has in a way designated the orientation of any ethical discussion on all bioethical issues. At this point, a brief overview of the relevant discussion in bioethics is necessary.

There is a group of bioethicists who believe that the proper treatment of suffering and its impact on the life of a terminally ill patient requires its categorisation into different kinds. They believe that this categorisation offers the appropriate grounds for designating the suitable therapeutic treatment. For example, some of them focus on the development of a taxonomy of factors that contribute to suffering such as physical symptoms, psychological symptoms and existential concerns that may serve as a framework for diagnosis, therapeutic intervention and ongoing scientific communication.[37] Others are interested in the categorisation of the different experiences of suffering, which fall into the categories of agent-narrative suffering, such as fear and angst, or of neuro-cognitive suffering, such as insomnia or bone pain.[38] However, in all these endeavours one finds not a single reference to what all this means for human life. On the contrary, they categorise suffering and use it as a conceptual tool for justifying the hastening of death, not only within the context of the doctrine of double effect. Thus, while this categorisation undoubtedly makes it easier on the practitioners, it results in a paradox and an unjustified outcome. Though it connects this categorisation with the administration of death,[39] namely the end of a human life at least in its biological aspect, it ignores any connection between this categorisation and the meaning of the life of a patient.

In addition, taking into account the 'treatment' of suffering in bioethical arguments, there is an unspoken assumption that suffering is either a constituent part of human existence[40] or the common enemy

37. Cherny, Coyle and Foley, 'Suffering in the Advanced Cancer Patient: A Definition and Taxonomy', pp. 57-63.

38. Jansen and Sulmasy, 'Proportionality, Terminal Suffering and the Restorative Goals of Medicine', pp. 323-25.

39. Jansen and Sulmasy believe that the distinction between the different types of suffering makes the application of the principle of proportionality regarding the imposing of the high risk of hastening the patient's death more accurate and justified (ibid., pp. 329-35). Others go a little bit further and argue that there are a number of principles and imperatives, such as the principle of professional or institutional mission, that are interwoven into the obligation to relieve suffering (Roy, 'The Relief of Pain and Suffering: Ethical Principles and Imperatives', pp. 4-5). The self-evident notion that generates such assumptions is the interest in a discussion that intentionally leads to a casuistry for the appropriateness or not of an intervention at the end of life.

40. Eberl explains how the consideration of suffering as a constituent of human nature is founded on the tradition of the natural law and the teaching of Aquinas

of humanity, given that all human beings suffer[41] and, therefore, it has to be fought for the sake of man, even at his expense. Such approaches towards suffering have been repeatedly challenged throughout this book and may be questioned further.

The discussion of the patristic tradition has shown that suffering, though it is experienced in human life as a natural effect because of the loss of the 'supernatural' communication of man with God in paradise, does not constitute an essential element of human existence. On the contrary, it belongs to the 'accidents', that is those elements that do not belong to the definition of man and cannot be considered as fundamental parts of human existence. In such a context, neither the distinction among the different kinds of suffering nor the connection of suffering with inalienable principles and imperatives can provide convincing arguments regarding the end of a human being. What really counts is the understanding of the accidental character of suffering and, therefore, the necessity for the subordination of such arguments to other priorities such as the voluntary development of the relationship of man with God and his fellow men. In other words, other elements of human existence have to be highlighted as crucial for one's own destiny. This does not mean that the role of suffering in human life is underestimated. On the contrary, suffering must be placed in a meaningful context that secures the dignity of a human being[42] and not a medically defined substantiality of suffering.[43]

A life is valuable not because of suffering but because of the anticipation of the life to come. For the Christian tradition, the end of suffering, though it accompanies the end of biological existence, is not viewed as a convincing orientation for one's own choices. On the contrary, what is really important is the overcoming of corruptible

(Eberl, 'Aquinas on Euthanasia, Suffering and Palliative Care', pp. 338-41).

41. '. . . [I]n our society, the evil is not so much death as physical suffering. Evil tends to merge with physical suffering.' (Manent, *A World Beyond Politics?*, p. 191).

42. Despite the fact that the notion of dignity has a long history in the western civilization, it resulted to have no particular meaning (Kondylis, 'Würde', *Historisches Lexikon zur politisch-sozialen Sprache in Deutschland* [HLPSS]), pp. 645-77.

43. For a similar approach towards suffering, see Augoustidis, 'Ἰατρικῶς ὑποστηριζόμενη αὐτοκτονία: θεολογικὴ προσέγγιση', pp. 10-12. In the same vein, Campbell says: 'The individual who suffers patiently embodies an acceptance of his or her own limits and finitude and achieves dignity in death through a continuation of those traits of character displayed during life' (Campbell, 'Suffering, Compassion, and Dignity in Dying', p. 115). This idea culminates in the phrase: 'It is mistaken . . . to isolate dignity from the totality of a person's life story as though dignity in death were a secularised form of deathbed salvation' (ibid., p. 124).

biological existence for the sake of human life, namely the orientation towards the various dimensions of human life and not towards death. To avoid any misunderstanding, the overcoming of biological existence does not imply a metaphysical orientation but rather the focus on those aspects of human existence that are not affected by death. Such aspects are those that, while rooted in one's own individuality, profit from one's interdependence with the rest of human beings as well as with God. It is this interdependence that makes the overcoming of one's own biological existence possible. For a Christian, life is not fulfilled in an isolated kind of individuality but rather in a relational individuality, namely the Christian form of individualism. In such a context suffering is not the crucial parameter for one's own destiny. Indeed, a Christian confrontation of suffering can only be considered as a means towards the actualisation of a Christian individualism.

3. The Doctrine of Double Effect and the 'Peaceful' Passing: Towards a Consideration of a Patient's 'Best Interests'

The patient's 'best interests' constitutes another essential source for arguments for euthanasia. This discussion is accompanied by the question of whether the deliberate administration of death is profitable to man. However, this question is not accompanied by the proper designation of death and what death stands for. This failure results in a common thread in all responses to the question of what constitutes the 'best interests' of a patient. Thus, the proponents of euthanasia, while they consider the deliberate administration of death in the medical context as profitable to man, fail to see that such a rationale leads to the end of human existence and, therefore, to the loss of power claims that is necessary for the self-preservation of a human being. Similarly, the opponents of euthanasia say that the deliberate administration of death cannot profit man, though in another way.

Interestingly enough, there is an curious meeting point between the proponents and the opponents of euthanasia, which is the patient's 'best interests', that of its profitability to man or not. This is exemplified in the administration of death through either removing life-sustaining means or the application of the doctrine of double effect, a doctrine applied in order to justify the alleviation of pain, despite the fact that the death of a patient will predictably be hastened as a result. It is in such a context that an uncritical adoption of contemporary ideology on the part of Christians, an ideology that clearly stands behind such arguments, takes place.

Apart from the possible justified morality of a medical action regarding the hastening of death of a patient, the Christian understanding of the coming of death is missing. Thus, it is not unexpected that, despite the adoption of either the doctrine of double effect or the practice of turning off the life-support machine, there are always worries regarding their proper application in each case. Even Christians are imprisoned in this practice and consider death as an event isolated from the rest of a patient's own life as well as from the life of his fellow men. This imprisonment betrays, in the most obvious way, the subordination of the free being who was created according to the image of God to the power of corruptible human nature and, at the same time, man's hesitation regarding his own responsibility. What interests all people, including Christians, is the justification of their actions. In a society where what is right and what is wrong is simply a matter of laws, the interest towards the justification of an action in the medical context even among Christians is presented as a one-way choice. However, it is interesting to see some of the theological presuppositions for such a popular orientation among Christians.

Harakas, one of the most representative Orthodox Christian ethicists in the United States, argues that: 'The only "good death" for the Christian is the peaceful acceptance of the end of his or her earthly life with faith and trust in God and the promise of the Resurrection.' Within such a consideration of the Christian 'good death' not only the removal of extraordinary mechanical devices but also the use of painkillers such as morphine – which may have an undefined effect on the length of the patient's life – are permissible.[44] Both practices secure a peaceful passing and therefore they fulfil the necessary condition for a 'good death'.

Obviously, both practices in a way administer death but wish to avoid the attribution of any voluntary character to these medical actions. Indeed, the free man is afraid of his own freedom and has to find the proper 'camouflage' for his decisions. What actually matters in this context is the completion of the necessary procedures. It is for this reason that the definition of the 'good death' perfectly matches a procedural rationale (i.e. a procedure towards a peaceful acceptance of the end of one's earthly life). No doubt, the interest of those in favour of a 'peaceful' passing while in sleep is the absence of any indication for the violation of the well-established moral laws such as the preservation of the biological life of a human being. This concern is suspicious since it is

44. Harakas, *Contemporary Moral Issues Facing the Orthodox Christian*, pp. 166-80. These recommendations are along the same lines as those of the Holy Synod of the Church of Greece (The Holy Synod of the Church of Greece, *Βασικές θέσεις ἐπὶ τῆς ἠθικῆς τῆς Εὐθανασίας*, § 15 and § 50).

expressed even by those who criticise the application of DDE.[45] In other words, with or without the application of DDE, the 'peaceful' passing without the direct intervention of man has to be secured. It is then not surprising that such a rationale is accompanied by the belief that death 'is not natural to us'[46] as well as the idea that 'immortality is the natural condition of man'.[47] Therefore, death becomes something that stands outside man's nature and, consequently, outside man's authority.

It is evident that these beliefs undermine the patristic tradition, according to which death is the natural effect of the composite hypostasis in man, whereas what is not natural is the 'supernatural' communication of man with God. In addition, these beliefs underestimate the fact that man as a free being has to take his own responsibilities and not to turn away from them through the accomplishment of any justification procedures. In such a context, death is considered as the end of biological existence and as the 'second' effect of a 'justified' moral action. However, God has given life to man, a life that does not simply incorporate the biological life of man but also his life and relationship with God (God did not simply create a being that was called a human being but a being according to his own image) as well as the lives of his fellow men, with whom he shares the same nature and the endowment of the image of God in man. Any attempt to reach an isolated consideration of the biological existence of a human being does not correspond to what God has given man and to the 'best interests' of a Christian patient.

III. Concluding Remarks

Both the presentation of the fundamentals of Christian individualism and the critique of modern individualism with regard to the current debate on euthanasia justify the fact that this book does not belong to the tradition of principlism and the procedural consideration of human life and that it does not uncritically accept the preordained designation of the arguments

45. Beaufils, '*Ta foi t'a sauvé*', pp. 239-41.
46. Harakas, *Contemporary Moral Issues Facing the Orthodox Christian*, pp. 166-74. The idea that what is 'natural' is what is healthy and strong whereas what is 'unnatural' is exactly the opposite reminds one of the Enlightenment ideology of natural law. For a critic of this ideology, see Zizioulas, *Disease and Healing in Orthodox Theology*, pp. 133-56. Zizioulas explicitly says that what is most 'natural' is the presence of disease in human life (p. 139). It is clearly implied that death as a consequence of a disease is also a natural event in human life.
47. The Holy Synod of the Church of Greece, *Βασικές θέσεις ἐπὶ τῆς ἠθικῆς τῆς Εὐθανασίας*, § 5.

in bioethics and, particularly, those surrounding euthanasia. In addition, the foundation of a Christian individualism that constitutes, by definition, a bridge or a link between a particular tradition and a particular society shows that this book places itself firmly in both the Christian tradition and modern society, since it is faithful to the Christian truth about human existence in order to establish what should be the proper orientation of man within the Church and wider society.

For the Christian tradition, while each individual is sovereign over his own life, he is at the same time, willingly or not, dependent not only on other beings (even a radical individualism cannot ignore the dependence of people on others in the medical context) but also on the limits that his own nature sets on him (death is not desired but nevertheless it comes). In that sense, a human being is a dependent individual. What is essential is the designation of the exact character of the dependence of each individual.

According to Christian individualism there is always a double dialectic within the life of a human being. The first one signifies the relationship between man and God, a relationship that takes place not on a metaphysical level but rather within one's own existence. The second one designates the relationship between human beings that is based on the assumption that all human beings share the same nature and that all human beings can in fact substantiate, under particular circumstances, in their life, what really corresponds to the character of human nature – man has been created by God according to His own image and, therefore, man has been endowed with a divine character that, due to its subjection to the fallen state of humanity, is not always brought to realisation. This double dialectic is always subject to the proper use of free will or, in other words, to the proper 'treatment' of one's own individuality.

With this in mind, it is possible to place the discussion of the issues surrounding euthanasia that refer to the ethical character of the different kinds of deliberate administration of death in a meaningful context. This context makes it explicit that any decision on human life and death has to take into account the character of human existence, otherwise it may be self-destructive in the sense not of the elimination of one's own existence but principally of the outrage against one's own existence.

From a Christian point of view, decisions on euthanasia should not concern only the administration of the biological end of a human being. As with all decisions related to human life, similarly, decisions related to human death are not isolated actions but are rather connected with all aspects of humanity, such as the relationships with God and between human beings that exist by nature. In addition, the proper placing of death in human life is imperative. As long as the meaning of the biological death of a human being is not clear, decisions regarding euthanasia will lack substantial grounds for their proper justification. Therefore, a Christian consideration of these decisions must take into account both the internal (the inner state of humanity) and external (the relationships with God and one's fellow men) 'dependencies' of man, as well as the limits of the effect that biological death has on human existence.

Christians believe that a human being is more than his biological existence. Therefore, biological death is by no means an absolute evil once there are other things more important than it, such as communication with God. In addition, biological death cannot affect human existence as a whole for the self-evident reason that it threatens only a part of it and that the end of the biological aspect of a human being does not coincide with his end. Consequently, death is considered as a positive event, for it marks the transition from the partial experience of the union with God to the fulfilment of union with God.

Regarding the internal 'dependencies' of human existence, man is a free and a self-determined being. However, he is not able ultimately to avoid biological death. He wishes to but his corruptible nature is not governed by his free will in his fallen state. Nevertheless, it is not human nature that has to reign over the human will and, consequently, over human existence. On the contrary, it is the destiny of the free will to rule over human nature with a view to union with God. No doubt, there is dialectic between what happens due to the corruptible character of humanity and the limited power of the free will. In such a context, the deliberate administration of death to one's own self may be considered as a decision that safeguards the proper order (as was given by God) in taking decisions, namely the leadership of soul over body. However, such an assertion, given the fallen condition of the free will, is not justified. Similarly, letting things happen as they come at least shows a voluntary acceptance of the 'rationale' of the fallen state of humanity and, at the same time, a voluntary resignation from one's own responsibility towards the union and communication with God.

From a Christian point of view, decisions at the end of life cannot be taken by a human being alone but rather in collaboration with God. In this way, any misappropriation of the divine power over human life and death is avoided. Moreover, man must submit his will to the divine will. These two actions are not necessarily dissociated and incompatible. It is the outcome of such a dialectic that would justify a decision actuated by a willingness to die. However, in such a context, a decision that appears to favour euthanasia challenges in the most declarative way the vision of euthanasia as it is appointed by bioethics. For the Christian tradition upon which this book is based, euthanasia makes sense only as part of what is considered as a Christian good death, namely a death that is desirable on the grounds that it serves one's own orientation towards God and others. It is worth noting that such an orientation is evident in the character of man and, particularly, in the external 'dependencies' of that character.

Regarding the external 'dependencies' of a human being, the individual is freely dependent not only on a divine Being by whom he was created but also on the rest of humankind – both those close to him (the physician and the relatives in the medical context) and on those he does not know. In that sense, the external 'dependencies' of a human being do not only entail the members of one's immediate family or the wider community in which one has chosen to live and to be part of. They also involve all those who belong to other communities because of the common nature that brings them closer. In such a context, the decision of a Christian regarding his own biological death is a matter of concern for all human beings. This is not an imposed practice but rather a free decision. For a Christian individual, decisions on euthanasia (the use of the term 'euthanasia' in this context is used despite its ties with the rationale of modern bioethics, a rationale that is challenged in this book) are decisions that take into account their implications for one's relationships with God and one's fellow men, namely relationships that include the whole universe. In other words, Christian individualism follows exactly the opposite process of de Tocqueville's presentation of individualism in modernity.

Through such a procedure, a Christian patient arrives at the crucial point that both Christ and the martyrs experienced and considers whether his or her decision would be profitable to his or her relationship with God, and what the impact of a particular decision would be on the rest of humankind. The obligation of the martyrs was to preserve their unity with God and not their biological existence. They had also to safeguard the recourse to a life-bearing death along with the preservation of their spiritual integrity and dignity. Given the interdependence between spiritual and bodily life, they were oriented towards the service of the former rather than the latter. For the Christian understanding of human existence, voluntary death, either spiritual or bodily, is not a novelty but a common and recommended practice. What is foreign to the Christian tradition is the deliberate administration of death in a medical context that considers man dismantled of the most constituent elements of his own existence and the rest of society.

Consequently, the 'rationality' of the medical context, in which the current debate on euthanasia has developed, is not justified to consider issues on human life and death and, as a consequence, it cannot, by any means, justify any argument regarding either the deliberate administration of death or the actions that cause death as a side effect, even in those cases where such actions appear rational and unavoidable. Such an assertion does not ignore the well-established practice in hospitals and the power claims of the sovereign rationality that prevails in them; the sovereign rationality in the medical context will continue to shape our biological existence in many ways. On the contrary, this assertion provides the basis for opening a discussion on understanding the inconsistencies in the arguments being used in the current reasoning on the character of human existence. The ending of the two chapters devoted to the patristic tradition on the cardinal role of worship, with special reference to baptism and the Eucharist, designates the context in which the willingness to die makes sense. In other words, this book challenges the monopoly of 'universal' principles, the 'universality' of which has been revealed as an illusion, and proposes a constant dialectic between the 'universal' and the 'particular'. To avoid any misunderstanding, such a proposal does not 'proceed in the abstract' and is not against any kind of participatory bioethics that 'is partly imbedded [*sic*] in and partly a reflection of an action for social change that links normative theory with the practical conditions that allow change to occur'.[48] However, it prefers, on the one hand, to elucidate the temptation of Christians to confuse the originality of the message that the Church brings to this world with the sovereign ideologies within contemporary society, with a view to the sharing of power in the public arena,[49] and, on the other, to provide a theological approach that can prove fruitful in decision-making on issues surrounding euthanasia, although what such responsibility would entail is not supplied in prescriptive detail.[50] However, the epilogue that follows may shed more light on this.

---

48. Cahill, *Theological Bioethics*, p. 6.
49. Bekos, 'Introduction', in Hauerwas, Χριστιανισμός και Αμερικανική πολιτική, pp. 7-33.
50. See also Reed, *The Genesis of Ethics*, p. 324.

Epilogue
Euthanasia – Self-sacrifice or Murder?

The present study on Christian ethics has attempted to cover a wide range of issues relevant to bioethics and, particularly, to the issue of euthanasia. A prerequisite of this attempt has been, among others, the discussion of more general issues such as the character of those theories that are related to human existence, since bioethics and euthanasia are directly concerned with human life. Therefore, the current book should not only be viewed as an approach towards a particular bioethical issue, but also as an endeavour at reaching a proper understanding of the fundamentals of ethical discourses today. Moreover, throughout this work one of the most central hypotheses found was the necessary consideration of the current ethical issues as integrated parts of the wider modern society and not as topics isolated from ordinary human life.

This book has attempted to challenge three fundamental imperatives of modern moral thought, in general, and of bioethics, in particular. The first one is the belief that within a culturally fragmented society there is no place for 'particular' moralities, an imperative that is based on the argument that a 'particular' morality lays the foundation for sectarian views of human existence, whereas a 'common' morality is in position to serve a moral consensus and, therefore, the harmonious functioning of society. Contrary to this belief, this book has shown that this argument is based on an illusion arising from ignoring the fact that all theories of human existence are subjective, polemical and, consequently, 'particular' by definition, and share a common ground regarding their basic structure, namely their interest towards self-preservation through power claims over their enemies.

The challenge to this imperative has offered the ground for contesting the second imperative, namely individualism, according to which the individual is considered as a being that takes care of itself and that is finally subsumed in egoism. It is on this ground that the context in which moral issues such as those that emerge in medical circumstances is designated. This book, always with reference to a 'particular' morality such as Christian theology, has presented a series of reasons for questioning the legitimacy of the particular moral arguments mainly elaborated in bioethics. Also it challenges the adequacy of the dominant bioethical arguments to cope with a variety of fears of the moral agents involved, such as the disguised power claims of those in power over those who are in a subservient position. In contrast to the individualism of modern society, the Christian form of individualism, without underestimating the importance of each person's own individuality, proposes a vision of human existence that, though it stems from a 'particular' morality, encompasses all human beings. Christian individualism is in fact a universalistic account of man's individuality. Generally speaking, a Christian is conscious that he is not only a member of the Christian community that takes the life of Christ as its basis and that is made up of its faithful members, but also that he is part of the universe that is not necessarily Christian and with which there is an interdependence.

The proposal of Christian individualism leads to the challenge to the third imperative, namely the imperative of consensus for the sake of globalisation at the cost of the 'particular' moralities. The universalistic account of the individuality of each person within the context of the Christian tradition gives rise to a moral perspective that in fact is an innovation for the history of human existence. Such a perspective secures not only one's own individuality, for the individual remains the cornerstone for decision-making, but also one's own narrative. These are always oriented towards the service of all humans, including one's own existence. In short, Christian individualism brings man face to face with his own responsibilities as well as the responsibilities of others. He has to participate in both. St Paul is very clear when he suggests that 'each of you should be concerned not only about your own interests, but about the interests of others as well' on the grounds of the deliberate choice of Christ to die for humankind:

> You should have the same attitude toward one another that Christ Jesus had, who though he existed in the form of God did not regard equality with God as something to be grasped, but emptied himself by taking on the form of a slave, by looking

> like other men, and by sharing in human nature. He humbled himself, by becoming obedient to the point of death – even death on a cross![1]

However, a few more things on the character of such a responsibility can be said, making the epilogue of a work primarily devoted to the issues surrounding euthanasia more substantial and pragmatic.

At the beginning of this book it was pointed out that euthanasia in its modern form occupies an in-between point between the extreme expressions of the range of social relationships that, according to Kondylis, correspond to the dipole of friendship/enmity. At the end of this book it is important, on the one hand, to discuss the character of euthanasia today, pinpointing, at the same time and in contradiction, the perception that seems to correspond to the Christian tradition. On the other hand, it is imperative to show the Christian ethos that should dominate and that should be adopted in order to confront such ethical dilemmas. This will be done by associating the main points of this book.

As was noted before, Christianity views individuality in ecumenical terms, since a person's individuality is not exhausted within the framework of society or a narrative. What is the way to reveal such a Christian character of individuality and, more particularly, in relation to euthanasia?

The answer to this question should not be derived from the description of a role for the Christian narrative, with the prospect of constructing so-called cosmopolitanism[2] – an ethic that 'relies on the ability to listen and to talk to people whose commitments, beliefs, and projects may seem distant from our own'.[3] On the contrary, the answer should focus on a kind of cosmopolitanism that is not confined to the ability to speak and listen to the other but that wants and tries to embrace the life of humanity as a whole, with the prospect of successfully managing the bioethical dilemma of euthanasia.

It was noted in the general introduction that euthanasia is nothing more than an expression of the possibilities that mortality offers to the acting subject who can use these possibilities at certain, usually chosen, moments both for other objects and for himself, since everyone knows or finds what he should do to bring his own death or the death of someone else's when this is wanted.[4] For Kondylis the extreme expressions of mortality, as the possibility of causing death, are self-sacrifice

1. Philippians 2: 4-8.
2. Appiah, *The Ethics of Identity*, p. 257.
3. Ibid., p. 246.
4. Kondylis, *Das Politische und der Mensch*, p. 241.

(friendship) and murder (enmity). If this is how things are, in which direction is euthanasia heading? Towards self-sacrifice or murder? Let us pose the question differently. How close is euthanasia to self-sacrifice or to murder, respectively?

If self-sacrifice is defined as the sacrifice of someone for the other, then it is difficult to allege that euthanasia is a social event that has anything to do with such a sacrifice. This does not mean that euthanasia is murder and that it is interconnected with the concept of someone killing someone else. Also, this does not mean a lot for its supporters since euthanasia could be detected at a point close to the extreme expression of enmity that is the murder.

Kondylis thinks that the anthropological parameter of mortality is an objective anthropological fact that 'can become a motive for many different expectations, attitudes and behaviours',[5] like self-sacrifice, murder or suicide, and which constitute interference to the social relation.[6] If the social relation coincides with the very being of society and belongs as a component of its meaning, whereas the politic is the particular social relation that makes the social as a whole its object and that must possess cohesion and order, one may draw the following conclusions.

First, euthanasia under no circumstances can become an object of discussion that is defined in terms of the characteristics of the clinic, since in such a framework of discussion the encounter of life or death issues can only lead to mismanagement. Second, euthanasia cannot become an object of discussion of a particular, narrow academic discipline such as bioethics, which has a particular ideology. In the preceding analysis it has been shown that this discipline is characterised by a weakness to encompass society as a whole, as well as a refusal to formulate any persuasive connection between human nature and the social relation and the political ethos, since it prefers bio-politics and not the formulations of an ethic that may be applied to the social situation as a whole. Third, the immediate consequence of the above is the conclusion that the dominant arguments of both the supporters (autonomy, dignity) and the opponents (the sanctity of life or the 'peaceful passing') have an ideological character – in the sense that they constitute hermeneutical beliefs and values that are dogmatically supported[7] – as they claim an overall power (though they are bonded to legislation, medical practices or the need to safeguard a direct or indirect involvement in the causation of death by someone to someone else or by someone to himself).

5. Ibid., p. 244.
6. Ibid., p. 246.
7. Popper, 'The Death of Theories and of Ideologies', p. 300.

We proceed to the main question regarding the character of euthanasia and whether, in the case of human mortality, it is either expressed as self-sacrifice or as murder, as friendship or as enmity. We will provide two answers that, as we will show, cannot be separated.

The first answer mostly matches the secular approach to the matter. Kondylis says that the verification of an act as friendly or hostile – an act cannot be characterised as something else – is connected with the question regarding what a mortal person can do to a mortal person and whose answer can be pleasant acts and/or useful, as well as unpleasant and/or harmful. The evaluation of an act as 'good' or 'bad' is excluded because man is not absolutely 'bad' when he kills and not absolutely 'good' when he loves.[8] Therefore, by avoiding the obstacle of evaluating euthanasia from the perspective of a particular spiritual tradition and, consequently, the danger of being accused of sectarian practices, we could say that euthanasia in its modern definition represents an unpleasant and harmful practice since it has been founded on an ideology that refuses to recognise its consequences for society as a whole and, therefore, for the human species.

The second answer corresponds in the main to the approach of Christian ethics presented in this book. A Christian individual cannot understand the logic that euthanasia expresses since the arguments that accompany it do not touch him or have any meaning for him. On the contrary, in euthanasia he recognises another form of the alienation of man that does not only go unnoticed by our society but that marks it in a negative perspective that may serve the needs of mass democracy but not the need of man for self-understanding and for understanding the reality that surrounds him. It is obvious that such a practice deprives man of his most fundamental right, that of freedom. As a consequence, he turns against man who, as a creation of God, aims to reinstate the relations with himself and with others, that is reality as a whole, something that characterises human nature.[9] In such an analysis, euthanasia seems to be more or less – this is not of too much importance – associated with the extreme expression of enmity that is murder.

The Christian tradition is a spiritual tradition founded on the cultivation of *philia* and love and it can only remain at the very opposite plane to the practice of euthanasia. The bioethical dilemma in euthanasia exists because the ethos that would clarify things is absent from modern

8. Kondylis, *Das Politische und der Mensch*, p. 244.
9. St Basil's thought on this issue is characteristic: 'nothing characterizes our nature more than to be in communion with one another, to be in need of one another and to love our species' (PG 31, 917A).

society. The ethos that is needed is the ethos of cosmopolitanism, but which is oriented to human existence and society as a whole. As was shown in the description of the Christian view of individuality with its all-encompassing perspective, the Christian tradition guarantees such an ethos, which is not equated with the effort to convert everyone into a Church member. A Christian cosmopolitanism marks the efforts of the Christian believer to start from his own narrative and to aim at grasping and taking into consideration the whole sociontic field.

The *intellectus archetypus* required to overcome the finite character of the human intellect, and which could be used to move away from the partial character of every conceptual framework in order to understand reality, may not exist.[10] However, for every Christian such a prospect is possible and comprises a permanent preoccupation and responsibility, in that he is certain that his weakness will be completed by the power of God. This is the kind of ethos that has been revealed through the study of the theology of St John Damascene and St Symeon the New Theologian.

10. Kondylis, *Das Politische und der Mensch*, p. 188.

Afterword
by Ulrich Volp

Everybody would agree that, with recent medical advances, today's world expects some of us to arrive at decisions and to solve ethical problems which simply did not exist a generation or two ago. This can be frightening, indeed give rise to fearful agony in the light of the need for a solitary, if not lone, decision. One strategy is to approach these deliberations by collecting criteria for or against one side, and it would appear that it tends to be a particular thought or criterion which eventually swings the decision in one or the other direction. However, it is the virtue of a book such as this one to remind us that this process is far more complex, and that any decision maker is anything but the solitary decider as he or she sometimes appears to be. He or she will be helped, if not manipulated, by contemporary bioethics and their justifications but, even more so, by what is considered to be 'the facts': the medical situation, the presumption of the nature of the state the human being has attained and, indeed, by what a human being is, what constitutes his or her humanity – often described today in fairly technical medical terms.

John Bekos' descriptive approach in the first part of this book shows the dynamics behind this reasoning and firmly situates them in the history of thought, society and politics of the twentieth and twenty-first centuries. The second part exposes the patristic tradition to a similar analysis and demonstrates its complex ethical reasoning which draws on an even older tradition of wisdom and ethical decision, starting from the Genesis narrative of God creating human beings and introducing death into their existence, and not ending with Aristotle and Porphyry. It is no accident, however, that we feel Bekos is more inclined to appreciate the honesty with which John Damascene describes his method as similar to that of the bees and their *alvaria* making use of the different said traditions. Both Damascene and Symeon are revealed as thinkers deeply concerned about the whence and what of anthropology, *viz.*, they investigate the present state of humanity in general and, indeed, what a human being is, what constitutes his or her humanity, and his or her death – described in biblical and philosophical terms. Thus, we are confronted with a forceful alternative not only to contemporary bioethics, but to the anthropological concept present in today's intensive care units (ICUs), a concept that describes the indicative mode of a human being's condition and thereby suggests imperatives of ethical decision. The force of these anthropologies can only be understood in the light of the absence of a convincing anthropological alternative since the Western theological anthropologies – from Augustine to Thomas Aquinas and Martin Luther – seem to have lost their persuasiveness for the time being. This alone would make an insight into the Greek anthropologies of the eighth to eleventh centuries a valuable addition to today's ethical discourse. However, it seems to be a common misunderstanding that Eastern and Western thought differs in that they arrive at different answers to the same questions. Instead, their theology differs substantially, because they ask different questions – despite the fact that the great Fathers of the East and the West built their thoughts on the same biblical texts and the same philosophical tradition. Western thinkers, such as Tertullian, Cyprian, Augustine and Luther, were interested in salvation and its feasibility rather than the constitution of the cosmos, in Christ's work of salvation rather than his person, the Church as an institute of salvation rather than its constitution through worship and remembrance or imitation of martyrdom, ethos rather than *logos*. Western theological 'anthropology' is sometimes almost synonymous with the doctrine of justification (leading up to the controversy about autonomy and heteronomy), whereas the Greek Fathers rather associated it with the Christological question of Christ's humanity and divinity. Obviously, Augustine's greatness owes a good deal to having successfully incorporated some of the Greek ideas, but he is still, I dare say, primarily concerned with decidedly 'Western' questions rather than those troubling Eastern minds of his period.

In some respects this book repeats the process witnessed in Augustine's time when the thinking of the Greek Fathers was brought into play in order to answer Western questions: Bekos exposes a question urgently asked and brought about by the technology driven health system of the contemporary 'West' – euthanasia in the sense used in this book – to the anthropological thinking of the East as exemplified by John Damascene and Symeon. This process is mind-blowingly revealing as to how deeply rooted contemporary bioethics are in the Western theological and anthropological traditions: the concept of a 'brain death' being a criterion for the existence or non-existence of a human being could perhaps only emerge in a tradition focussing on what human beings do, rather than what they are, a tradition which is but ignorant of the concept of a hypostatic union of body and soul so ingrained in Greek thinking. However, by confronting contemporary bioethics with a complex anthropological concept developed over one and a half millenia (from Plato and Aristotle to Symeon), this book also asks the fundamental question of the relationship between anthropology – what constitutes a human being and his or her humanity – and an ethical decision over the life of such a being. How does the indicative mode evolve into an imperative? This is a question which requires further thought for anybody being faced with the difficult decisions I mentioned in the beginning. I sincerely wish that this book should be taken as admonition and exhortation for this thought process: the anthropological roots of our thinking, the traditions which shaped Christian society and thought, be they Latin or Greek, constitute a more promising point to start than the indicatives of the ICU.

Ulrich Volp
Chair for Ecclesiastical History and History of Doctrine (Patristics)
Johannes Gutenberg University Mainz
Germany

Bibliography

i. English translations of patristic writings used in the present study

St John of Damascus, *Writings: The Fount of Knowledge*, F.H. Chase (trans.) (Washington, DC: Catholic University of America Press, 1958)

St John of Damascus, *On the Divine Images: Three Apologies Against Those Who Attack the Divine Image*, D. Anderson (trans.) (Crestwood, NY: St Vladimir's Seminary Press, 2000)

Symeon the New Theologian, *The Discourses*, C.J. de Catanzaro (trans.) (New York: Paulist Press, 1980)

Symeon the New Theologian, *The Practical and Theological Chapters and the Three Theological Discourses*, P. McGuckin (trans.) (Michigan: Cistercian Publications, 1982)

St Symeon the New Theologian, *On the Mystical Life: The Ethical Discourses, Vol. 1: The Church and the Last Things*, A. Golitzin (trans.) (Crestwood, NY: St Vladimir's Seminary Press, 1995)

St Symeon the New Theologian, *On the Mystical Life: The Ethical Discourses, Vol. 2: On Virtue and Christian Life*, A. Golitzin (trans.) (Crestwood, NY: St Vladimir's Seminary Press, 1996)

St Symeon the New Theologian, *On the Mystical Life: The Ethical Discourses, Vol. 3: Life, Times and Theology*, A. Golitzin (trans.) (Crestwood, NY: St Vladimir's Seminary Press, 1997)

ii. References

Afentoulidou, I. 'Οἱ ὕμνοι τοῦ Συμεὼν τοῦ Νέου Θεολόγου: σχέσεις τῶν ἐπιγραφῶν μὲ τοὺς ὕμνους', *Βυζαντινά*, 22 (2001), 123-47

Agamben, G. *Homo Sacer: Sovereign Power and Bare Life*, D. Heller-Roazen (trans.) (Stanford: Stanford University Press, 1998)

Alfeyev, H. *St Symeon the New Theologian and Orthodox Tradition* (Oxford: Oxford University Press, 2000)

Anagnostopoulos, B. 'Ἡ περὶ τῆς Θεοτόκου διδασκαλία τοῦ Ἰωάννου τοῦ Δαμασκηνοῦ', *Εὐχαριστήριον, Τιμητικὸς Τόμος Ἀμίλκα Σ. Ἀλιβιζάτου* (Athens, 1958), 570-78

Andriotis, N.P. *Ἐτυμολογικὸ λεξικὸ τῆς κοινῆς νεοελληνικῆς* (Thessaloniki: Manolis Triantafyllidis Foundation, 1983)

Appiah, K.A. *The Ethics of Identity* (Princeton: Princeton University Press, 2005)

Aquinas, Thomas, *The Summa Theologica*, Fathers of the English Dominican Province (trans.) (New York: Benziger Bros, 1947-1948)

Arendt, H. *On Violence* (San Diego: Harcourt Brace & Co., 1970)

Ariès, P. *Essais sur l'histoire de la mort en occident: du moyen âge à nos jours* (Paris: Editions du Seuil, 1975)

Aristotle. *Nicomachean Ethics*, R. Crisp (ed. and trans.) (New York: Cambridge University Press, 2000)

Armstrong, D.M. *A Materialist Theory of Mind* (London: Routledge, 1993)

Augoustidis, A. 'Ἰατρικῶς ὑποστηριζόμενη αὐτοκτονία: θεολογικὴ προσέγγιση', proceedings of the Scientific Conference, *The Church and Bioethics: The Word of Science and the Word of Religion* (Chambésy, Geneva), 11-15 September 2002, unpublished manuscript

Augustine, *The City of God against the Pagans*, trans. R. W. Dyson (Cambridge: Cambridge University Press, 1998)

Baker, A.B. 'The Application of the Criteria of the Just War Theories in the Resolution of Medical-Ethical Dilemmas at the Bedside', *Linacre Quarterly*, 62 (4) (1995), 3-19

Bathrellos, D. *The Byzantine Christ: Person, Nature, and Will in the Christology of St Maximus the Confessor* (Oxford: Oxford University Press, 2004)

Battin, P.B. *The Least-Worst Death: Essays in Bioethics on the End of Life* (New York: Oxford University Press, 1994)

Beauchamp, T., and Childress, J. *Principles of Biomedical Ethics* (Oxford: Oxford University Press, 2001)

Beauchamp, T. 'A Defense of the Common Morality', *Kennedy Institute of Ethics Journal*, 13 (3) (2003), 259-74

Beaufils, D. '*Ta foi t'a sauvé*': *Approche orthodoxe de la maladie et de la mort* (Paris: Desclée de Brouwer, 1996)

Bekos, I. 'Τὸ κακὸ σήμερα', *Σύναξη*, 94 (April-June 2005), 4-12

Bekos, I. 'The Image of God in Man According to St John Damascene: Implications on Issues Surrounding Euthanasia', in F. Young, M. Edwards and P.M. Parvis (eds), *Studia Patristica, Vol. XLII* (Leuven: Peeters, 2006), 285-90

Berkman, J. 'How Important is the Doctrine of Double Effect for Moral Theology? Contextualizing the Controversy', *Christian Bioethics*, 3 (2) (1997), 89-114

Bole, T.J. 'The Theoretical Tenability of the Doctrine of Double Effect', *The Journal of Medicine and Philosophy*, 16 (5) (1991), 467-73

Boyle, J. 'Who Is Entitled to Double Effect?', *The Journal of Medicine and Philosophy*, 16 (5) (1991), 475-94

Boyle, J.M. 'Toward Understanding the Principle of Double Effect', in P.A. Woodward (ed), *The Doctrine of Double Effect: Philosophers Debate a Controversial Moral Principle* (Notre Dame: Notre Dame University Press, 2001), 7-20

Breck, J. 'Bioethical Dilemmas and Orthodoxy', *Σύναξη*, 68 (1998), 5-20

Breck, J. *The Sacred Gift of Life: Orthodox Christianity and Bioethics* (Crestwood, NY: St Vladimir's Seminary Press, 1998)

Breck, J. 'Bio-Medical Technology: of the Kingdom or of the Cosmos', *St Vladimir's Quarterly*, 32 (1) (1988), 5-26

Brock, S. 'Iconoclasm and the Monophysites', in A. Bryer and J. Herrin (eds), *Iconoclasm: Papers Given at the Ninth Spring Symposium of Byzantine Studies* (Birmingham: Centre for Byzantine Studies, University of Birmingham, 1975)

Cahill, L.S. 'Theological Contexts of Just War Theory and Pacifism: A Response to J. Bryan Hehir', *The Journal of Religious Ethics*, 20 (2) (1992), 259-65

Cahill, L.S. *Theological Bioethics: Participation, Justice, and Change* (Washington, DC: Georgetown University Press, 2005)

Calhoun, L. 'The Metaethical Paradox of Just War Theory', *Ethical Theory and Moral Practice*, 4 (2001), 41-58

Campbell, C.S. 'Suffering, Compassion, and Dignity in Dying', *Duquesne Law Review*, 35 (1) (1996), 109-24

Castoriadis, C. *Ὁ θρυμματισμένος κόσμος* (Athens: Ypsilon, 1990)

Castoriadis, C. *Le monde morcelé* (Paris: Editions du Seuil, 1990)

Cavanaugh, T. 'Double Effect and the Ethical Significance of Distinct Volitional States', *Christian Bioethics*, 3 (2) (1997), 131-41

Changeux, J.-P., and Ricouer, P. *What Makes Us Think? A Neuroscientist and a Philosopher Argue about Ethics, Human Nature and the Brain* (Princeton: Princeton University Press, 2000)

Cherny, N.I., Coyle, N., and Foley, K.M. 'Suffering in the Advanced Cancer Patient: A Definition and Taxonomy', *Journal of Palliative Care*, 10 (2) (1994), 57-70

Chevalier, C. *La Mariologie de St Jean Damascène* (Rome: Pontificium Institutum Orientalium Studiorum, 1936)

Childress, J. 'Just-War Criteria', in T.A. Shannon (ed), *War or Peace? The Search for New Answers* (New York: Orbis Books, 1980), 40-58

Childress, J. 'Just-war theory: The Bases, Interrelations, Prioritics, and Functions of Their Criteria', *Journal of Theological Studies*, 39 (3) (1978), 427-55

Christou, P. 'Εἰσαγωγή', in P. Christou (ed), *Βίος τοῦ Συμεὼν ὑπὸ Νικήτα Στηθάτου-Κεφάλαια-Εὐχαριστίαι* (Thessaloniki: Gregorios Palamas, 1983)

Cipolla, C.M. *Before the Industrial Revolution: European Society and Economy, 1000-1700* (London: Routledge, 1993)

Clouser, K.D., 'Bioethics', in T.L. Beauchamp and L. Walters (eds), *Contemporary Issues in Bioethics* (Belmont: Wadsworth Publishing Company, 1989)

Committee on Medical Ethics, Episcopal Diocese of Washington, DC. *Assisted Suicide and Euthanasia: Christian Moral Perspective: The Washington Report* (Harrisburg, PA: Morehouse Publishing, 1997)

Corlett, A.J. 'Is There a Moral Duty to Die?', *Health Care Analysis*, 9 (1) (2001), 41-63

Descartes, R. *Meditations on First Philosophy*, D.A. Cress (trans.) (Indianapolis: Hackett Pub. Co. Inc., 1979)

Donchin, A. 'Autonomy, Interdependence, and Assisted Suicide: Respecting Boundaries/Crossing Lines', *Bioethics*, 14 (3) (2000), 187-204

Doucet, H. *Les promesses du crépuscule: réflexions sur l'euthanasie et l'aide médicale au suicide* (Geneva: Labor et Fides, 1998)

Duffy, J. 'Hellenic Philosophy in Byzantium and the Lonely Mission of Michael Psellos', in K. Ierodiakonou (ed), *Byzantine Philosophy and its Ancient Sources* (Oxford: Clarendon Press, 2002), 139-56

Dworkin, G. *The Theory and Practice of Autonomy* (Cambridge: Cambridge University Press, 1988)

Dyck, A.J. 'Ethics in Medicine', unpublished manuscript

Dyobouniotes, K. *Ἰωάννης Δαμασκηνός* (Athens, 1903)

Eber, G. 'Orthodox Christian Bioethics', *Christian Bioethics*, 1 (2) (1995), 128-52

Eberl, J.T. 'Aquinas on Euthanasia, Suffering and Palliative Care', *The National Catholic Bioethics Quarterly* (Summer 2003), 331-54

Engelhardt, H.T. *The Foundations of Bioethics* (New York: Oxford University Press, 1996)

Engelhardt, H.T. 'Respect for Life and the Foundations of Bioethics', in D. Noble and J.D. Vincent (eds), *The Ethics of Life* (Paris: UNESCO, 1997), 21-36

Engelhardt, H.T. *The Foundations of Christian Bioethics* (Lisse: Swetz & Zeitlinger Publishers, 2000)

Engelhardt, H.T. 'The Many Faces of Autonomy', *Health Care Analysis*, 9 (3) (2001), 283-97

Ermoni, V. *St Jean Damascène* (Paris: Librairie Bloud & Cie, 1904)

Farantos, M. *Δογματικὴ καὶ ἠθική: εἰσαγωγικά* (Athens, 1973)

Faucon, P. 'Infrastructures philosophiques de la théodicée de Jean Damascène', *Revue des Sciences Philosophiques et Théologiques*, 69 (1985), 361-87

Fletcher, J. *Morals and Medicine* (Princeton, NJ: Princeton University Press, 1979)

Florovsky, G. *The Byzantine Fathers of the Fifth Century (Belmont, MA: Nordland, 1987).*

Fortino, E.F: 'Sanctification and Deification', *Diakonia*, 17 (3) (1982), 192-200

Foucault, M. *The Birth of the Clinic: An Archaeology of Medical Perception* (New York: Vintage Books, 1994)

Foucault, M. *The History of Sexuality: An Introduction* (New York: Vintage Books, 1990)

Fountoulis, I. *Λειτουργικὰ Θέματα* A (Thessaloniki, 1977), 101-16

Frede, M. 'John of Damascus on Human Action, the Will, and Human Freedom', in K. Ierodiakonou (ed), *Byzantine Philosophy and Its Ancient Sources* (Oxford: Clarendon Press, 2002), 63-95

Fuchs, T. 'The Notion of "Killing": Causality, Intention and Motivation in Active and Passive Euthanasia', *Medicine, Healthcare and Philosophy*, 1 (1998), 245-53

Fuchs, E., Lalive d'Epinay, C., Michel, J. P., Scherer, K. R, & Stettler,. 'La notion d'autonomie: une reformulation interdisciplinaire', *Cahiers Médico-Sociaux*, 41 (1997), 161-80

Gillon, R. 'Persistent Vegetative State, Withdrawal of Artificial Nutrition and Hydration, and the Patient's "Best Interests"', *Journal of Medical Ethics*, 24 (1998), 75-76

Gondreau, P. *The Passions of Christ's Soul in the Theology of St Thomas Aquinas* (Münster: Aschendorff Verlag, 2002)
Grisez, G. *The Way of the Lord Jesus I: Christian Moral Principles* (Quincy, IL: Franciscan Press, 1997)
Gunderson, M. 'A Right to Suicide Does Not Entail a Right to Assisted Death', *Journal of Medical Ethics*, 23 (1997), 51-54
Guroian, V. 'Euthanasia and Care for the Dying in the Orthodox Tradition', in J.T. Chirban (ed), *Ethical Dilemmas: Crisis in Faith and Modern Medicine* (Lanham, MD: University Press of America, 1993), 35-47
Habermas, J. *The Theory of Communicative Action I: Reason and the Rationalization of Society*, trans. T. McCarthy (London: Heinemann Educational Books Ltd, 1984)
Habermas, J. *Moral Consciousness and Communicative Action*, trans. C. Lenhardt and S.W. Nicholsen (Cambridge: MIT Press, 1990)
Habermas, J. *Die Zukunft der menschlichen Natur: Auf dem Weg zu einer liberalen Eugenik?* (Frankfurt am Main: Suhrkamp Verlag, 2001)
Haldon, J.F. *Byzantium in the Seventh Century: The Transformation of a Culture* (Cambridge: Cambridge University Press, 1990)
Harakas, S. *Contemporary Moral Issues Facing the Orthodox Christian* (Minneapolis: Light & Life Pub. Co., 1982)
Hatzinikolaou, N. 'Ἀρχὲς ὀρθόδοξου βιοηθικοῦ προβληματισμοῦ', proceedings of the conference, Principles and Values for the Constructing of Europe, Athens, 4-6 May 2003, in https://www.bioethics.org.gr/013_Sinedriofr.html [accessed 12 June 2019]
Hauerwas, S. *Suffering Presence: Theological Reflections on Medicine, the Mentally Handicapped, and the Church* (Notre Dame, IN: University of Notre Dame Press, 1986)
Hauerwas, S. *Christian Existence Today: Essays on Church, World and Living in Between* (Grand Rapids, MI: Baker Books House Co., 1988)
Hauerwas, S. *Dispatches from the Front: Theological Engagement with the Secular* (Durham, NC: Duke University Press, 1994)
Hauerwas, S., and Pinches, C. *Christians among the Virtues: Theological Conversation with Ancient and Modern Ethics* (Notre Dame, IN: University of Notre Dame Press, 1997)
Hauerwas, S. Χριστιανισμός και Αμερικανική πολιτική: Μια κριτική της χριστιανικής Αμερικής, trans. and ed. I. Bekos (Athens: En Plo, 2007)
Hausherr, I. *Un grand mystique byzantin: vie de Syméon le nouveau théologien, 940-1022* (Rome: Pontificium Institutum Orientalium Studiorum, 1928)
Hays, B.R. *The Moral Vision of the New Testament: Community, Cross, New Creation* (Edinburgh: T&T Clark, 1996)
Heyd, D. 'The Meaning of Life and the Right to Voluntary Euthanasia', in A. Carmi (ed), *Euthanasia* (Berlin: Springer-Verlag, 1984), 169-74
Holl, K. *Gesammelte Aufsätze zur Kirchengeschichte II* (Tübingen: J.C.B. Mohr, 1928)
Holy Synod of the Church of Greece, *Βασικές θέσεις ἐπὶ τῆς ἠθικῆς τῆς Εὐθανασίας*, in http://www.bioethics.org.gr/Euthanasiagr.pdf [accessed 12 June 2019]

Hussey, J.M. *The Orthodox Church in the Byzantine Empire* (New York: Oxford University Press, 1986)

Interparliamentary Assembly on Orthodoxy, 'The Declaration of the Basic Principles of Bioethics Based on the Orthodox Tradition', 9th Annual General Assembly, Bucharest, June 2002, in http://eiao.org/archives/1683 [accessed 12 June 2019]

Janin, R. *La géographie ecclésiastique de l'empire byzantin* (Paris: L'Institut français d'études byzantines, 1969)

Jansen, L.A., and Sulmasy, D.P. 'Proportionality, Terminal Suffering and the Restorative Goals of Medicine', *Medicine and Bioethics*, 23 (4-5) (2002), 321-37

John Paul II, *Evangelium Vitae*, in http://w2.vatican.va/content/john-paul-ii/en/encyclicals/documents/hf_jp-ii_enc_25031995_evangelium-vitae.html

Jonas, H. *Philosophical Essays: From Ancient Creed to Technological Man* (Englewood Cliffs, NJ: Prentice-Hall, 1974)

Jonas, H. *The Imperative of Responsibility: In Search of an Ethics for the Technological Age* (Chicago: University of Chicago Press, 1984)

Jonas, H. *Philosophische Untersuchungen und Metaphysische Vermutungen* (PUMV) (Frankfurt: Suhrkamp, 1994)

Jonas, H. *The Phenomenon of Life: Toward a Philosophical Biology* (Evanston, IL: Northwestern University Press, 2001)

Jonsen, R.A. *The Birth of Bioethics* (Oxford: Oxford University Press, 1998)

Jubilee Bishops' Council of the Russian Orthodox Church, *Bases of the Social Concept of the Russian Orthodox Church* (2000), in http://orthodoxeurope.org/page/3/14.aspx [accessed 12 June 2019]

Kaldellis, A. *The Argument of Psellos' Chronographia* (Leiden: Brill, 1999)

Kallis, A. 'Johannes von Damaskus', in M. Greschat (ed), *Gestalten der Kirchengeschichte: Alte Kirche II* (Stuttgart: Verlag W. Kohlhammer, 1984), 289-301

Kant, I. *Groundwork of the Metaphysic of Morals*, trans. H.J. Paton (New York: Harper & Row, 1964)

Kant, I. *Critique of Pure Reason*, trans. P. Guyer and A.W. Wood (Cambridge: Cambridge University Press, 1998)

Karahalios, G. 'Michael Psellos on Man and His Beginnings', *The Greek Orthodox Theological Review*, 18 (1&2) (1973), 79-96.

Karayiannopoulos, I. *Ἡ Μεσαιωνικὴ δυτικὴ Εὐρώπη: Εἰσαγωγὴ στὴ μελέτη τῆς ἱστορίας της, τοῦ κοινωνικοῦ καὶ οἰκονομικοῦ της βίου* (Thessaloniki: Vanias, 1996)

Karmiris, I. 'Ἡ δογματική διδασκαλία τοῦ Ἰωάννου Δαμασκηνοῦ', in *Θρησκευτικὴ Ἐγκυκλοπαίδεια III* (Athens, 1940)

Karmiris I. *Τὰ δογματικὰ καὶ συμβολικὰ μνημεῖα τῆς Ὀρθοδόξου Καθολικῆς Ἐκκλησίας I* (Athens, 1960)

Kass, L.R. 'Appreciating the Phenomenon of Life', *Hastings Center Report*, 27 (7) (1995), 3-12

Kass, L.R. *Life, Liberty and the Defence of Dignity: The Challenge for Bioethics* (San Francisco: Encounter Books, 2002)

Kazhdan, P.A., and Epstein, A.W. *Change in Byzantine Culture in the Eleventh and Twelfth Centuries* (Berkeley: University of California Press, 1985)

Kazhdan, A. *A History of Byzantine Literature (650-850)* (Athens: The National Hellenic Research Foundation, 1999)

Kierkegaard, S. *Repetition* (Princeton, NJ: Princeton University Press, 1946)

Koder, J. 'Γιατί ο Συμεών ο Νέος Θεολόγος έγραφε τους ύμνους του', Νέα Εστία, 1794 (November 2006), 806-19

Kondylis, P. *Macht und Entscheidung: Die Herausbildung der Weltbilder und die Wertfrage* (Stuttgart: Ernst Klett Verlag für Wissen und Bildung, 1984)

Kondylis, P. *Der Niedergang der bürgerlichen Denk- und Lebensform: die liberale Moderne und die massendemokratische Postmoderne* (Weinheim: VCH Acta Humaniora, 1991)

Kondylis, P. *Ἀπὸ τὸν 20ᵒ στὸν 21ᵒ αἰώνα: Τομὲς στὴν πλανητικὴ πολιτικὴ περὶ τὸ 2000* (Athens: Themelio, 1998)

Kondylis, P. *Das Politische und der Mensch: Grundzüge der Sozialontologie Band 1 (Soziale Beziehung, Verstehen, Rationalität)* (Berlin: Akademie Verlag, 1999)

Kondylis, P. 'Würde', *Historisches Lexikon zur politisch-sozialen Sprache in Deutschland*, Band 6, 1984, pp. 645-677

Konstantinidis, C. 'Τεχνητὴ γονιμοποίησης καὶ θεολογία', *Ὀρθοδοξία*, 33 (1958), 66-79, 174-90, 329-35 and 451-68; and *Ὀρθοδοξία*, 34 (1959), 36-53 and 212-30

Konstantinidis, C. *Ἡ ἀναγνώριση τῶν μυστηρίων τῶν ἑτεροδόξων στὶς διαχρονικὲς σχέσεις Ὀρθοδοξίας καὶ Ρωμαιοκαθολικισμοῦ* (*The Recognition of the Sacraments of Heterodoxies in the Diachronic Relations between Orthodoxy and Roman Catholicism*) (Katerini, Greece: Epektasi, 1995)

Koritansky, J.C. 'Alexis de Tocqueville (1805-1859)', in H. Heuermann (ed), *Classics in Cultural Criticism II* (Frankfurt am Main: Verlag Peter Lang GmbH, 1990), 15-38

Kotter, B. *Die Schriften des Johannes von Damaskus I-V* (Berlin: Walter de Gruyter, 1969-1988)

Krivocheine, B. 'The Writings of St. Symeon the New Theologian', *Orientalia Christiana Periodica*, 20 (1954), 298-328

Krivocheine, B. *St Symeon the New Theologian: Life-Spirituality-Doctrine, 'In the Light of Christ'* (Crestwood, NY: St Vladimir's Seminary Press, 1986)

Kushe, H. 'Euthanasia', in P. Singer (ed), *A Companion to Ethics* (Oxford: Blackwell, 1997), 294-302

Leemans, J., Mayer, W., Allen, P., and Dehandschutter, B. *Let Us Die That We May Live* (London: Routledge, 2003)

Lemerle, P. *Le premier humanisme byzantin: notes et remarques sur enseignement et culture à Byzance des origines au Xe siècle* (Paris: Presses universitaires de France, 1971)

Levinas, E. *Totality and Infinity: An Essay on Exteriority*, trans. A. Lingis (Pittsburgh: Duquesne University Press, 1969)

Levinas, E. *Otherwise than Being or Beyond Essence*, trans. A. Lingis (Pittsburgh: Duquesne University Press, 1981)

Levinas, E. 'Dialogue with Emmanuel Levinas', in R.A. Cohen (ed), *Face to Face with Levinas* (Albany, NY: State University of New York, 1986), 13-33

Little, M. 'Assisted Suicide, Suffering and the Meaning of a Life', *Theoretical Medicine and Bioethics*, 20 (1999), 287-98

Locke, J. *An Essay Concerning Human Understanding* (Oxford: Clarendon Press, 1979)

Loewy, E.H., and Loewy, R.S. '*Lebensunwertes Leben* and the Obligation to Die: Does the Obligation to Die Rest on a Misunderstanding of Community?', *Health Care Analysis*, 7 (1) (1999), 23-36

Loewy, E.H. 'The Role of Suffering and Community in Clinical Ethics', *The Journal of Clinical Ethics*, 2 (2) (1991), 83-89

Lossky, V. *In the Image and Likeness of God* (Crestwood, NY: St Vladimir's Seminary Press, 1974)

Louth, A. *St John Damascene: Tradition and Originality in Byzantine Theology* (Oxford: Oxford University Press, 2002)

MacIntyre, A. *After Virtue: A Study in Moral Theory* (Notre Dame, IN: University of Notre Dame Press, 1984)

MacIntyre, A. *Whose Justice? Which Rationality* (London: Gerald Duckworth & Co. Ltd, 1988)

MacIntyre, A. *Three Rival Versions of Moral Enquiry* (Notre Dame, IN: University of Notre Dame Press, 1990)

MacIntyre, A. 'What Has Christianity to Say to the Moral Philosopher', in A.J. Torrance and M. Banner (eds), *The Doctrine of God and Theological Ethics* (London: T&T Clark, 2006)

Manent, P. *The City of Man*, trans. M.A. LePain (Princeton, NJ: Princeton University Press, 1998)

Manent, P. *A World beyond Politics: A Defense of the Nation-State*, trans. M.A. LePain (Princeton, NJ: Princeton University Press, 2006)

Mango C. 'Historical Introduction', in A. Bryer and J. Herrin (eds), *Iconoclasm: Papers Given at the Ninth Spring Symposium of Byzantine Studies* (Birmingham: Centre for Byzantine Studies, University of Birmingham, 1975)

Mantzarides, G. *Εἰσαγωγὴ στὴν Ἠθική: Ἡ Ἠθικὴ στὴν κρίση τοῦ παρόντος καὶ τὴν πρόκληση τοῦ μέλλοντος* (Thessaloniki: P. Pournara Press, 1995)

Marquis, D.B. 'Four Versions of Double Effect', *The Journal of Medicine and Philosophy*, 16 (5) (1991), 515-44

Matsoukas, N. 'Φιλοσοφία καὶ δογματικὴ διδασκαλία τοῦ ἁγίου Ἰωάννου Δαμασκηνοῦ', in *Ἐπιστημονικὴ Ἐπετηρίς Ἀριστοτελείου Πανεπιστημίου*, 14 (1969), 253-324

Matsoukas, N. 'Εἰσαγωγή', in Matsoukas (ed), *Ἰωάννου Δαμασκηνοῦ, Κατά Μανιχαίων Διάλογος. Πρὸς τοὺς διαβάλλοντας τὰς ἁγίας εἰκόνας λόγοι τρεῖς* (Thessaloniki: P. Pournara, 1988), 9-36

McGuckin, J.A. 'The Theology of Images and the Legitimation of Power in Eighth-Century Byzantium', *St Vladimir's Theological Quarterly*, 37 (1) (1993), 39-58

McKenny, G.P. *To Relieve the Human Condition: Bioethics, Technology and the Body* (Albany, NY: State University of New York Press, 1997)

Meany, J.J. *The Image of God in Man According to the Doctrine of St John Damascene* (Manila: San José Seminary, 1954)

Metz, T. 'Recent Work on the Meaning of Life', *Ethics*, 112 (4) (2002), 781-814

Meyendorff, J. *Byzantine Theology: Historical Trends and Doctrinal Themes* (New York: Fordham University Press, 1979)

Mill, J. S. *On Liberty and Utilitarianism* (New York: The Liberal Arts Press, 1956)

Mitsopoulos, N. *Θέματα ὀρθοδόξου ἠθικῆς θεολογίας* (Athens: OEDB, 1993)

Moffatt, A. 'Schooling in the Iconoclast Centuries', in A. Bryer and J. Herrin (eds), *Iconoclasm: Papers Given at the Ninth Spring Symposium of Byzantine Studies* (Birmingham: Centre for Byzantine Studies, University of Birmingham, 1975), 85-92

Nagel, T. 'War and Massacre', *Philosophy and Publis Affairs*, 1 (3) (1972), 123-44

National Commission for the Protection of Human Subjects of Biomedical and Behavioral Research. *The Belmont Report: Ethical Principles and Guidelines for the Protection of Human Subjects of Research* (Washington, DC: Department of Health, Education and Warfare (USA), 18 April 1979)

Nellas, P. 'Η θεολογία τοῦ "κατ' εἰκόνα"', *Κληρονομιά*, 2 (b) (July 1970), 293-320

Niarchos, C.G. 'Aristotelian Influences on John of Damascus' Theory of Essence (Substance) and Hypostasis', in *Méthexis: Etudes Néoplatoniciennes Présentées au Professeur Evanghélos Moutsopoulos* (Athens: CIEPA, 1992), 193-206

Nietzsche, F. *The Will to Power*, trans. W. Kaufmann (New York: Vintage Books, 1967)

Nozick, R. *Anarchy, State, Utopia* (New York: Basic Books, 1974)

Papadopoulos, S. *Πατρολογία II* (Athens, 1990)

Peach, L.J. 'An Alternative to Pacifism? Feminism and Just-War Theory', *Hypatia*, 9 (2) (1994), 152-72

Pellegrino, E.D., and Thomasma, D.C. *A Philosophical Basis of Medical Practice* (New York: Oxford University Press, 1981)

Phidas, V. 'Ζητήματα βιοηθικῆς ἐκ τῶν ἐπιστημονικῶν παρεμβάσεων διὰ τὴν ἀποτροπὴν τοῦ θανάτου' ('Bioethical Issues with Respect to Scientific Interventions to Avert Death'), proceedings of the Scientific Conference, *The Church and Bioethics: The Word of Science and the Word of Religion* (Chambésy, Geneva), 11-15 September 2002, unpublished manuscript

Phidas, V. *Droit canon: une perspective orthodoxe* (Chambésy, Geneva: Centre Orthodoxe du Patriarcat Oecuménique, 1998)

Phidas, V. *Ἐκκλησιαστικὴ ἱστορία I & II* (Athens, 1992)

Phidas, V. *Βυζάντιο: Βίος-Θεσμοί-Κοινωνία-Τέχνες* (Athens, 1997)

Pirenne, H. *Les villes du moyen âge* (Paris: Presses Universitaires de France, 1992)

Popper, K. 'The Death of Theories and of Ideologies', in Ecole Libre de Philosophie « PLETHON » (ed), *La réflexion sur la mort*, 2e Symposium International de Philosophie (Athens: Estia, 2002), 296-329

Potter, V.R. 'Biocybernetics and Survival', *Zygon*, 5 (1970), 229-46

Potter, V.R. 'Bioethics, the Science of Survival', *Perspective in Biology and Medicine*, 14 (1970), 127-53

Potter, V.R. *Bioethics: Bridge to the Future* (Englewood Cliffs, NJ: Prentice-Hall, 1971)

Potter, V.R. *Global Bioethics* (Michigan: Michigan State University Press, 1988)

Powers, M. 'Contemporary Defences of the Doctrine of Double Effect', *Revue Internationale de Philosophie*, 49 (3) (1995), 341-56

Putman, H. *Mind, Language and Reality* (London: Cambridge University Press, 1995), 291-303

Quinn, W.S. 'Actions, Intentions, and Consequences: The Doctrine of Double Effect', *Philosophy and Public Affairs*, 18 (4) (1989), 334-51

Rachels, J. *The End of Life: Euthanasia and Morality* (Oxford: Oxford University Press, 1986)
Rawls, J. *A Theory of Justice* (New York: Oxford University Press, 1973)
Reed, E.D. *The Genesis of Ethics* (Cleveland: The Pilgrim Press, 2000)
Richter, G. *Philosophische Kapitel: Johannes von Damaskus* (Stuttgart: Anton Hiersemann, 1982)
Ricoeur, P. *Fallible Man*, trans. C. A. Kelbley (New York: Fordham University Press, 1986)
Ricoeur, P. 'Nature and Freedom', in D. Stewart and J. Bien (eds), *Political and Social Essays* (Athens: Ohio University Press, 1974)
Ricoeur, P. *Oneself as Another*, trans. K. Blamey (Chicago: University of Chicago Press, 1992)
Ricoeur, P. 'Intellectual Autobiography', in L.E. Hahn (ed), *The Philosophy of Paul Ricoeur* (Chicago: Open Court, 1995), 3-53
Ricoeur, P. *Le Juste 2* (Paris: Editions Esprit, 2001)
Romanides, J. *Τὸ προπατορικὸν ἁμάρτημα* (Athens: Domos, 1992)
Ross, W.D. *The Right and the Good* (Indianapolis: Hackett Pub. Co., 1988)
Rossum, J. 'Priesthood and Confession in St Symeon the New Theologian', *St Vladimir's Theological Quarterly*, 20(4) (1976), 220-28
Roy, D.J. 'The Relief of Pain and Suffering: Ethical Principles and Imperative', *Journal of Palliative Care*, 14 (2) (1998), 3-5
Rozemond, K. *La Christologie de St Jean Damascène* (Murnau am Staffelsee: Buch Kunstverlag Ettal, 1959)
Ryle, G. *The Concept of Mind* (Chicago: Chicago University Press, 2002)
Schaeder, H. 'Die Christianisierung der Aristotelischen Logik in der byzantinischen Theologie, repräsentiert durch Johannes von Damaskus (ca. 750) und Gregor Palamas (ca. 1359)', *Kerygma und Dogma*, 8 (1962), 293-309
Schmitt, C. *Political Theology: Four Chapters on the Concept of Sovereignty*, trans. G. Schwab (Cambridge: MIT Press, 1986)
Schneewind, J.B. *The Invention of Autonomy: A History of Modern Moral Philosophy* (Cambridge: Cambridge University Press, 1998)
Scouteris, K. 'Ἡ ἱερότης τοῦ ἀνθρωπίνου προσώπου καθ' ἑαυτὴν καὶ σὲ σχέση πρὸς τὰ βιοηθικὰ διλήμματα' ('The Sacredness of the Human Person in Itself, with Reference to the Bioethical Dilemmas'), proceedings of the Scientific Conference, *The Church and Bioethics: The Word of Science and the Word of Religion* (Chambésy, Geneva), 11-15 September 2002, unpublished manuscript
Shuman, J.J. *The Body of Compassion: Ethics, Medicine and the Church* (Eugene, OR: Wipf & Stock, 1999)
Siasos, L. *Πατερικὴ κριτικὴ τῆς φιλοσοφικῆς μεθόδου* (Thessaloniki: P. Pournara, 1989)
Singer, P. *Practical Ethics* (Cambridge: Cambridge University Press, 1993)
Singer, P. *Rethinking Life and Death* (Oxford: Oxford University Press, 1994)
Singer, P. *Writings on an Ethical Life* (New York: HarperCollins, 2000)
Sotiropoulos, C. *Συμεὼν ὁ Νέος Θεολόγος: Βίος-Ἔργα-Διδασκαλία* (Athens, 1986).
Sotiropoulos, C. *Οἱ νηπτικοὶ Πατέρες περὶ τῆς κατὰ Χριστὸν τελειώσεως τοῦ ἀνθρώπου* (Athens, 1991).

Steinbock, B., and Norcross, A. (eds). *Killing and Letting Die* (New York: Fordham University Press, 1994)
Stiefenhofer, D. *Des Heiligen Johannes von Damaskus: Genaue Darlegung des Orthodoxen Glaubens* (Munich: Verlag Josef Kösel & Friedrich Pustet, 1923)
Studer, B. *Die Theologische Arbeitsweise des Johannes von Damaskus* (Murnau am Staffelsee: Buch-Kunstverlag Ettal, 1956)
Svoronos, N. 'Παρατηρήσεις γιὰ τὴ συμβολὴ τοῦ Βυζαντίου στὴν πνευματική ἐξέλιξη τῆς Δυτικῆς Εὐρώπης: Ἡ περίπτωση τοῦ Ἰωάννου Δαμασκηνοῦ', in *Βυζάντιο καί Εὐρώπη* (Athens: European Cultural Center of Delphi, 1987), 115-52
Tatakis, B. '*La philosophie byzantine*', in E. Bréhier (ed), *Histoire de la philosophie*, Fasc. Suppl. II (Paris : Presses Universitaires de France, 1949)
Tauber, A. 'From the Self to the Other: Building A Philosophy of Medicine', in M.A. Grodin (ed), *Meta Medical Ethics: The Philosophical Foundations of Bioethics* (Dordrecht: Kluwer Academic Publishers, 1995), 157-95
Tauber, A. 'Historical and Philosophical Reflections on Patient Autonomy', *Health Care Analysis*, 9 (2001), 299-319
Tocqueville, A. de. *Democracy in America*, trans. A. Goldhammer (New York: The Library of America, 2004)
Tsirpanlis, C.N. 'The Problem of Free Will and Evil in St John of Damascus', in C. Tsirpanlis, *Greek Patristic Theology: Basic Doctrines in Eastern Church Fathers* (New York: EO Press, 1979), 65-86
Turner, H.J.M. 'St Symeon the New Theologian and Dualist Heresies: Comparisons and Contrasts', *St Vladimir's Theological Quarterly*, 32 (4) (1988), 359-66
Vachicouras, G. *Ἡ ἔννοια τοῦ θανάτου κατὰ τὸν ἅγιο Γρήγοριο Νύσσης* (Katerini, Greece: Epektasi, 1999)
Veatch, R.M. *A Theory of Medical Ethics* (New York: Basic Books Inc., 1981)
Veatch, R.M. 'The Foundations of Bioethics', *Bioethics*, 13 (3/4) (1999), 206-17
Veatch, R.M. 'Is There a Common Morality?', *Kennedy Institute of Ethics Journal*, 13 (3) (2003), 189-92
Vovelle, M. *La mort et l'occident de 1300 à nos jours* (Paris: Gallimard, 1983)
Waldenfels, B. 'Levinas and the Face of the Other', in S. Critchley and R. Bernasconi (eds), *The Cambridge Companion to Levinas* (Cambridge: Cambridge University Press, 2002), 63-81
Walzer, M. *Just and Unjust Wars* (New York: Basic Books, 1977)
Walzer, M. *Thick and Thin: Moral Argument at Home and Abroad* (Notre Dame, IN: University of Notre Dame Press, 1994)
Ware, K. 'The Mystery of God and Man in St Symeon the New Theologian', *Sobornost*, 6 (4) (Winter 1972), 227-36
Williams, G.H. 'The Neo-Patristic Synthesis of Georges Florovsky', in A. Blane (ed) *Georges Florovsky: Russian Intellectual and Orthodox Churchman* (Crestwood, NY: St Vladimir's Seminary Press, 1993)
Williams, R. 'Afterword', in S. Hauerwas and S. Wells (eds), *The Blackwell Companion to Christian Ethics* (Oxford: Blackwell, 2006)
Zakythinos, D. '*La grande brèche dans la tradition historique de l'Hellénisme, du septième au neuvième siècle*', in *Χαριστήριον εἰς Ἀναστάσιος Κ. Ὀρλάνδον* (Athens: Library of the Archaeological Society, 1966), 300-27

Zizioulas, J. 'Εὐθανασία: Ἀποφάσεις κατὰ τὸ τέλος τῆς ζωῆς', proceedings of the conference on *Euthanasia: Decisions at the End of life*, organised by the Medical Association of Athens, *Ἐνημέρωση τῶν Γιατρῶν*, 157 (Dec 2000-Jan 2001), 15-18

Zizioulas, J. 'Ἀσθένεια καὶ θεραπεία στὴν Ὀρθόδοξη Θεολογία' ('Disease and Healing in Orthodox Theology'), proceedings of the conference, *Θεολογία καὶ ψυχιατρικὴ σὲ διάλογο* (Athens: Apostoliki Diakonia, 1999), 133-56

Zizioulas, J.D. *Being as Communion* (Crestwood, NY: St Vladimir's Seminary Press, 1985)

Zografidis, G. Βυζαντινὴ φιλοσοφία τῆς εἰκόνας: Μιά ἀνάγνωση τοῦ Ἰωάννου Δαμασκηνοῦ (Athens: Ellinika Grammata, 1997)

Index